LOVE IN THE TIME OF AIDS

LOVE
IN THE
TIME
OF
AIDS

INEQUALITY, GENDER,
AND RIGHTS IN SOUTH AFRICA

MARK HUNTER

Indiana University Press
Bloomington and Indianapolis

This book is a publication of

Indiana University Press
Office of Scholarly Publishing
Herman B Wells Library 350
1320 East 10th Street
Bloomington, Indiana 47405 USA

www.iupress.indiana.edu

☉ The paper used in this publication meets the minimum requirements of the American National Standard for Information Sciences—Permanence of Paper for Printed Library Materials, ANSI Z39.48-1992.

Manufactured in the United States of America

Library of Congress Cataloging-in-Publication Data

Hunter, Mark.
    Love in the time of AIDS : inequality, gender, and rights in South Africa /
Mark Hunter.
      p. cm.
    Includes bibliographical references and index.
    ISBN 978-0-253-35533-1 (cloth : alk. paper) — ISBN 978-0-253-22239-8 (pbk. : alk. paper) 1. Man-woman relationships—South Africa. 2. Equality—South Africa. 3. AIDS (Disease)—South Africa. I. Title.
    HQ952.H86   2010
    30670968'090511—dc22

                                 2010011262

1 2 3 4 5 6 7 8 20 19 18 17 16 15

For
Atiqa and Leila

CONTENTS

ACKNOWLEDGMENTS

It was 1988 when I first visited South Africa to volunteer for a year at a township school in Mthatha called Ikhwezi Lokusa. Six years later South Africans freed themselves from apartheid, and in that year, 1994, I returned amid the celebrations. Virtually every year since then I have lived in or visited the country, forming deep links with its people and places that I cannot acknowledge enough in these pages.

In 1997–98, I studied at the School of Development Studies, University of KwaZulu-Natal, and this institution has been my academic home since then. Bill Freund and Vishnu Padayachee have consistently offered me advice and support. I also owe an enormous debt to the History Department at UKZN. Almost every argument in this book was chewed over by its superb seminar series. Tribute for sustaining this space must be paid to Keith Breckenridge, Vukile Khumalo, Vanessa Noble, Julie Parle, Marijke du Toit, and Thembisa Waetjen. And I must give special thanks to Catherine Burns and Jeff Guy. Catherine has provided copious advice along the way, and I am one of the many people who have benefited from her selfless support of her colleagues. I have learnt an enormous amount about KwaZulu-Natal through my friendship with Jeff, whose passion for history is immense. To Rob Morrell, a UKZN colleague until recently, thanks for encouraging me to write several articles on masculinities and for your ongoing advice, friendship, and support.

Lynn Thomas read the complete manuscript with an incredibly detailed but supportive eye. Jeff Guy, Katharine Rankin, and Jon Soske gave incisive comments too. Percy Ngonyama diligently checked for mistakes in isiZulu, and Ankita Jauhari provided research assistance in Toronto. I also thank Indiana University Press's reviewers, Shula Marks and Richard Parker, and the anonymous reviewer from the University of KwaZulu-Natal Press. At Indiana University Press, Dee Mortensen supported my work very early on and I appreciate her skilled and professional treatment of a "first-book author." Later, I valued Shoshanna Green's marvelous editorial skills.

Also, I must thank some more institutions where this work was presented: Duke University (Concilium on Southern Africa); University of Cape Town (AIDS and Society Research Unit); University of Toronto (Women and Gender Studies Institute); University of Michigan (Afroamerican and African Studies); University of Western Ontario (Geography); University of KwaZulu-Natal (School of Development Studies, HEARD); University of the Western

Cape (History). I also benefited from the "Retheorising Sexuality" conference held at the Rockefeller Foundation's Bellagio Center and organized by Peter Aggleton, Paul Boyce, Henrietta Moore, Richard Parker, and Jeffrey Weeks.

Libby Ardington helped me to find the family with whom I stayed in Mandeni, for which I am most grateful. During my stay, I had a key collaborative relationship with the Africa Centre for Health and Population Studies in Hlabisa. I thank Mike Bennish, Carol Camlin, Kobus Herbst, Vicky Hosegood, and Ian Timaeus. Thembeka Mngomezulu and I jointly conducted interviews in Hlabisa, and I gained a great deal from her insights into rural South Africa.

It is hard to imagine a more pleasant environment to conduct archival work in than the Killie Campbell Africana Library, and thanks go to Hloni Dlamini and Neli Somers for their help. At the Durban Archives I was ably assisted by Ntombifuthi Khuzwayo, Stanley Mnguni, Unnay Narrine, Rishi Singh, and Sicelo Zulu.

Many other South Africans and Africanists contributed their insights, encouragement, and friendship over the years. They include Richard Ballard, Franco Barchiesi, Debby Bonnin, Shirley Brooks, Ben Carton, Kerry Chance, Sharad Chari, Jennifer Cole, Sindy Damoyi, Andy Gibbs, Marie Huchzemeyer, Vashna Jagarnath, Deborah James, Bridget Kenny, Vukile Khumalo, Astrid van Kotze, Francie Lund, Andrew Macdonald, Thenjiwe Magwaza, Pranitha Maharaj, Mike Mahoney, Ntsiki Manzini, Hein Marais, Gerry Maré, Molly Margaretten, Sarah Mathis, Mandisa Mbali, Sane Mdlalose, Bheki Ka Mncube, David Moore, Mike Morris, Thulani Ntuli, Sarah Nutall, Julie Parle, Raj Patel, Kathleen Pithouse, Richard Pithouse, Deborah Posel, Dorrit Posel, Eleanor Preston-Whyte, Smitha Radhakrishnan, Graeme Reid, Glen Robbins, Ben Roberts, Steven Robins, Jenny Robinson, Jeff Sallaz, Melanie Samson, Fiona Scorgie, Nafisa Essop Sheik, Ari Sitas, Jabulani Sithole, Caroline Skinner, Stephen Sparks, Alison Todes, Imraan Valodia, Cheryl Walker, Liz Walker, Samantha Willan, and Ilana van Wyk.

While I was undertaking my Ph.D. research, the growing strength and influence of the Treatment Action Campaign reminded me that there was still much within the AIDS world to contest. In Mandeni, the TAC's chairperson, Richard Shandu, led the way; beyond that, I was just one of many people inspired by the courage and leadership of Zackie Achmat.

In Mandeni I enjoyed volunteering at the Mandeni loveLife youth center and learnt much from its dedicated staff and volunteers. David Harrison, loveLife's former CEO, provided a trenchant criticism of my interpretation of the organization in chapter 10. Although he might not agree with the final version, I appreciate his openness in debating loveLife with me.

At the University of Toronto, I had many enjoyable and enlightening discussions about South Africa with my Geography comrade Thembela Kepe. Linzi Manicom's work on gender has long influenced my own and I am very grateful for our conversations. I also benefited from interacting with many others, including Anne-Emmanuelle Birn, Michael Bunce, Deb Cowen, Amrita Daniere, Girish Daswani, Matt Farish, Michael Lambek, Tania Li, Ken MacDonald, Minelle Mahtani, Scott Prudham, Katharine Rankin, Ted Relph, Sue Ruddick, Rachel Silvey, and Andre Sorensen.

Lesley Lawson took a large red pen to an early draft of this book and helped me to restructure it. As well as proposing the book's title, she pushed me to reflect on whether I really needed all the academic concepts I used: to recognize that what is theory to one person is elitist jargon to another. I have tried throughout to retain both a sense of my own social location and the voices of my informants/interlocutors, all in a way that is critically engaged with social theory. There is no doubt that I have failed to achieve this aim! But acknowledging it helps to explain some of the stylistic decisions I have made in this book.

It would take a South African passionate about the country to supervise and support a dissertation whose political and intellectual center of gravity so obviously wanders beyond the U.S. institution for which it was written. In Gillian Hart I had not only such a person but someone who allowed my study to twist and turn in sometimes uncertain ways. Gill also undertook the unenviable task of guiding a foreign student financially and practically through the Berkeley Ph.D. system with great skill and commitment. After the completion of my Ph.D. I have enjoyed her continued support and friendship.

Michael Watts and, before her move from Berkeley, Ruthie Gilmore also inspired my work and provided invaluable critical comments along the way. And Michael Burawoy's contribution to my studies went well beyond that which might be expected from an "outside" dissertation committee member. The work of another sociologist, Ann Swidler, also helped to steer me in the direction of "love" at a key moment, and I appreciated the encouragement she gave to my project. I had the privilege of studying alongside a number of remarkable students, including Joe Bryan, Ben Gardner, Dan Graham, Jenna Loyd, and Chris Niedt.

Funding for the research and writing of this book came from many sources: a Wenner-Gren Dissertation Research Grant, an International Predissertation Fellowship from the Social Science Research Council and the American Council of Learned Societies with funds provided by the Ford Foundation, an SSRC International Dissertation Research Fellowship, a Rocca Fellowship, an Allan Sharlin Research Fellowship, and a Berkeley Human Rights Summer Fellowship. I am grateful to all.

I enjoyed a year as a Mellon Postdoctoral Fellow at Dartmouth College that helped to get the book off the ground. Thanks to Mark Davidson, Mona Domosh, Jennifer Fluri, Susanne Freidberg, Frank Magilligan, Christopher Sneddon, Richard Wright, and especially Andy Friedland.

My greatest debts have accumulated in KwaZulu-Natal. I offer profound thanks to my "family" in Mandeni who hosted me with good humor and enormous warmth, and to the family in Hlabisa with whom I also stayed for a shorter time. In Mandeni, my research assistant, whose name, like the families,' I have kept back to protect the identities of informants, was the person with whom I worked the closest while conducting research. With great skill and insight, she arranged and facilitated numerous interviews. Without her remarkable ability to constantly find fascinating people with whom to talk, this project would have been much weaker. Without the willingness of Mandeni's residents to be subjected to numerous questions, some directed toward the most intimate parts of their lives, this project would not have been possible at all. Ngiyabonga kakhulu kunina nonke eMandeni. Sahlala ndawonye, sakhala ndawonye, sahleka ndawonye. Ngafunda okuningi ngendlela enhle yokuphila. Ngiyathemba ukuthi lencwadi izosiza ngandlelathize kwisimo esinzima sengculaza—Umzingeli.

To my wife, Atiqa Hachimi, my deep thanks for your support, love, and honest criticisms as I agonized over this book. Thank you for your willingness to be part of my worlds in Mandeni and Durban during our stays in South Africa. Our daughter, Leila, lit up our lives after her birth in 2008 and kept us smiling with love in the time of writing.

Author's note: All royalties from this book will be donated to the Treatment Action Campaign.

A NOTE ON RACIAL TERMS

It is inherently problematic to use and therefore reiterate the language of "race." Paradoxically, however, as the new constitution of South Africa embraced non-racialism, race categories took on a new salience in order to make it easier to understand and redress past inequalities. Four racial categories are therefore still widely used today in South Africa: African, white, Indian, and coloured.

While we can't, yet, do without a racial vocabulary, the meaning of racial terms and the very idea of "race" are never stable. Even after the 1950 Population Registration Act was passed to classify citizens in the apartheid era, some people moved between races. The population census itself frequently changed its conception of "races" (or "population groups"). The category "Africans" was defined in various ways over the years: "Natives" (1951); "Bantu" (1960); "Blacks" (1980); "African/Black" (1996); and "Black African" (2001).

Although deconstructing race is not the primary aim of this book, understanding AIDS' history leads me to show the contingent joining of race and intimacy; the deep entanglement of ethnicity, gender, and race; and the increasing inequalities within (but reductions in inequalities between) racially defined groups. In particular, the recent growth of a middle class that encompasses all "races" erodes the very strong historical link between race and class—though the poorest South Africans are still virtually all "African."

Most of my informants/interlocutors differentiate themselves in isiZulu from other apartheid-designated "races" by using the term "black" (*abantu abamnyama*, black people, or simply *abantu*, people). This category is contrasted, for example, to *abelungu*, white people. However, with the rise of the black consciousness movement in the late 1960s and 1970s, the term "black" also came to refer to all people of color; I therefore use the term only in contexts where its meaning is clear. My informants also use the four official racial categories, which I draw upon in the book.

I use lowercase for "coloured" and "white" but uppercase for "African" and "Indian" since, although the concepts the latter index are also socially constructed, the words are derived from the names of continents. To improve the book's readability I use somewhat sparingly qualifiers like "white-designated," as well as scare quotes themselves.

ACRONYMS

AIDS	Acquired Immune Deficiency Syndrome
ANC	African National Congress
ARVs	antiretroviral (AIDS) drugs
GEAR	Growth Employment and Redistribution
HIV	Human Immunodeficiency Virus
IFP	Inkatha Freedom Party
MCP	multiple concurrent partners
RDP	Reconstruction and Development Programme
SAPPI	South African Pulp and Paper Industries, Limited
STI	sexually transmitted infection
TAC	Treatment Action Campaign
UNAIDS	Joint United Nations Programme on HIV and AIDS
US$	United States dollars (throughout the book the rand/dollar exchange rate is taken to be 8:1)

LOVE IN THE TIME OF AIDS

ONE

Gender and AIDS in an Unequal World

In 2006, Jacob Zuma, then sixty-four and South Africa's former deputy president, was accused of rape. Zuma, who had entered anti-apartheid politics after growing up in rural KwaZulu-Natal, faced charges from a woman he had known for some time—her father was a fellow member of the African National Congress before his death. "Khwezi" (Star), as she was called by her supporters, was only half Zuma's age and an HIV-positive AIDS activist.

The trial—in the words of one newspaper headline, "23 Days That Shook Our World"—appeared to crystallize fundamental gulfs in South Africa's young democracy.[1] Outside the court, and watched by the hungry media, some of Zuma's supporters burnt photographs of Khwezi and yelled, "Burn the bitch!" Inside the courtroom, Zuma controversially drew on Zulu customs to claim that he could acquire sex relatively easily and was therefore no rapist: "*Angisona isishimane mina*," he stated (I don't struggle to attract women/I am not a sissy). He also argued that in Zulu culture a man who left a woman sexually aroused could himself be charged with rape. Zuma's defense, in other words, was that he was no rapist, just a traditional patriarch with a large sexual appetite.[2]

Separated by police from Zuma's supporters, gender activists shouted strong support for Khwezi. They argued that prominent politicians should be upholding, not undermining, the post-apartheid constitution's commitment to gender rights. The international and national press generally agreed: the South African *Mail & Guardian*, for instance, described Zuma's statements as "Neanderthal."[3] The trial's importance, commentators noted, was paramount in a country that was purportedly the rape and AIDS capital of the globe.[4]

Yet, despite this controversy, Zuma's political career went from strength to strength after his acquittal. Three years later, and following a bitter leadership battle within the ruling ANC party, a popular "Zunami" led to his election as president with 66 percent of the vote. How did a self-proclaimed sexist, a man charged with rape (and later corruption), become so popular in a country that overthrew the most oppressive, the most rights-denying, the most illiberal, system of racial rule—apartheid?

Zuma's story came to intrigue me in part because he frequently made assertions about the naturalness of Zulu patriarchy that my research tried to destabilize. Certainly, the obstacles Khwezi and thousands of women like her faced in pursuing a rape charge revealed deep male biases in supposedly liberal legal institutions and in society at large. For many within AIDS circles, the Zuma trial was an iconic moment that laid bare the extent of gender inequalities in the country.

But what also fascinated me was countless women's undoubted enthusiasm for Zuma. Living in my field site, Mandeni, KwaZulu-Natal, in April 2006 during the rape trial, I spoke with numerous *isiZulu* speakers about the leader; conversations were especially pertinent because he hailed from Nkandla, a rural area only some seventy kilometers to the northwest. In contrast to dominant criticisms, many women I knew told me that Zuma was a respectable man and celebrated the fact that he had several wives. This sentiment was repeated across the country.[5]

Subsequent events were to show that public adulation for Zuma had limits, if these could also be framed in terms of a gendered sense of respectability. In early 2010 it came to light that he had fathered a child out of wedlock with the thirty-nine-year-old daughter of a prominent soccer administrator. Facing sustained criticism, he was forced to apologize publicly.

Nevertheless, the undoubted support of many women for the Zunami provides a revealing entry point into gender in the midst of an AIDS pandemic. Zuma's court testimony in 2006 is a good place to start; it imparts some subtle clues as to his esteem and, by association, the intricate gendering of the South African postcolony. More than simply a titanic struggle between men and women or rights and tradition, the trial represented something of a meeting point for divergent meanings of gender and intimacy.

Consider first Zuma's statement that he had offered to pay *ilobolo* (bridewealth) to marry Khwezi after she accused him of rape. The English-speaking press poured scorn on this statement, but ilobolo enjoys such gravitas that the isiZulu press did not present Zuma's comments in such negative terms.[6] Indeed, to dismiss ilobolo as simply a patriarchal tradition or a sign of the commodification of relationships (i.e., a bribe) is to miss the way it marks respectability—even more so today than formerly because of the rarity of marriage among young, often unemployed, South Africans. As capitalism bit deeper into the twentieth century, ilobolo connected work to kin and wages to love in profoundly important ways.

Commentators also seized on Zuma's use of the phrase *"isibaya sikababa wakhe"* (her father's cattle kraal) to refer to a woman's genitalia. Yet the term draws meaning not simply because it signifies men's unbridled control over women. The reference to a cattle kraal warns that a daughter's impregnation will reduce the ilobolo cattle a father receives. In the course of my research, many older people used the phrase and some compared it favorably with a brash contemporary youth culture out of which emerged songs with titles such as "Sika Lekhekhe" (literally "cut the cake," where *ikhekhe* is slang for a woman's genitalia).[7] Zuma's use of the cattle metaphor spoke—rather ironically, given the context—to an era when society valued not simply sexual pleasure nor sexual conquest but childbirth and kinship.

These points might appear trivial in the face of terrible acts of male power in South Africa today. But they provide important glimpses into the quite profound shifts that have taken place in South Africans' intimate lives over the last generation and which I detail throughout this book. This does not in any way assume that sexual violence should not be an important point of focus—obviously it is the most common reading of the rape trial and a major theme in the study of gender and AIDS in South Africa today. But they raise questions about how fundamental shifts in political economy and intimacy are embodied in other ways. The Zuma rape trial certainly represents masculine views on gender and sex—but it also raises important questions about love, children, labor, and kinship.

AIDS and the Political Economy and Geography of Intimacy

This book is an ethnography of one place, Mandeni, KwaZulu-Natal, and presents arguments about why AIDS emerged so quickly in South Africa. In giving considerable attention to gender, I oppose claims by men like Zuma that culture is static by showing how even some of the most celebrated Zulu "traditions" emerged in the colonial period. At the same time, the profound mismatch between criticisms of Zuma and his popularity among many South Africans, including women, suggests that we must sharpen our analysis still further. To this end, I combine ethnography and history to illuminate the deep connections between political economy and *intimacy*—a broader term than sex that extends analysis into fertility, love, marriage, and genital pleasure. This allows me, in turn, to argue that profound recent transformations in intimacy at a time of chronic unemployment and reduced marriage rates must be taken more seriously. The key question then is not *whether* gender is central to understanding AIDS but *how* the pandemic is gendered. This story is centered on one of the areas worst affected by HIV in the world: in 2008 a shocking 39 percent of women tested positive for HIV in antenatal clinics in the KwaZulu-Natal province.[8]

I tell this story by bringing political economy into constant tension with the everyday lives and emotions of those most marginalized in society. The embodiment of inequalities that drives AIDS today is undeniably a form of "structural violence," to use a term popularized by anthropologist-doctor Paul Farmer.[9] Yet, as Scheper-Hughes and Bourgois note, the concept of structural violence often fails to move from a political-economic context into everyday worlds to capture "how victims become victimizers and how that hides local understandings of structural power relations."[10] By constantly viewing the economic and the intimate as dialectical—that is, in an ever-changing relationship to one another and other socio-spatial processes—I show how new patterns of inequality became embodied among marginalized South Africans.[11] An example of how I take this forward is the book's attention to changing understandings and embodiments of love as the country's political economy transformed.

Inseparable from mapping transformations to gender and intimacy is my attempt to provide a more detailed analysis of AIDS' social roots.[12] The most influential political-economic explanation for AIDS in South Africa is men's long history of circular migration to the gold and diamond mines. Yet this fails to capture key contemporary trends, especially the rise of unemployment and the greater mobility of women. Indeed, the dramatic pace of the pandemic and its specific social geography raise searching questions about the country's new fault lines. From 1990 to 2005, the national prevalence of HIV rose from less than 1 percent to nearly 30 percent among pregnant women.[13] And surprisingly little attention is given to AIDS' geography, despite the fact that four studies have now suggested that the highest HIV rates are found in informal/shack settlements, areas that house some of the poorest South Africans.[14] Such an analysis yields the argument that the scale of the AIDS pandemic was neither an inevitable consequence of apartheid nor simply a product of former president Mbeki's much-criticized questioning of the causal link between HIV and AIDS. A politics of AIDS that connects disease to its social and geographical roots, one already forged in South Africa by health activists, can help reverse infection trends.

In brief, to explain South Africa's rapid rise in HIV prevalence, the book's central argument is that intimacy, especially what I call the *materiality of everyday sex*, has become a key juncture between production and social reproduction in the current era of chronic unemployment and capital-led globalization. In other words, as unemployment has cast a cruel but uneven shadow on the country, certain aspects of intimacy have come to play a more central and material role in the "fleshy, messy, and indeterminate stuff of everyday life."[15] In South Africa, the recession of the mid-1970s signaled a decisive shift from labor shortages to unemployment, and this pattern continued throughout the 1980s and after apartheid ended. Joblessness and labor market casualization engendered an extraordinary social gap between a shrinking group of mostly male core workers and the rest of the population.[16] Of particular importance, women's rapid movement into the labor force, while at first partly driven by industrial employment, has not been matched by employment growth in recent years. Along with reduced marriage rates, these labor market changes represent a generational shift that can be crudely summarized as follows: from mostly men *earning a living* and supporting a wife to many men and women *making a living* in multifarious ways.[17]

How can we conceptualize intimacy, an intensely personal and embodied part of life, in relation to making a living in economically hard times? A rich literature on social reproduction now connects the economy, gender, and matters of everyday life: in the realm of intimacy, longstanding themes include how wives' domestic and sexual labor subsidizes capitalist production and how sex workers provide men with not only sex but "the comforts of home."[18] From the 1980s, the ascendancy of free-market economics, together with the relative decline of nuclear families, yielded new research themes. In the current "globalization" era, commentators point out, life for many, especially women, is more insecure: states have rolled back social provisions and a "vagabond" capital is ever more able to shirk support for aspects of social reproduction from health benefits to pensions.[19]

The concept of social reproduction helps to situate South Africans' bodies within wider processes, including colonialism, capitalism, and state practices. However, the dialectic relationship between political economy and intimacy I forefront emphasizes constant, intricate changes to bodily practices that a historical-ethnographic approach can best illuminate. This ethnography, begun only six years after democracy, uses life stories and observations to show how young South Africans navigate, while simultaneously producing, intimate relationships at a time of growing inequalities but political freedom.

As unemployment rose, young South Africans found it especially hard to find work: by 2005 a staggering 72 percent of women and 58 percent of men aged between fifteen and twenty-four were unemployed.[20] In part because of rising unemployment and increasing female mobility, marriage in South Africa has undergone perhaps one of the sharpest reductions in the world, with the proportion of Africans living in a married union halving from the 1960s; in many ways marriage has today become a middle-class institution.

I emphasize in some detail how intense gendered conflicts—a kind of structural distrust—result in part from the almost complete demise of marriage and the tensions inherent in navigating alternative life paths. And this analysis allows me to argue that, from roughly the 1980s, something of a perfect storm of political economy, gender, and household and family trends resulted, just as HIV found its way into South Africa. I summarize these processes as the *changing political economy and geography of intimacy*. As I explain later, this concept is an analytical tool to highlight certain recent shifts in intimate relations that affected the rapid onset of AIDS; rather than charting unambiguous historical ruptures, much of my empirical evidence will focus on more contradictory tensions that are necessary to understand this and other abstractions.

I also need to state very clearly that I do not conceptualize declining marriage rates as some kind of reduction in morality, ending of love, or "breakdown" of the heterosexual family. These unhelpful tropes have been widely repeated in South Africa and elsewhere for many decades. They tend, as I argue throughout this book, to underestimate how racial rule not only weakened certain aspects of the patriarchal family but also promoted new "patriarchal bargains" between men and women.[21] To understand South Africa today it is, therefore, vital to avoid a picture of apartheid as a blunt force that drove a linear decline of sexual morals; instead we must ask how a range of social processes reconfigured money, morality, dependency, power, pleasure, and pain in different social milieus. Similarly, while I consider political economy in detail, poverty is not, on its own, an adequate explanation for AIDS, since many affected people can be relatively well off.[22]

Instead, I argue that we must pay more attention to how the coming together of low marriage rates and wealth and poverty in such close proximity —common features across Southern Africa where HIV rates are the highest— can today drive gender relations and material sexual relationships that fuel AIDS. Sex workers explicitly selling sex are obviously at high risk of contracting HIV. Yet, more significant to the scale of South Africa's AIDS pandemic, I argue, are boyfriend-girlfriend "gift" relationships that involve material benefits for unmarried women but also feelings of love and a wide range of moral and reciprocal obligations. This is the scenario that I describe as *the materiality of everyday sex.*[23]

Gender and the Paralyzing Binary of Rights and Tradition

I return now to the gendering of AIDS. It took until the 1990s for gender to be given any real consideration in AIDS policy circles. Yet women constitute 60 percent of all HIV infections in sub-Saharan Africa, an area harboring 68 percent of the global 33.4 million infections.[24] Rape is one reason for this discrepancy, and the Zuma rape trial vividly showed the failure of legal institutions in South Africa to protect women from male violence. Women are also biologically more susceptible to AIDS: the female genital tract has a greater exposed surface area than the male genital tract. Moreover, younger women have less mature genital tissue and thus are even more susceptible to infection.[25] In addition, the most widely promoted technology used to protect against sexually transmitted infections (STIs), the male condom, depends on men's willingness to use it.

Given the above, feminist activists have played a critical role in drawing attention to the gendering of the AIDS pandemic. Long struggles have been waged in favor of female condoms and microbicides, the latter being compounds inserted by a woman into her vagina to reduce the chances of STI (including HIV) transmission; these are still in the trial stage. Transnational campaigns have, in turn, forged important alliances against sexual violence. Activists have also played a critical role in challenging the "imperial moralities" of George Bush's PEPFAR fund (President's Emergency Plan for AIDS Relief); this initiative favored organizations that promoted sexual abstention and forced recipients to sign pledges opposing abortion.[26]

Many such campaigns on AIDS and gender have been framed in terms of "rights." From the 1960s the U.S.'s civil rights movement, and from the 1970s the gay rights movement, won important gains, in part by arguing that rights must be extended to marginalized groups. And in respect to AIDS, George Bush's moral conservatism, for instance, could be presented as denying women basic sexual and reproductive rights.

Yet while rights represent an enormously powerful and important agenda, I follow scholars who argue that we must consider their deeply paradoxical nature.[27] This is particularly pertinent in South Africa, where the remarkable advent of democracy gave rights-talk a stark immediacy in both the policy world and South Africans' everyday lives. Symbolized by Nelson Mandela's personal forgiveness, democracy replaced apartheid with a new flag, a new anthem, strong narratives of nation-building, and a form of citizenship underpinned by human rights. But this embrace of liberal democratic rights also gave credence to the view that what went before democracy was somewhat backward ("Neanderthal," to use the *Mail & Guardian*'s description of Zuma)—or at the very least not worthy of reexamination in the modern era. And terrible acts of male power, which some men justify through "tradition," also help to portray gender as a zero-sum phenomenon, with rights leading the battle for equality. I make three further points on gender and rights below.

First, as many observers have noted, middle-class citizens typically have the greatest means to enforce liberal rights. To put it crudely, a rights-based agenda runs the risk of downplaying the political-economic roots of AIDS. In respect to gender, Shireen Hassim has chronicled how the women's movement ultimately had more success in enshrining formal legal rights than in creating substantive (redistributive) gender change during South Africa's democratic transition.[28] The 1996 constitution did go beyond an orthodox liberal framework. Designed to redress the racist past, it protected certain socio-economic rights, including housing and health; citizens have drawn on these proactively, with some success. Exactly how rights play out in the realm of AIDS, however, demands more critical analysis.

A second closely related point is that gender-rights approaches do not always recognize the multiple inequalities with which gender is entangled. As Linzi Manicom argues, post-apartheid discourses of gender and citizenship can work to cast gender as the only means through which women can achieve social justice. At the time of South Africa's political transition, she argues, feminist writings on citizenship were "rendered in the grammar of liberal democracy," and this produced "*gendered* political subjects in ways that emphasize gender over other contending social identifications."[29] This point raises questions about the extent to which a poorer South African woman might share the same notion of citizenship and rights as a richer woman; indeed, it suggests that the very meaning of womanhood may vary across vast social differences. It alerts us that gender-rights language today can downplay the inseparability of being a female-bodied person and simultaneously being racialized, classed, and sexualized in profoundly important, and often very diverse, ways.

My third point is the need to subject "rights" as well as "tradition"—their frequent nemesis—to rigorous historical and ethnographic interrogation. Colonialism brought liberalism to Africa but also "indirect rule," a form of governance whereby settlers devolved day-to-day power to "traditional" structures led by chiefs. As the anthropologists Jean and John Comaroff describe, this history means that "built into the very scaffolding of all postcolonies" is both a modernist culture of rights-based legality and simultaneously the ability of citizens to make powerful claims by evoking cultural difference.[30]

Importantly, the post-apartheid government did not question, and indeed sought to further institutionalize, this binary. In 1996, two years after the apartheid regime ended, South Africa's new constitution advanced a series of rights, including some concerning gender and same-sex relations. At the same time, the constitution granted citizens the right to practice their tradition (for instance, Zuma had the right to testify in court in isiZulu and defend himself as someone simply practicing Zulu customs). Separate institutions were established along these binary lines, for instance a Human Rights Commission and a House of Traditional Leaders. Here are two poles in society that work to solidify consciousness into one of two camps.

Yet South Africans always exceed this tradition/rights binary in revealing ways. The isiZulu verb *ukulunga*, from which the word *amalungelo* (rights) derives, is actually more akin to the phrase "to be right," and therefore holds wider meanings than modern universalistic notions of rights. One dictionary, for instance, defines *lunga* as "Get or be in order, fit correct, be as it should be . . . Be morally good, be righteous."[31] Hence, while gender rights typically occupy the headlines today, I stress how they always come together with gendered expectations of "rights and wrongs." And only historical analysis can allow us to see how the era of modern liberal rights contains within it the sediments of these past expectations and contestations.

My historical ethnography involved long periods of living in an informal settlement and studying the history of intimacy in this and surrounding areas, especially Sundumbili township, one of many planned settlements built for "Africans." Particularly in my early years of research, when the constitution was being widely publicized, I was struck by how frequently rights were discussed by young people. Their creative and varied employment of rights made me somewhat doubtful about rights' claims to speak to universal norms and to be able to prevail over the AIDS pandemic. Moreover, to my surprise, older women recalled that "traditional" institutions like Inkatha had actually brought them some rights, albeit tied up with the preservation of hierarchies based on *inhlonipho*, or respect.[32]

Yet, while skeptical of some claims attached to rights, I do not see them as simply a mechanism that "governs" (somewhat passive) bodies—a view that can downplay the ways in which rights are both mutable and highly contested. The strength of ethnography is its ability to reveal the "micro processes lodged in moments of transformation."[33] I show, for instance, how women draw on rights to actively contest intimate relations, including the use of condoms. At the same time, I also demonstrate how rights-based AIDS messages can also be spectacularly turned on their head: some women can argue that rights and equality brought them the right to have multiple boyfriends—an entitlement that men often claim is solely theirs.

A number of studies on gender rights do, of course, take these intricacies and paradoxes into consideration.[34] But we can pause and consider the significance of South Africa's realization of rights just at the time that it confronted AIDS, a disease already saturated with racialized and spatialized meanings. And we should note how, from the outset, traditional/modern binaries have framed questions of "African AIDS": many of the earliest explanations for high

HIV prevalence in Africa blamed it on so-called "traditional" practices such as "dry sex" or "witchcraft."[35] Might African patriarchy become a new kind of exotic and backward set of practices on which AIDS is blamed?

Relevant to this question is the enormous influence development agencies and Western academics have in framing AIDS interventions in poor countries. More than twenty years ago, Chandra Mohanty famously drew attention to the tendency of Western accounts to create a homogonous category of "Third World Women," to whom modernizing interventions can be directed.[36] More recently, Amina Mama warned that a large "gender and development" industry can lead to "gender technocrats touting a new kind of export product."[37] These critiques raise an important question: what essences of womanhood do intervention campaigns draw on? And here Wendy Brown cautions that discourses of rights can, ironically, be deeply masculinist in assuming an "ontologically autonomous, self-sufficient, unencumbered subject."[38]

Let me put these points in a different way, since they might seem a particularly problematic matter for a man, and a white man at that, to raise. At a time when gender is, at last, receiving attention from national governments and international organizations, there are worrying signs that cursory and decontextualized understandings of gender are being instituted. The prominence of rights in South Africa's recent democratization makes it especially important that we critically evaluate their implementation. To use a policy example, one prominent section in UNAIDS' *2008 Report on the Global AIDS Epidemic* is called "Gender Inequality and Harmful Gender Norms."[39] AIDS practitioners, it suggests, must zero in on harmful gender norms and remove or modernize them. Phrases like "traditional expectations related to masculinity" give the impression that to do so, all that is needed is a good dose of Western liberalism.

This approach can be deeply dehistoricizing and analytically weak. Does women's support for Zuma constitute a harmful gender norm? What do we mean by empowerment? Should we ever use such loaded words as "tradition" to talk about historical practices? Of course, the AIDS pandemic stimulated much rich work on gender, some of which I draw on in this book. And rights are not always tied up with problematic views of gender. Yet, especially in a new liberal democracy like South Africa, they represent a key vocabulary whose paradoxes are rarely questioned within the AIDS policy world.

Some Concepts: Gender, Intimacy, the Household, and Love

In developing a historical-ethnographic approach to AIDS, I conceive of political economy and intimacy as being mutually constituted within multiple geographies. Migration patterns, work, the T.V., and many other factors affect the way both male-female and same-sex couples engage today in their intimate lives. These dynamics intersect especially closely with meanings and practices around gender, and I have already argued that more attention to history must be given when using this concept. As Joan Scott says, a central question must be *"how* hierarchies such as those of gender are constructed and legitimized . . . a study of processes, not of origins, of multiple rather than single causes."[40]

Scott also insists that gender history is not equivalent to women's histories, and work on masculinities takes up this challenge. Raewyn Connell's influential concept of "hegemonic masculinity" captures the ongoing cultural politics of gender, but I also hope to contribute to her lesser-used analysis of cathexis, or the emotional side of male power.[41] Of course, women's emotional attachment to men has long formed an important part of feminist writings, including in Simone de Beauvoir's landmark discussion of love in *The Second Sex.*[42] One contribution I hope to make, however, is to bring men and women as well as masculinities and femininities into the same conceptual frame.[43]

I use "gender," then, to represent a social hierarchy formed in relation to perceived biological differences in reproductive organs (differences themselves historically-geographically constructed). At its simplest level, this hierarchy advantages certain people (mostly but not always male-bodied persons) and disadvantages others (often female-bodied persons). It is contested but also constantly reiterated, including through institutions like the labor market that, around the world, tend to advantage men. And gender is never simply "acted on" in simple ways. For instance, the employment of gender "rights" narratives helps to produce what we mean by gender rather than affecting a stable, predefined entity. It is now relatively common in the academy (although less so in AIDS work) to conceive of gender as cross-cut by other forms of difference: for instance, race, class, and sexuality. But none of these categories, such as sexuality, are preformed, and we must be attentive to their usefulness in different contexts.[44] I cannot deal in depth with these questions but hope to approach some of these tensions, at least in a way helpful to my project, through an historical analysis of gender and intimacy.

My intention in using the word "intimacy" is not to downplay the high levels of violence perpetrated by men on women in South Africa and elsewhere. However, the more I tried to understand the history of AIDS, the more my focus expanded outward from what Foucault famously described as the "fictitious unity" of "sex."[45] The broader concept of intimacy allows me to give attention to shifting notions of masculinities and femininities, questions around fertility, same-sex as well as female-male relations, matters of pleasure, and the vastly understudied sphere of love.[46] Indeed, when South Africanist historians have differentiated between sex and intimacy, for instance in considering inter-racial marriage (and not simply sex), their work has revealed much about the intricate contours of racial rule.[47] Yet AIDS writings have tended to fixate on "sex" without considering in any detail what is meant by the term—or ade-quately considering its constitution through historical-geographical change.

Another reason I use the word "intimacy" is that until quite recently "sex-uality" was a term without much meaning in my research site. Of course the notion of "having a sexuality" is relatively new everywhere it exists, and is tied to the rise of medical discourses and disciplines like sexology. But the central focus of this study is not on the production of the discourse of "sexuality," nor on any "indigenous" alternative, nor on the way people take up (subject) positions through such discourses. While I hope to contribute to the study of the history of sexuality in South Africa, this book's aim is more restricted: to explore a wide range of changes that led to patterns of intimate practices and meanings that now drive AIDS.

Erotic practices are enormously varied and I agree with those who argue that studies of intimacy in Africa are generally heteronormative.[48] At the same time, I accept the prevailing view that most South Africans become infected with HIV through male-female sex. I try to deal with this tension in the fol-lowing way. While giving most attention to male-female intimacy, I consider same-sex relationships throughout—if perhaps not to the extent merited by previous silences. I argue, for instance, that sexual networks comprise not only male-female but also male-male linkages (and no doubt female-female ones, although I have less evidence for this). And I follow scholars who argue for caution when we interpret past practices of male-male "sex," in part because marriage to women remained important to many of these men. One contri-bution of this book, therefore, is to provide a particularly detailed study of male-female intimacy and gender that recognizes, although it does not always pursue in detail, connections between male-female and same-sex intimacy.

Following from the above, I must use the words "sex" and "sexuality" with some caution. Of course I cannot avoid these concepts, especially "sex," which is an English word widely incorporated into isiZulu conversations today. Indeed, as the book moves through the twentieth century I increasingly use "sex"—like many South Africans—to mean penis-vagina penetration and to signify a discourse that ties erotic pleasure to an individual's identity.

In considering the "household" (rather than simply the "family") I hope to capture the fluid, interconnected geographies of reciprocity and attachment that exist as people make a living in different ways and places.[49] In general terms, I use "household" to mean either a single person or a group of people who share significant elements of life, from remittances to daily meals. Households can therefore be made up of married couples, a lone migrant worker, cohabiting male-female or same-sex couples, and many other arrangements. More than one household can live in a single dwelling, and households can stretch between homes in different locations. If the definition sounds somewhat broad, this is because there is a complex array of household types in South Africa today.

Giving attention to the household helps to clear some space between intimacy and the narratives of "family decline" or "family degeneration" that particularly surround the lives of black South Africans. Households are not sites of morality that simply "break down" but dynamic institutions formed in relation to the labor market, kinship, racial segregation, the state, and much more. Historicizing the contingent relationships between race, the household, and intimacy is especially important when stereotypes of "African promiscuity" are still common.[50] And this history helps to bring to light the socio-spatial dynamics that underpin the fact that "African" South Africans are most likely to be infected with HIV today.[51]

Indeed, hardly mentioned today, but with uncanny parallels to the present moment, is the migration of thousands of poor white women to towns from rural areas in the first half of the century who, facing meager industrial wages, were pushed into "prostitution." This trend is described in great detail in psychiatrist Louis Freed's book *The Problem of European Prostitution in Johannesburg*, published in 1949. As Freed showed, sexually transmitted infections were, in fact, prevalent among all "races" in South Africa prior to the introduction of penicillin in the 1940s and 1950s.

Certainly, it took a series of labor and welfare laws aimed at promoting poor white families and the state's massive employment of Afrikaners (propelled by the election of the apartheid government in 1948) to pull many poor white women out of this sexual economy. Here, we must note, "education" took the form not of the "safe-sex" campaigns aimed at individuals that are common today, but of massive state investment in schooling for whites that underpinned their preferential position in the labor market during the apartheid era.

Today, the racial structuring of households finds expression in the fact that unemployment is at 4.6 percent among whites and 42.5 percent among Africans; 59 percent of the white population is married, whereas the figure among Africans is only half that (30 percent).[52] Of course, there are fundamental differences between the challenges faced by a government answerable

to only a white minority and those faced by one elected by the greater population. Yet, as we shall see, the state's interventions after apartheid were relatively
modest, and gender was only peripherally important in areas, such as housing,
where it had been significant.

Indeed, just as the country faced the massive new threat of AIDS, the
state argued that laissez-faire economic policies were necessary in the era of
"globalization." Its generally technocratic interventions failed to conceptualize work with housing, production with social reproduction, and economy
with health. Nor did AIDS intervention campaigns—often funded from
overseas—typically address these connections. Yet, as AIDS programs came
and went, the disease's structural roots arguably worsened: in the first ten
years of democracy unemployment rose by 7 percentage points to 47 percent
among women and by an equal amount to 31 percent among men.[53] And one
recent United Nations study found that South African cities have the most
unequal distribution of income in the world.[54]

LOVE IN THE TIME OF AIDS?
ROMANTIC LOVE AND PROVIDER LOVE

Over the last several years a rich literature on love has emerged, in part
in response to the AIDS pandemic.[55] Yet Africa is still often thought of, and
written about, as loveless.[56] More than a century ago, (male) settlers in Natal
claimed that they had a moral mission to liberate love from the supposedly
restrictive clutches of patriarchal African society. In 1878 Bishop Colenso,
compiling his Zulu dictionary, illustrated his definition of the word *uthando*
(love) with the phrase "the Government says that girls should choose through
love, and not be compelled to husbands" (*uHulemente ute izintombi azitshaye
ngotando, zingabotshelwa emadodeni*).[57] This promotion of love, while presented
in moral terms, dovetailed with settlers' economic interests: facing stark labor
shortages, many imagined that African men were living idly in homesteads,
"buying" wives who were entrapped in polygamous marriages.

Generations later, the anthropological literature on African kinship and
ilobolo tended to present marriage as a mechanical exchange of women
between kinship groups. The famous structural-functionalist anthropologist
Radcliffe-Brown wrote in 1962 that "the African does not think of marriage
as a union based on romantic love." Affection, he argued, "is the product of
the marriage itself."[58] Also grounding their work on the belief that love was
absent in "traditional" society, the small number of writers who did study love
in Africa tended to see it as a quintessentially modern force fighting against
restrictive traditions; they saw individualistic practices, such as the modern
companionate marriage, and new communication forms, such as the love let-

ter, as undermining the dense kinship bonds that characterized traditional African society.[59]

This sense of love as a liberatory force is, in fact, common in many settings. Pioneering historians of romantic love in the West traced a centuries-long shift toward individuals' greater marital choice (as opposed to kin's influence) and growing companionship within marriage. Lawrence Stone, who coined the term "affective individualism," afforded probably the most well-known account.[60] While this work typically concentrated on the sixteenth to nineteenth centuries, writers on the twentieth century have pointed to the centrality of consumption to a commercialized form of romantic love that gained enormous popularity.[61] Celebrating a further shift at the end of the century—a kind of extreme version of romantic love's individualism—sociologist Anthony Giddens posited the emergence of "confluent love," a contingent "rolling contract" whereby women and not just men could leave "relationships" at any time.[62]

This rich literature on love clearly has relevance in South Africa. The remarkable spread of Christianity in particular helped to promote monogamy over polygamy and provide, in missions, a place of refuge for the relatively small number of women forced into marriages they explicitly opposed. Quite a lot of historical sources exist to show how a version of romantic love took shape in the twentieth century: these include church documents, magazines read by a new Christian elite, and love letters.

The critical study of romantic love also brings into sharp relief how social change can reconstitute selfhood—the very notion of individualism that permeates the concept of marital "choice." Indeed, as an increasing number of Christians in South Africa took their wedding vows the "I" of their voices differed from the "I" in a pre-Christian world. Studying romantic love therefore helps to problematize ahistorical notions of "agency."

Yet romantic love has important analytical limits. As critics of the Western literature on romantic love argue, studies' reliance on written sources such as diaries and love letters can bias them in two ways. First, it tends to skew attention toward the literate middle classes. Second, it tends to promote a teleological framework whereby modern societies become progressively more loving—a framing especially problematic in the case of "Africa," a space long seen as backward. These biases, in turn, serve to downplay love's expression in practical acts of cooperation and mutual assistance that predate literacy.[63] In other words, the dazzling light of romantic love can blind us to more mundane but nevertheless vital forms of connection.

The importance of recognizing practical acts of love in a colonial context leads me to put forward a second type of love, what I call *provider love*. This book argues that expressions of love enacted through cooperation and mutual assistance—practices that are simultaneously material and meaningful, even if they are not articulated in writing—are crucial to the intertwined histories of love and exchange in twentieth-century South Africa. Provider love is enmeshed in a set of profoundly important gender expectations that came to hinge on men's rapidly growing dependence on wage labor at a time of racial rule. A man fostered provider love by paying ilobolo and subsequently supporting a wife (or wives); in turn a woman contributed love by maintaining the marital home.

Today, the existence of sex-money exchanges often leads to claims that sex has become "transactional" or "commodified." Yet the concept of provider love allows us to take more seriously young South Africans' assertions that their intimate relationships are, at some level, about love without dismissing the material realities of life. It helps, for instance, to address the following questions: why do gift exchanges that encompass sex take place mostly between "boyfriends" and "girlfriends" and not "prostitutes" and "clients"? Why do many people divide multiple concurrent partners into a "main" lover and plural "secondary" lovers? And why in many instances do lovers not use condoms to protect themselves from potential HIV infection?

Moving beyond the idea of love "coming to Africa," this book therefore focuses on two forms of love that, as I will show, are deeply interwoven: romantic love and provider love. Attention to the former foregrounds more individualized patterns of courting and marriage. It also shows how love became a dynamic force in the remaking of selves even if marital choice was common before colonialism. Attention to the latter allows us to see the changing ways in which men have provided love in South Africa as love became embroiled with vastly different forms of male assistance: from a position where men were the providers in marital households to one today where men can support multiple unmarried girlfriends.

About the Book

It is necessary to give several caveats. Although I try to deconstruct racialized notions of sexuality, I am aware of the difficulties of doing so. In Mandeni, my research site, South Africans classified as African under apartheid make up about 95 percent of the population. At one time, I considered broadening my scope to include studying intimacy in the nearby white, Indian, and coloured areas to prevent this project from being simply focused on "African sexuality." In the end such a project, with so few secondary sources to launch it from, was so daunting as to be unfeasible. Instead, I tried to unravel connections between "races," and pushed deeper historically when I felt uneasy at the politics of writing a contemporary ethnography of intimacy. I also undertook research outside of Mandeni, working with a research group in rural Hlabisa, an area from which many residents of Mandeni had migrated. This provided invaluable insights into the lives of rural migrants. In fact, on a day-to-day basis, many residents have much closer links with the KwaZulu hinterland than areas a few miles to the east or south.

More generally, as some writers have powerfully argued, AIDS and sex are not the same thing: racialized assumptions can exaggerate the importance of sex (and heterosexual sex especially) to the spread of AIDS.[64] In addressing intimacy, I leave open, and largely unexamined, vital questions around the importance of co-factors in the AIDS pandemic. Particularly, poor nutrition and the prevalence of other sexually transmitted infections connected to poverty undoubtedly play a role: an HIV-positive person with another STI, for instance, has a three to five times higher chance of infecting a sexual partner with HIV.[65] Tremendous inequalities in health services also affect the disease's progression: 15 percent of the population has access to private health care facilities while the remainder, most of whom are black, depend on an overburdened public health service.[66]

Writing about terrible social conditions faced by millions of shack dwellers today, Sbu Zikode, the leader of *Abahlali baseMjondolo* (the Durban-based shack dwellers movement), said in 2006, "Our bodies itch every day because of the insects. . . . You must see how big the rats are that will run across the small babies in the night."[67] Zikode's testimony stands as a vital reminder of the need to understand the spatiality of multiple causes of AIDS. These matters are under-researched and I look, therefore, at only one dimension of AIDS—intimacy.

The book is divided into three parts: Revisiting Intimacy and Apartheid; Intimacy after Democracy; and Interventions. Key arguments are contained in this structure. We must not understand apartheid as a "degeneration" of family life but explore how racial capitalism intersected with and worked through the male-led home. Then we need to consider how AIDS coincided with the emergence of a democratic South Africa which, in turn, collided with the global ascendancy of free-market economics. Finally, we must consider interventions and politics in the context of both the first and second sets of findings.

The next chapter will introduce my primary research site, Mandeni. Chapter 3 traces how male migrancy and Christianity transformed ideas of intimate "traditions" in the early twentieth century. Here, I stress the emergence of new connections between wage labor, men's roles as providers, and emotions. Chapter 4 moves to an urban setting and explores ideas of respectability in Sundumbili township and the importance of state-granted housing to the male provider identity. As chapter 5 shows, from the 1970s women increasingly challenged men's role as head of household; many moved into the informal/shack settlement surrounding Isithebe Industrial Park and carved out a living as "industrial women." But women's independence was relatively short-lived as unemployment rose. Moving into the post-apartheid period, chapter 6 foregrounds social and spatial shifts that "left behind" the majority of South Africans both literally and figuratively.

The next four chapters elucidate the contemporary cultural politics of intimacy. I look at how women draw on rights in unanticipated ways (chapter 7), the reworking of masculinities (chapter 8), and connections between money, sex, and love (chapter 9). The conclusion (chapter 10) explores the politics of AIDS interventions through two different AIDS organizations that emerged in Mandeni, the activist group Treatment Action Campaign and the youth-AIDS NGO loveLife.

Several aims of this book have already been described, but an overarching one derives directly from the people who tolerated my many intrusions into their lives. I was often asked at the end of interviews what I was doing about the AIDS situation in Mandeni. The short answer was, very little—or perhaps that I was working with the Treatment Action Campaign or helping a local gender violence NGO to raise funds, both of which I did at varying times. My longer answer, however, was that I would try and write a dissertation and possibly a book that linked the poor economic conditions, especially the devastatingly high unemployment rates, to the prevalence of AIDS. Massive unemployment was the explanation for the pandemic overwhelmingly given to me by residents. The connection between AIDS and unemployment turned out to be fraught with complexities I never anticipated, but it is one that none of my informants ever doubted exists—and neither do I.

TWO

Mandeni:
"The AIDS Capital of KwaZulu-Natal"

If you drive north from Durban up the N2 highway you might smell central Mandeni before you see it. You know you are getting close when you cross the Thukela River, which formerly divided the British colony of Natal from the independent Zulu Kingdom. Then, turning onto a northwest-bound road, you will pass the former white town of Mandini. Its name is actually a misspelling of "Mandeni," an older word for the area and now the name of the local municipality.

Continue driving and you be assaulted by a nasty, sulphurous smell just as the fuming chimneys of a paper mill come into view. If you wish to take in some spectacular apartheid landscape, close your car windows and turn north from here. To your right you'll be admiring the lush sugar-cane farms of the former white-designated land; but glance left and you'll see the former KwaZulu homeland/bantustan—a sprawling African township and thousands of shacks. Then, at a place called Isithebe, you'll see a giant industrial complex of more than 180 factories.

Arriving suddenly in the 1970s and 1980s, Isithebe's heavily subsidized factories were part of an apartheid social engineering project aimed at deterring black South Africans from entering large white towns. Isithebe's industrial success made the area something of a jewel in the apartheid crown.

By 1997, however, the popular magazine *Drum* had declared Mandeni the "AIDS capital of the province [KwaZulu-Natal]."[1] This is a terrible reputation, especially since KwaZulu-Natal is the country's most AIDS-affected area, where nearly four out of ten pregnant women today test positive for HIV, the virus that leads to AIDS.[2]

The province of KwaZulu-Natal came into being after the merger of the KwaZulu homeland and Natal Province in 1994. It is now the most populous of South Africa's nine provinces, hosting 9.4 million of the country's 44.9 million people.[3] After a series of boundary and name changes, Mandeni's present borders were drawn in 2000.[4] I consider in this book primarily the area I call "central Mandeni," which incorporates the vast bulk of the municipality's

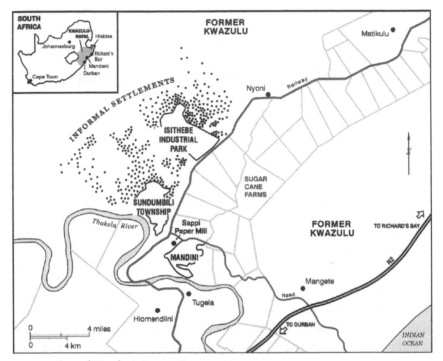

MAP 2.1. Central Mandeni, Present Day

population. I give most attention to two areas, Isithebe informal/*jondolo* settlement, which hosts a mostly migrant population, and Sundumbili township, which houses more permanent urban residents. Mandeni's history forms the backbone of this book and I summarize it only briefly here.

Like all of South Africa, Mandeni bears the heavy scars of colonial land dispossession. Some twenty years after the British defeated the Zulu Kingdom in 1879, Zululand became part of the colony of Natal. Then, in 1904, in one vicious swoop, the Zululand Land Delimitation Commission designated 40 percent of Zululand's most fertile land for the use of white settlers. This arbitrary land theft is marked by the large swathe of sugar cane farms that today cut through Mandeni's heart.

In 1910 Natal became part of the Union of South Africa, the modern South African state. With a national economy centered on minerals extraction, most men growing up in Mandeni in the early twentieth century expected to work in the country's rich gold and diamond mines. Policies of racial segregation entrenched male migration patterns and kept most Africans' permanent homes in rural "reserves." In Mandeni, most of this reserve land was supervised from the district capital, Eshowe, by white officials, although tax collection and customary law was administered on a day-to-day basis by government-approved chiefs. Few local men worked on the fertile white-owned sugar plantations in Mandeni: cane was typically cut by migrant male workers from Mpondoland or Mozambique (then under Portuguese control).[5]

This rural landscape became industrialized in 1954 when SAPPI (South African Pulp and Paper Industries, Limited) built a large paper mill on the banks of the Thukela River. Yet an even more significant boost to industry in the area came in 1971 when the state targeted this homeland space for "industrial decentralization" and established Isithebe Industrial Park. By 1990, 23,000 people in Isithebe were employed, half of them women.

In the 1990s, however, as the state removed industrial subsidies, the industrial park went into decline, and after 1994, when the new government reduced trade tariffs, it faced crippling competition from international producers. Women, in particular, continued to move to Mandeni in great numbers, to stay in informal settlements, but could not find employment.

Today, around 95 percent of Mandeni's residents are African, nearly 2.5 percent are Indian (mostly descendants of indentured laborers), around 2 percent are white (mostly descendants of Europeans), and 0.5 percent are coloured (a category roughly denoting "mixed-race").[6] Until democracy in 1994, these racial categories largely determined where a person would live. Tugela, a small trading area south of the Thukela River, was the main area where Indians were forced to reside. Coloureds were restricted to Mangete; this area had its origins in the Zulu king Cetshwayo's granting of land to the white *inkosi* (chief) John Dunn (who had forty-nine African wives).[7] To the south of SAPPI, the white town of Mandini was built. To the north, the township of Sundumbili was established for Africans; this was located in a former "reserve" that became part of the KwaZulu "homeland" in the 1970s. In addition to this geography, I briefly explore women's migration to Isithebe from Hlabisa, an area about 120 kilometers northeast of Mandeni.

I lived to the north of Isithebe Industrial Park in the informal/jondolo/shack settlement. I explain these terms in more detail in chapter 5 but, in brief, I generally use the term "jondolo settlement" when referring to Isithebe but "informal settlement" when discussing other unplanned areas across South Africa marked by informal houses. I do so to try and balance the need to indicate the similarity of unplanned settlements (which is captured by the term "informal settlement") and the fact that *umjondolo* (pl. *imijondolo*) is a vernacular term for temporary accommodation whose connotations go well beyond the word "informal."

The conversations, interviews, and observations I draw stretch over almost a decade of research in the region (2000–2009) and include more than a year and a half living in isiZulu-speaking settings. I stayed in Mandeni in 2000, 2001, and 2006 for between one and four months and did my main fieldwork while living in Mandeni extensively from 2002 to 2005, while also conducting archival work in Durban. I undertook further follow-up work in Mandeni in 2007 and 2009. I also lived with a family in rural Hlabisa for one month in late 2003.

During my time in Mandeni, I learnt an enormous amount from the large family with whom I stayed, although from the outset I agreed not to write about their lives. I lived slightly away from their main house, in a small concrete-block umjondolo structure that backed onto a row of imijondolo rented by rural migrants. Eating and socializing with the family, I got to see family members finish school, bear children, and search for work. None married. In turn, and revealing of our quite different paths, the family watched me finish a degree, find work, marry, and then become a father. Despite our very different personal trajectories—ones echoed in South Africa as a whole—the family's warmth led me to spend five Christmases (2000, 2002, 2003, 2004, and 2005) in Isithebe. Every Christmas Day we danced to deafening music for hours until we eventually succumbed to Mandeni's excruciating summer heat.

Outside of this family, I got to know many other Mandeni residents, some also for nearly ten years. I hung out at shebeens (informal drinking places), attended funerals, visited friends, went to church services, volunteered at a youth center, and much more. I also conducted three hundred or so formal interviews with around two hundred people for this project; some I interviewed as many as five times. Nearly all the interviews were conducted in isiZulu and I translated most of them myself, occasionally with some help from isiZulu speakers on certain passages.[8] I support these ethnographic methods with historical records, including court cases, government documents, and past ethnographies.[9]

My study of AIDS came about somewhat by chance. I first began living in Isithebe's informal settlement in 2000 as part of a seven-month "predissertation" stay in South Africa. At the time, I was relatively oblivious to the area's association with high HIV rates and intent on continuing with my master's degree research on labor issues in the area (this degree was completed in 1998 at the University of KwaZulu-Natal). I also hoped to improve my isiZulu, and I asked a former colleague familiar with Mandeni to help me find a family in the area with whom to stay; it just so happened that this family resided in Isithebe. From here I started asking residents about employment, labor rights, and industrial change.

Yet living in the community soon meant meeting residents with various ailments, including tuberculosis, stomach pains, and skin problems such as *ibhande* (a local term for shingles because the illness creates a feeling that a person's body is being constrained by a band). Looking more closely at AIDS statistics and the youthfulness of the area's population, I began to ask, with a sense of guilt and inadequacy, whether it could really be true that perhaps half of the people I knew were HIV positive. Before antiretroviral (ARV) medicines became available in 2004 I wondered about the morality of spending money on my research when I could be using it to pay for medicine. I debated with myself what I would do if someone I was close to, such as a member of my adopted family, fell ill from AIDS and my small monthly research budget might contribute to supplying life-saving drugs (although it could have done so only in quite a minor way at that time, because of ARVs' exorbitant cost).

I returned to Berkeley in 2001 completely mentally exhausted. I remembered that this was not the first time South Africa had imparted such a feeling: in 1989, then eighteen years old, I returned to Britain from a year volunteering in a township school in the former Transkei "homeland." At that time, witnessing apartheid first-hand spurred me to ditch my undergraduate degree course in physics to study politics and development studies and embrace anti-apartheid student politics. So again, twelve years later, this beautiful, captivating—but shockingly unequal—country was transforming my plans. It wasn't long before I decided to study AIDS and connect the subject to my first interest in the area, political economy.

Over the years, I spent a lot of time exploring the nooks and crannies of Mandeni's social geography. However, I do not consider this ethnography to be simply "local." My understanding of Mandeni is influenced by a conceptualization of space as "produced" and "relational"; in other words, I conceive of places as being power-laden and formed in relation to other places.[10] In the social sciences, the label "local" can be used to suggest that research sites have firm boundaries. But geographers have long stressed that the local is part of a web of dynamic social processes stretching to scales that include the national and the global; a study of the local can therefore cut through, and help to clarify, larger-scale social processes. The themes I stress make this an especially important conceptualization. As feminist geographers have argued, there has long been a bias toward seeing gender and social reproduction as somehow "local" and the economy as "global."[11]

It is through this conception of space that I also consider Zuluness.[12] As a consequence of apartheid's efforts to divide black South Africans into discrete ethnic groups (Zulu, Xhosa, etc.), questions of ethnicity are politically charged in the country. IsiZulu, a central but not exact signifier of Zulu identity, is

South Africa's most spoken home language and the majority of its speakers live in KwaZulu-Natal, although many live too in Gauteng Province. Though considering a wider geography obviously has some advantages, by concentrating on one place, one language, and one (produced) ethnicity, I am able, I hope, to provide a fine-grained account of social change. This is, by necessity, a global and not a local historical ethnography, and Zuluness itself, as I show, is deeply entangled with the colonial process. I do not defend place-based ethnographies as the only way to understand these issues, but I hope that this study provides insights into the tremendous shifts in intimacy over the twentieth century. But more on Mandeni later: for now some reflections on the wider context of AIDS in South Africa and the world.

AIDS in South Africa

The disease that is now called AIDS first came to light in 1981 after a cluster of cases of rare skin cancer were found among gay men in the U.S. Similarly, in South Africa, the first reported cases of AIDS in the early 1980s were among white gay men. By 1986, however, a study commissioned by the Johannesburg-based Chamber of Mines found that nearly 4 percent of Malawian migrants were HIV positive.[13] Soon afterward, it became clear that HIV was disproportionately affecting Africans, the group who faced the most severe discrimination under apartheid. Moreover, while more women than men were HIV positive, the relatively small aggregate gender differences in infection signaled that male-female sexual intercourse was an important transmission mechanism.

All HIV and AIDS statistics are socially produced and mediated by existing categories; the obvious example of this in South Africa is the category of "race," which hides much within its seemingly impermeable boundaries. But the figures were unequivocal in showing a tremendous rise of HIV infections in the 1990s. By 2003, just before the government embarked on a program to provide antiretroviral drugs that greatly retard HIV's progression to AIDS, around 770 people *per day* died from AIDS.[14]

Compared to other pathogens, HIV is difficult to transmit. From the mid-1980s, health officials around the world warned about the dangers of a virus that eroded the immune system, leaving the body vulnerable to opportunistic infections. But in the West the disease remained largely contained within "high risk" groups like hemophiliacs, gay men, and people who inject drugs. Indeed, the HIV epidemic remained most centered on sub-Saharan Africa: warnings that parts of Asia are on the verge of a huge epidemic have not yet been proven accurate. While it is difficult to anticipate future trends, the more than five and a half million people living with HIV in South Africa represent a greater number of infections than exist in the whole of Asia.[15]

The bulk of AIDS funding, however, has not gone toward understanding the social-spatial drivers of the pandemic. Most resources have been spent on biomedical research, including efforts to develop (profitable) treatments and a vaccine (this still appears to be far away). Ethnographic studies are especially burdened by the widespread belief in health circles that they lack the scientific authority of epidemiology—a key tool used by public health authorities to monitor disease patterns, usually through sophisticated statistical techniques. Too often, weak explanations for HIV's high prevalence in Africa left unchallenged racist stereotypes of "African promiscuity" deeply embedded in the Western psyche and the legacy of colonialism. Surely, some asked, AIDS was just a consequence of lascivious African sexuality—or, in more sophisticated terms, of an "African system of sexuality"?[16]

To counter racist stereotypes, some South Africanist scholars sought to emphasize AIDS' political-economic roots. While drawing attention to important themes, the analysis, as I show, was often only partial. To expose the long-standing connections between racial capitalism and STIs, many researchers drew comparisons between AIDS and the syphilis pandemic that peaked in the 1940s and was so famously outlined in Sidney Kark's 1949 article "The Social Pathology of Syphilis in Africans."[17] Kark showed in this piece how migrant labor restricted Africans from settling in urban areas and forced men into long absences from their rural homes. Housed in overcrowded compounds, some men engaged in sexual relationships with urban-based women and then passed on infections to their wives in rural areas.

The projecting forward of the male migrancy model probably reached its peak with the release of the South African film *Yesterday* in 2003. The film, widely lauded in AIDS circles, tells the story of a young uneducated KwaZulu-Natal mother who falls ill and discovers her mineworker husband has infected her with HIV.[18] Of course, male migration undoubtedly played a critical role in the early stages of the pandemic and still plays a part today. However, because the institution symbolized the negative influence of racial rule, including the breaking up of families, it became an easy target to blame for AIDS. The male migrancy model did not adequately address what I call the changing political economy and geography of intimacy. Table 2.1 summarizes some of the differences between the spread of sexually transmitted infections today and in the 1940s/50s, the era when Kark connected male migration to syphilis.[19] It must be noted that this is a very crude summary of the themes in this book.

More recently, an increasingly popular explanation for AIDS—one with value, if it tends to exalt a single cause—is that of sexual networking, the connecting of individuals through sex. Scholars argue that more important than people's simply having multiple sexual partners is the existence of concurrent relationships (as distinguished from the practice of serial monogamy).[20] This is because HIV viral load (the amount of virus in the blood) and thus a person's infectiousness is at its highest during the first few months and the latest stages of infection. HIV can therefore be passed on much more easily by a person who is newly infected and has a high viral load (and such people are usually asymptomatic). In dense sexual networks, everyone is linked to the newly infected person.

In the last few years this practice has taken on an acronym, MCP (multiple concurrent partners or partnerships), and intervention programs have been launched. And the argument is sometimes made that Africans, even rich Africans, have multiple partners more often than other groups—that "race" and "culture" are therefore more important than poverty to sexuality and AIDS. Yet the categories of race and culture, if used uncritically, afford a false unity to the social history of AIDS. Even if rich African men like Jacob Zuma argue that Zuluness is synonymous with men having multiple partners, poverty and apartheid helped to construct what gets called Zulu "culture" (often by men). Statistical surveys favored by epidemiologists might show a correlation between race and AIDS, but race can never be thought of as an unambiguous category: it manifests numerous dynamic processes, ones always entangled with differences due to age, class, gender, and much more.

It is for these reasons that I show in some detail how the production of the masculine *isoka* (playboy) figure—and, more broadly, the nature of the "sexual double standard"—can only be understood by considering changes wrought by colonialism, apartheid, and chronic unemployment. And I insist that without addressing the structural reasons why men and women have more than one sexual partner, any behavioral intervention campaign is unlikely to provide a major breakthrough, even if some writers argue that similar campaigns had success in Uganda, where HIV rates were reduced significantly in the 1980s.[21]

One of my arguments is that the "materiality of everyday sex" is a key driving force behind multiple concurrent partners. Most studies of concurrency acknowledge this point but they rarely describe in any detail connections between sex-gift exchanges and broader aspects of everyday life. It is, for instance, widely accepted that wealth inequalities can drive relationships between younger women and older, usually richer, boyfriends: recent data shows that intergenerational sex is relatively common and that nearly four times as many women as men aged twenty to twenty-four are HIV positive (21.1 percent compared to 5.1 percent).[22] At the same time, the gender and

TABLE 2.1.
Summary of the Changing Political Economy
and Geography of Intimacy

SOCIAL CONTEXT	1940s/1950s	TODAY
Labor/Class	A high demand for the labor of African men, some demand for the labor of African women. Very low wages.	Chronic unemployment, especially among Africans. Rising class divisions.
Household	Marriage increasingly unstable but still common in both rural and urban areas. Wedlock seen as a joint but contested project of "building a home." Rural households largely dependent on remittances from married men.	Very low marriage rates and great hostility between young men and women. Growth in the number of smaller households. Rural areas dependent on state pensions, child support grants, and remittances from both men and women.
Geography	Men in circular migration patterns, some women moving to urban areas. Many informal settlements "removed" by apartheid planners.	Both men and women in multiple migration patterns, including circular migration. Growth of informal settlements, typified by small imijondolo.
Penetrative Sexual Relations	Some migrant men have multiple partners. Some women dependent on men in extramarital relationships. Premarital relationships not generally characterized by the exchange of sex for money.	Many women dependent on men, sometimes multiple men, in a situation where most people are not married. Exchanges of money for sex are common, although defined not as "prostitution" but as gifts from "boyfriends" to "girlfriends."

generational politics that encase these relationships are poorly understood. By presenting a single analysis that combines political economy, masculinities and femininities, and money and love, I show that "transactional sex" is not a discrete practice that can be simply acronymed ("TS") and then modified. It is deeply embedded in the country's changing political economy and attendant social meanings.

Mandeni and AIDS

If Mandeni is the "AIDS capital of KwaZulu-Natal," KwaZulu-Natal has the highest HIV rates in South Africa, and South Africa has the highest number of HIV positive people in the world, locating an AIDS study in this setting has obvious relevance.[23] Three reasons are commonly given for KwaZulu-Natal's status as the worst affected of the country's nine provinces: its hosting of the large port city of Durban, the fact that most isiZulu speakers do not circumcise, and the history of intense political violence between Inkatha and ANC supporters in the region in the 1980s and early 1990s.[24] All of these explanations are plausible. But my research yields two further possible reasons that need to be given more attention: under apartheid, present-day KwaZulu-Natal was the area where industrial decentralization was most successful. It was also the region where shacks grew the quickest in the 1970s and 1980s. Both histories left patterns of inequality and demographic shifts that are perhaps more extreme in this province than elsewhere.

My main aim, however, is to make an argument not about Mandeni in relation to the KwaZulu-Natal region but about the country as a whole. I believe that this history of Mandeni can tell a wider, if necessarily partial, story about why AIDS emerged so quickly in South Africa. Many of the key forces shaping twentieth-century South Africa find expression in Mandeni: racialized land dispossession, industrial growth and decline, the building of a formal African township, the rise of informal/shack settlements, and extreme population mobility. I use throughout the book national statistics and reports demonstrating that the themes I explore qualitatively—unemployment, migration, reductions in marriage, the rising number of shacks—are very much a part of South Africa's modern history. And numerous studies of sex and intimacy in contemporary South Africa, some of which I quote, reveal themes similar to the ones I stress. These include high levels of sexual violence and what I call the materiality of everyday sex.

It is generally believed that the "heterosexual" AIDS pandemic began in equatorial Africa and then moved east and south until it reached South Africa in the 1980s.[25] I cannot generalize about whether the issues I explore are relevant to explaining AIDS elsewhere in the continent of Africa or in the wider world. The pandemic is incredibly varied: prevalence is less than 1 percent in Senegal, whereas in Southern Africa HIV rates of 20 or 30 percent are not uncommon.[26] I would, however, stress the importance of an approach that takes the political economy of intimacy as foundational in understanding patterns of HIV prevalence.[27] Of course, many other factors come into play. Christianity, as I show, helped to rework intimate worlds in South Africa, and low HIV rates in predominantly Islamic countries invite further attention to questions of faith. But religion itself, while important, can't be simply seen as operating outside of political economies, demographics, and an array of intimate practices.

Although I have not conducted comparative research, the themes I discuss in this book are perhaps especially pertinent to the most AIDS-affected region of the world, Southern Africa: here, the historical inequalities caused by mining and a highly developed form of capitalism come together with some of the lowest marriage rates in the world. Indeed, one recent study found a strong correlation between HIV and non-marriage—and it particularly noted the low marriage rates in Southern Africa.[28] This does not mean that marriage simply "protects" against HIV; on the contrary, many wives are infected by their husbands and, in these cases, messages that promote monogamous love and not condom use can put women at risk if their husbands have extramarital affairs.[29] There is certainly not, therefore, a straightforward link between marriage and HIV infection.[30] But whether HIV infection takes place within or outside a marital union, we must conceive of marriage in any setting as an institution that incorporates material flows, moral obligations, lived geographies, power relations, and pleasures and pains. And we must ask how, if marriage is absent, these processes and practices are reconfigured in ways that can both decrease and increase the chance of HIV transmission.

Postcolonial Politics of Researching AIDS

> *The racial becomes the spatial. The social construction of race becomes one with the physical occupation of space. The racialized becomes the segregated, and racial meanings become inscribed upon space.*
>
> —ALLAN PRED, *Even in Sweden*

When I first stayed in Mandeni in 2000, the area was still reeling from political violence. In the early 1990s, as democracy neared, the ANC and the

Zulu nationalist Inkatha Freedom Party (IFP) clashed and hundreds of people lost their lives. In 1999, half a decade after elections, the last scholars to undertake social research in Mandeni before me were advised to leave the area for their own safety. This history came abruptly to my attention early on in my research in 2000. I arrived one day at what I thought would be an informal interview with a member of the IFP and, instead, found myself being grilled by six senior members, several of whom were notorious "warlords." They wanted to know how I could help them raise money for the upcoming local elections. The fact that we met in the township police station told its own story about the state's biases toward the IFP in the apartheid days.

Yet as political violence and therefore my need to appear unaffiliated with any organization faded, AIDS activism began a remarkable rise in South Africa. This was born from multiple roots: the pain of thousands of AIDS deaths; the injustice of patent laws that made life-saving drugs too expensive for most South Africans; and a government that questioned basic AIDS science. These troubling happenings triggered the rise of the Treatment Action Campaign, a group which I worked with at times and whose politics shaped some of the themes in the book.

Over the years, I got to know many people well in Mandeni. One of the first I met was a man I call Thami.[31] He worked in Mandini, the town built for SAPPI's white employees, a place that most African residents call *emakwatasi* (quarters) today because of its association with African women being employed there as domestic workers. Thami was a popular car guard who carried shopping bags from the local supermarket to people's cars with a humor that availed him well with his mostly white clients. He lived a hundred meters from me in the jondolo settlement in one of the cheapest rented imijondolo, made of mud, stones, and wood.

In late 2000, Thami offered to introduce me to some of his friends, and we walked along the narrow dirt paths that separated the numerous rows of imijondolo scattered across the settlement; many were made from concrete blocks and were rented at around R60 to R80 per month (approximately US$9) rather than the R20 he paid his landlord.[32] I met his girlfriend and child and we shared some beers at a nearby store. One day, we continued up a steep bank to the home of his sister Sindiswa. His family had lived in Isithebe for generations and from the 1970s watched the place transform from a quiet rural area to an overcrowded informal settlement. Sindiswa, maybe twenty-five, was seated in a badly lit room watching her child playing in the corner. She asked her brother whether his white friend could secure her a job in one of the nearby factories; residents widely assumed that I had contacts in the adjacent industrial park.

Two weeks later, at 6:20, I woke up to a distressed knock on my door. "Sindiswa is ill," her brother said; "can you take her to the hospital?" Twenty minutes later, he was stewarding my car up the steep, muddy bank toward his sister's room. "Higher, higher," he cried, as the wheels on my old rusty Mazda spun vigorously. As he carried his sister out of the front door I began to realize why he had pleaded with me to park so close to the house: her slim, limp body was eyed with a mixture of sympathy and curiosity by the neighbors. He laid his sister on the back seat with her legs resting on their mother's knees, this elderly woman by now having joined us. Sindiswa's eyes were tightly shut and her breathing was shallow as she clung desperately to life.

After a twenty-minute drive, I swung the car aggressively through the large green gates at Stanger Hospital and parked in the courtyard next to several ambulances. One employee nodded toward an empty hospital bed that sat near the entrance of the casualty department. We lifted Sindiswa onto it. Large brown double doors were the last obstacle to the emergency room. Inside, a nurse came over and asked "Uphethwe yini?" (What does she have?). "Ikhanda" (Head) was the reply. The room was jam-packed with people and equipment, but the nurse craftily maneuvered the bed in between two others, plunging a syringe into Sindiswa's arm to withdraw a sample of blood. In the reception area, Thami's mother pushed me forward into the queue to register new patients: she was well aware that the staff were less likely to ask a white person why we had not taken Sindiswa to Mandeni's nearest hospital, a place with a far worse reputation than the institution at which we had arrived.

Despite our efforts, several weeks later Sindiswa sadly passed away.

Sindiswa's funeral—the first of many that I attended—was held at the family home in Isithebe. We listened sadly to the testimonies of friends and family and walked slowly around the coffin. Small donations were volunteered after mourners took a last glance at the corpse. Yet, as we waited for food and drink, the sad tones of remembrance were punctuated by sharp words of disagreement. The heated discussions were taking place next to the burial company's old hatchback car, and it was clear Sindiswa's family was having difficulty paying for the burial service. Several minutes later, this was confirmed when Thami asked me if the coffin could fit into my Mazda so I might drive it to the graveyard. I told him this would be impossible—it would have stuck out of the back and likely fallen out. Eventually he struck a deal with the funeral company and the coffin was appropriately conveyed.

I tell this story because at Berkeley, like all other graduate students, I filled in numerous forms on ethics that gave close attention to how I would gain "informed consent" from a neatly defined group of "research subjects." But the everyday ethical dilemmas I faced during my research project extended much further than these rather abstract exercises. Was I to take my car further up the slippery bank, put a coffin into it, use racial privilege to get someone to the front of a queue? After the funeral, my location in a web of racialized meanings was brought home to me even more shockingly when a woman I didn't recognize came up to me in the nearby supermarket and thanked me with tears in her eyes for attending the burial. I was taken aback and overcome with guilt. Why should I be thanked in such terms for attending a funeral? If anything, I was the one person present who had had resources to assist Sindiswa.

Yet the assumption that whites do not care about the lives of black South Africans is reiterated every day in Mandeni, in part because poverty still restricts most black South Africans to apartheid spaces. Death, for many isi-Zulu speakers, is a profoundly social act that puts the living in a relationship with *amadlozi* (the ancestors), and my modest act of respecting death seemed to be viewed as partially subverting social relationships instituted in the apartheid era. However, even if my long stay in the informal settlement partially disrupted racialized meanings, my wealth and ability to leave made me complicit in them. Within a few minutes I could walk from my umjondolo to the industrial park, and there I would be assumed to be a factory manager with power over hundreds of people's lives. This difficulty of not being complicit in the practices I criticize is a tension that ran through my research and runs through this book.

As for Thami . . . I kept in touch with him for several years. But on my return after one trip away I noticed he was no longer in his usual place in the car park. The new car guard said he had passed away. *"Wayegula"* (He was sick), he explained, in a way that suggested both a long illness and the inevitability of his death. A few months later, a storm took away the row of mud, stick, and stone shacks where he had last stayed—erasing this memory with the same tragic finality that attended the deaths of so many people who appear in this book.

PART 1

Revisiting Intimacy
and Apartheid

THREE

Providing Love:
Male Migration and Building a Rural Home

The inkosi's (chief's) court was a strange place to talk about sex. Seated on rows of benches that scraped noisily on the concrete floor, attendees were mostly senior men, a fact that reinforced the court's masculine aura. Trying my best to act deferentially by avoiding eye contact, I stole glances at the inkosi and observed his graying stubble and medium build. The court secretary ushered me forward when it was my turn to talk. The attendees seemed pleased that I spoke isiZulu, even though my speech was far from perfect.

"My research looks at why AIDS is so bad in South Africa," I said, and then asked for permission to conduct interviews in the chief's territory. The court fell into a brief pause. After several minutes of questions about my university affiliation and where I was staying in Isithebe, one of the *izinduna* (chief's officials) leapt in with a statement and everyone laughed. I realized he was talking about *ukusoma*, usually translated as "thigh sex" or "to have thigh sex." This practice was widely reported among young courting couples in Southern Africa and involves a man rubbing his penis between a woman's thighs; the woman's legs remain crossed to prevent vaginal penetration. The chief looked at me and, with some trepidation, I said that I had learnt about ukusoma after talking with elderly informants. The audience waited on the chief's response and, after a brief silence, he laughed, signaling that others could relax into amused glances.

The court's welcoming response and elderly informants' general willingness to discuss ukusoma with me—it became almost an ice-breaker—raised questions about the very meanings of "sex" and the politics of a white man's studying it. Was I a potential guardian of tradition, someone who might help reinvigorate old customs that protected young people from the dangers of modern life? Or was I, perhaps, a representative of modernity, someone the chief thought might provide scientific information about the dangers of AIDS to young people? On both counts, a large literature on the "invention of tradition" has now made it clear that we must approach tradition and modernity as dynamic concepts rather than static opposites. Insights into this theme come from Africanists' studies of ethnic mobilization, customary law, and the modernity of "traditions" such as witchcraft.[1] Yet much less is known about the production of traditions of courtship and love.

And what—to repeat—do we mean by "sex"? Following in particular Michel Foucault's *The History of Sexuality*, it is now widely accepted that "sexuality" is not a transhistorical phenomenon. It is only in the last few hundred years, Foucault argues, that sex in the West became a central part of being, or the self. This raises questions about how to understand forms of intimacy practiced in Southern Africa in previous milieus. Ukusoma, for instance, is usually seen today as a form of non-penetrative "sex." Similarly, "have sexual intercourse in a certain lewd way externally" was how Clergyman John Colenso defined *ukuhlobonga* (another word for ukusoma) in his 1861 dictionary.[2] Yet the reaction of the court I visited, like accounts I describe later, suggests that isiZulu speakers saw these intimate practices in quite a different register than modern notions of "sex."

And how do we understand historical changes to "sexuality"? Individuals in the West, according to Foucault, came to see themselves through new sexual discourses that emerged with (but cannot be reduced to) the rise of capitalism and the modern administration of populations. Yet South Africans faced the full force of imperial plunder. In contrast to the modernizing European state, the colonial state relied ultimately on oppressive power. And it promoted racial boundaries and ethnic identifications that were quite different from Western sexologists' categorizations of acts as "normal" or "abnormal," to use this example.[3]

In this chapter I develop a historical-ethnographic approach to explore intimate practices and, related but not equivalent, the domain of "sex" in South Africa's colonial setting. Although AIDS has stimulated rich studies on sexuality, development agencies like UNAIDS have typically approached sex "with a vocabulary that assumes a self-evident object."[4] Carol Vance's warning in 1991, therefore, that AIDS would likely strengthen a pluralist approach to sexuality (the study of many sexual cultures) that left core aspects of "sexuality" untouched remains relevant. Generations of anthropologists, Vance argued, showed great expertise in cultural relativism—that is, in showing divergences in culture—although they typically viewed aspects of sexuality such as "sex drive" as precultural.[5] To understand "sex," I will argue following this point, we need to simultaneously focus in on it and decenter it; to investigate its construction as an apparently distinct domain but also to explore under-researched arenas that helped to construct it and were constructed by it—the political economy of love and masculinities being emphasized here.

In what follows, I give particular attention to how colonialism, capital-ism, and Christianity—the three great forces of the early twentieth century—transformed intimacy in South Africa. I provide here a greatly simplified story, and I certainly do not want to suggest that colonialism, Christianity, or capitalism were singular forces that swept across the present-day KwaZulu-Natal region. The last twenty years of colonial and postcolonial studies have taught us that colonialism was constitutive of Western modernity and that the colonizer and colonized were never static categories.[6] What follows, then, is a broad-brush introduction to the region and, more than anything, a cry for the importance of studying history to understand the AIDS pandemic today.

At the heart of the political economy of intimacy during the early period of colonialism was a fundamental shift: the movement of the hitherto self-sufficient rural homestead into dependence on wage labor. Each region in present-day South Africa undoubtedly had its own specific dynamics. Nevertheless, sometime in the early twentieth century, perhaps in the 1920s or '30s, the rural household and many of its ritual and emotional practices, including marriage, became overwhelmingly dependent on male wage labor. This structural servility, into which urban-based households also fell, extended until the current period of unemployment and low marriage rates. The specific gendered contours of AIDS's rise cannot be understood without appreciating the historical connection between work and the marital household.

My simultaneous attention to political economy and intimacy influences the way in which I consider this history. The first section outlines not only the forces of individualism that came to Africa—and here romantic love was a powerful symbol—but the development of what I call provider love. This emo-tional bond between lovers was instigated by ilobolo (bridewealth), became directed toward building a marital home, and, in both forms, depended on men's wage labor.

The second part of the chapter is motivated by the need to question com-mon framings of gender and "tradition" in the era of AIDS. In South Africa's new liberal democracy, strong opinions are articulated both for and against "traditions." Yet, despite holding seemingly opposite views, both sides can reify "traditions" as historically static practices—as part of either a golden past or an era of patriarchal dominance. In contrast, I emphasize the importance of destabilizing any foundational claims on "traditions." I do so by showing how isoka, a symbolic figure justifying men's sole entitlement to multiple intimate partners (a kind of "sexual double standard"), was partly produced in the early part of the twentieth century.[7]

Provider Love

Any consideration of love must start by noting that marital choice and passion have existed in South Africa for as long as we can find records. Early dictionaries not only defined the isiZulu verb *ukushela* as "to woo" (of a man) but described the wooer as "burning with love, desire, enthusiasm"; moreover the Zulu verb *ukuqoma*, which means "to accept a lover" (of a woman), also meant simply "to choose."[8] Although "forced marriages" were noted by settlers, they do not seem to have been common or uncontested by Africans.[9] Yet, these points notwithstanding, migrant labor and Christianity reworked notions of intimate choice in fundamental ways.

The stimulus that pushed African men into migrant labor was the discovery of diamonds at Kimberley (1867) and gold at Johannesburg (1886). Mining capital at this time competed furiously with white-owned farms for labor; indeed, in the British colony of Natal labor shortages had already led sugar cane farmers to successfully lobby for indentured labor to be sourced from India. Although some Africans lived and worked in or on the outskirts of towns and villages, the majority over time were consigned to areas of rural land called "locations" or later "reserves." From there a growing number of young men embarked on circular patterns of migration to mines, where they worked for months at a time. This colonial cartography —land dispossession, state taxation, migrant labor, and reserves—redrew literal and imaginative maps in the nineteenth and early twentieth centuries. By 1950, the medical doctor and social researcher Sidney Kark found that 90 percent of men between twenty and twenty-five years old were temporarily absent from the rural area of Polela in Natal.[10]

In order to consider how migrant labor, together with agrarian decline, transformed the foundations of the homestead, we need to understand the centrality of the marital homestead to all aspects of life prior to the advent of colonial rule in Natal in the mid-1840s (later in Zululand).[11] Scattered across the land at this time, *imizi* (homesteads, sing. *umuzi*) were led by *abanumzana* (male heads of households), who could marry polygamously if resources permitted. If the household head was a polygamist, a homestead would include different *izindlu* (houses) to which wives were affiliated (the *indlunkulu* and *ikhohlo* being the first and second houses). It was in or near the umuzi that the kin buried their dead and undertook rituals to ensure the ongoing protection of the ancestors (*amadlozi*).

The inherent dynamism of the rural homestead demands attention. Most people today know Zuluness as a symbol of military power in Africa: this

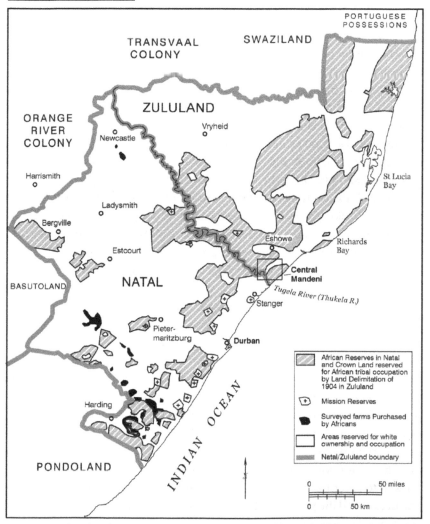

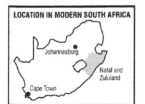

LOCATION IN MODERN SOUTH AFRICA

Johannesburg

Natal and
Zululand

Cape Town

PORTUGUESE
POSSESSIONS

TRANSVAAL
COLONY

SWAZILAND

ZULULAND

ORANGE
RIVER
COLONY

Vryheid

Newcastle

Harrismith

St Lucia
Bay

Ladysmith

Bergville

Eshowe

Richards
Bay

Estcourt

Central
Mandeni

BASUTOLAND

NATAL

Tugela River (Thukela R.)

Stanger

Pieter-
maritzburg

Durban

African Reserves in Natal
and Crown Land reserved
for African tribal occupation
by Land Delimitation of
1904 in Zululand

Harding

Mission Reserves

Surveyed farms Purchased
by Africans

Areas reserved for white
ownership and occupation

Natal/Zululand boundary

PONDOLAND

INDIAN OCEAN

0   50 miles

0   50 km

MAP 3.1. Natal and Zululand, 1905. The boundaries of the fragmented "reserves" where
Africans were required to live remained almost unchanged throughout the twentieth
century, even after the land became part of the KwaZulu "homeland" in the 1970s. As
indicated on the map, present-day "central Mandeni" cuts through both former reserve
and white-designated land. Map adapted from Davenport and Hunt, *The Right to the Land.*

image developed as a result of the rise of the Zulu Kingdom under Shaka in the early nineteenth century and its strong resistance to colonialism until its military defeat by Britain in Zululand in 1879. Yet without the continuing productivity of thousands of homesteads within the kingdom this military prowess would have been impossible. It was the agricultural labor of women and children and the stock-keeping skills of the abanumzana that allowed unmarried men to serve in the state army. And only when the Zulu king gave permission for both male and female *amabutho* (age-sets, regiments) to marry were new homesteads established. Tight control over marriage, then, was at the heart of what is widely believed to be Shaka's brutal military rule.

To enable marriage and the founding of a productive homestead, a groom's family had to give ilobolo—usually in the form of cattle—to a bride's family. In keeping with women's essential role in bearing children in a labor-intensive rural economy, ilobolo was closely connected to a woman's reproductive capacity. A wife "without issue" might see her ilobolo returned to her husband's family or be replaced for childbearing purposes by her sister.[12] Indeed, the centrality of children to ilobolo caused one anthropologist to define ilobolo not as "bride price" but as "child price."[13] Of course, it is insufficient to focus solely on this meaning of ilobolo: a smaller collection of gifts flowed from the bride's to the groom's family, for instance, and these signaled the important role of marriage in establishing kinship links.[14] Yet, at one level, childbirth was undoubtedly central to ilobolo and therefore to the set of arrangements we translate today as "marriage."

Marriage and ilobolo were enmeshed in a myriad of emotions and practices at this time, but of great importance was the notion of *hlonipha* or "respect" (hlonipha is the stem form, which denotes the concept; *ukuhlonipha* is the verb "to respect"; and *inhlonipho* is the noun form, "respect"). Hlonipha was an embodied set of acts of deference that maintained social hierarchies, typically from the young to the old, subjects to chiefs, or wives to husbands. To act with *inhlonipho* was to be bashful and shy, shun certain places, and avoid using certain words and phrases.[15] Everyday spaces were demarcated along these lines. Notions of *hlonipha*, for instance, ensured that women were rarely allowed to enter the center of the *umuzi*, the *isibaya* (cattle kraal). And these practices linked the present to the past because not practicing *inhlonipho* could upset *amadlozi* (the ancestors).

We shall see how hlonipha remained a potent and contested concept throughout the twentieth century, including as it became reshaped by Christianity. But past ethnographic studies emphasize the profoundly gendered nature of hlonipha. In his account of precolonial society, the prominent missionary Alfred Bryant noted that "the Zulu women are quite remarkable for their 'respectful' behavior . . . which affects them constantly in both speech and action."[16]

Courting, ilobolo, and notions of respect were in constant flux before the arrival of settlers.[17] But colonialism recast the gendered and generational basis of marriage and courting in important ways. By the early twentieth century, a brute new reality dominated the rural homestead: settler land dispossession and taxes diminished agricultural and cattle-rearing capacity, and with it a father's ability to provide ilobolo for his sons. At the beginning of the twentieth century—when rural areas still provided some sort of subsistence—roughly one in three men in Natal had more than one wife.[18] By 1936–37 cattle ownership in Natal averaged only 7.2 cattle, which was not enough to cover the ilobolo for even one son's marriage.[19] Now, virtually the only way a young man could marry—typically no more than one wife—was by embarking on migrant labor and saving money for several years. Marriage itself had always been an ambiguous and drawn-out process.[20] But now it was thrown into dependency on paid work.

Male migrancy placed husband-wife relations under great stress—and many critics of racial rule pointed this out over the years. Disturbing new questions, inseparably personal and material, reverberated through rural areas. Would migrant men continue to support their wives? Or would they instead *bhunguka*, abandon their rural homes? Would women remain in the rural homestead, or become disillusioned and leave for the growing urban areas? These tensions are reflected in numerous civil court judgments granting couples a "dissolution of a customary union."[21] And migrant labor also intensified generational stresses. As young men worked, they relied less on their fathers for ilobolo cattle and therefore the means to marry and attain manhood.[22]

Yet instead of viewing courting and marriage as degenerating inexorably in this period, I wish to emphasize certain continuities. These encompass the period from the early twentieth century, when the rural imizi became dependent on wage labor, to roughly the late 1970s–1980s, when unemployment reached very high levels. I heard constant support for this perspective when my elderly informants, male and female, repeatedly described their primary life project through the isiZulu metaphor *ukwakha umuzi* (to build a home / to build a homestead).

As migrant labor grew in importance, a man's constant movement to and from work became not only a factor in conjugal instability but a condition for family survival.[23] This sense of a fragile but definite "patriarchal bargain" is captured well by anthropologist Phillip Mayer's research in the Eastern Cape in 1978. Although recording a variety of situations, including women's greater independence, he said that in many areas "tensions within the sexes and generations were contained with a remarkable degree of success, given the long absences of the men. . . . As long as the husband played his part, by working and remitting what was deemed a fair proportion of his wages, most women were willing to labour for the *umzi* [*isiXhosa*, "homestead"] and to remain loyal wives." [24]

The key question, then, is not simply how capitalism undermined or commodified courting and marriage but how material and emotional worlds became reworked when men were absent from rural homes for so long. Central to this reworking was young men's newfound control over money, in the form of their wages, although this control was always subject to claims from chiefs and fathers. To achieve adulthood and the status of *umakoti* (wife), a woman now depended on a young man's ability to work and not his father's capacity to provide ilobolo. By the 1950s Sidney Kark was noting how migrant labor gave young men new powers in Natal: "the range of choice for girls is extremely limited at any particular moment of time owing to the scarcity of men at home. The men, on the other hand, have almost unlimited choice among the girls." [25] Anthropologist Isaac Schapera also recorded that migrants who returned to Bechuanaland had new powers to indulge in courting and penetrative intercourse (which I will return to later). [26]

I use the term "provider love" to suggest a set of material and emotional links that encompassed a woman being *lobola*'d (having bridewealth paid for her) and a marital couple "building a home." The strong connection between emotional bonds and migrant labor emerged as a major theme in interviews I conducted with elderly men and women. Indeed, most elderly informants elaborated how loving someone (expressed using the verb *ukuthanda*, which also means simply "to like") combined both passion and more mundane considerations. Women described how their desire for a man could result from their "falling in love" in a romantic sense or from the powerful action of love medicines. A male suitor might *hayiza* a woman (place her under a love spell), propelling her into uncontrollable screaming and ultimately into his arms. [27]

However, whatever the complex ways in which passion befell women, the experience of being seized by love was usually said to overlap with more practical considerations, and these considerations were closely connected to labor migration. Having recounted how love came uncontrollably to them, many elderly women recalled searching for a boyfriend who was hardworking, intended marriage, and would eventually provide steady support for the marital umuzi. The emotional body and the material world were inextricably linked—as they have been in all societies at all times.

Mrs. Ndlovu was eighty years old when she spoke with me at her home on the outskirts of Sundumbili township. Her comments give a sense of how an irrational "arrival of love" could be blended with more practical considerations that centered on a man's ability to pay ilobolo and provide for a wife. It is obviously not possible to consider this interview—and indeed any others in this book—as unmediated representations of the past. How much did the dominance of romantic love today affect her comments? There is no simple answer to this question, and many avenues of discussion could be followed. I offer here only my interpretation of her words and gestures. I asked Mrs. Ndlovu first about her husband:

> MH: Why did you like him?
>
> Mrs. Ndlovu: I don't know, love just arrived.
>
> MH: Were there other people who were *shela*-ing you?
>
> Mrs. Ndlovu: Yes . . .
>
> MH: When women started to qoma a man, what were the promises he would make, like "maybe I will marry you"?
>
> Mrs. Ndlovu: I could not love someone if I did not know what they were going to do with me [taking into account the rest of the interview, she is clearly referring to paying ilobolo]. . . . If a boy would come to me and tell me that he loves me, I would ask him what he can do for me, since he says that he loves me. Some would tell me that they would respond some other day, and then they would never return.

In much of Europe and North America, the emergence of capitalism and, relatedly, men's modern breadwinner role yielded a similar pattern of women's dependence on men.[28] But Mrs. Ndlovu suggests that migrant labor recast the very heart of marriage in South Africa, ilobolo. As men earned wages, ilobolo came to signify the wage-earning potential of a largely absent young man. And this new sense of ilobolo became intertwined with emotions that were talked about as love. Without this history—one that has tended to be neglected—we cannot understand an apparent paradox that I return to later: women's frequent defense of ilobolo over the course of the twentieth century.

For men, emotional bonds understood as love were also entangled with the joint but contested project of "building a home." Many elderly men with whom I spoke recalled going to great lengths to woo a girlfriend. From men's perspective, key to finding a wife was watching an actual or potential girl-friend's behavior to see if she showed respect (had *inhlonipho*) and was hard-working (*khuthele*). To most men, these attributes signaled her potential as someone who might *vusa umuzi kababa* (build up a father's homestead), a powerful metaphor that emphasizes a son's duty to continue his father's lineage.

Mrs. Ndlovu described the attributes men valued:

> MH: What would happen if a man had to choose between a hard-working and a beautiful girl?
>
> Mrs. Ndlovu: Everyone would notice a girl who worked hard at home, and the boys would place great value on a hardwork-ing girl who respected her parents.

Men and women thus looked for some of the same things in a marital partner: if a woman fell in love with a man who had the potential to provide ilobolo, a man looked for a hardworking and respectful woman who would fulfill her side of the patriarchal bargain. Of course physical attraction played a part for both men and women. But as the missionary Alfred Bryant succinctly put it in 1949 when describing men's choosing of women, "To such physical beauty must too be added the moral virtues of gentle submissiveness and willing service, agricultural and domestic diligence, and healthy generative organs."[29]

Romantic Love

I have outlined above the key features of what I call provider love. Yet this is closely related (both in the events of the past and in the way they are remembered today) to romantic love. One immediate example of how provider and romantic love came together is the way that migrant labor gave a man the economic ability to push aside the wishes of kin and make his own choice of who he would marry.

But romantic love, of course, cannot be reduced to either capitalism or money. Central to its growing stature was the influence of missionaries who opposed polygamy and promoted new ideas of marital choice and companionship within marriage. A measure of Christianity's influence can be seen in the fact that by the end of the twentieth century 76 percent of Africans identified themselves as Christians.[30] The influence of Christianity, even on those who did not identify with the religion, was nothing short of profound.

While the earliest African Christians lived on separate mission reserves, the widening dispersal of churches and mission-run schools reduced the geographical and social distance between *amakholwa* (Christians) and *amaqaba* (heathens). Eshowe District, where much of Mandeni is located, is an area of approximately 70 by 30 kilometers, and in 1951 it had an African population of 45,600.[31] Missionary enterprise in the area dates from the mid-nineteenth century, but most Western churches were established in the Eshowe District between 1910 and 1930, and by 1950 there were sixty-three churches in six denominations (in order of the denomination's total number of local churches, these were Norwegian Mission, Roman Catholic, Anglican, American Lutheran, Salvation Army, and Methodist).[32] In part because Christian marriages came to be increasingly seen as *phucukile* (civilized), a growing number of rural marriages were solemnized with Christian rites: in 1951, 33 percent of Africans in the country's towns and 18 percent in rural areas were married in civil, mostly Christian, marriages.[33]

Christianity and schooling were two sides of the same coin during this period: many churches established schools for their congregations. And literacy, in turn, opened up rural lives to new ideas and practices of intimacy. By the mid-twentieth century images of romantic love circulated widely in magazines and newspapers that could be brought to rural areas from growing towns.

Perhaps more than any other new practice, the individual and self-reflective practice of penning a love letter came to symbolize modern changes to courting.[34] Love letters did not foreclose collective discussions about love. Yet they allowed young women and men to increasingly bypass kin and those charged with supervising courting, especially the older girls called *amaqhikiza*. These figures—remembered with some humor by most informants—had acted as intermediaries between young lovers and were especially recalled for their role in guarding young women's chastity.

During one interview, Tholakale, a widow in her sixties, gave me a powerful example of how women could embrace Christianity's emphasis on marital choice, and in the process remake their selves. I interviewed Tholakale five times. Her rural homestead was one of the many today led by a widow who supports her children and grandchildren on a government pension. One day, discussions turned to levirate marriage, in which a man enters the homestead of his deceased brother and enters into marital relations with his widow (the isiZulu word, *ukungena*, literally means "to enter"). Tholakale vigorously opposed ukungena, presenting it as a harsh and unjust tradition. Usually when we chatted during interviews she replied directly to me. However, during this discussion, she turned to my full-time female research assistant and her friend and addressed them both. She told them passionately of times in the past when ukungena had forced women to marry men they hardly knew, stories that were met with cries of *"Hhayi-bo!"* (No way!) by my research assistant and her friend.

Many of my informants also recalled that a monogamous Christian union helped to foster closer "love" relations after marriage. As anthropologist Absolom Vilakazi put it in his 1962 ethnography of a rural isiZulu-speaking community, "When people get married by Christian rites, they are told they should live with each other, bear each other's weaknesses and that each shall give up father and mother and cling to his or her spouse." According to Vilakazi, this gave a woman "greater freedom for her and greater intimacy with her husband."[35] Yet, as older women's frequent criticisms of men demonstrate, these idealistic statements need to be qualified. Men's philandering, in particular, could threaten marriages that emphasized companionship.

Indeed, competing notions of masculinity influenced, and became shaped by, men's encounters with romantic love. Mr. Sibiya, born in 1933 in northern KwaZulu-Natal but now living in Sundumbili township, was educated at a mission school up to Standard 6, a high level of schooling for that time (eight years). His mother had been a Christian, although his father identified as a traditionalist and not someone who followed Western religion. Showing how Christianity and literacy could be positioned as unmasculine, Mr. Sibiya recalls that his peers looked down on his attendance at a mission school. They warned him, "If you study, what are you going to do? It is necessary that you *lusa izinkomo* [herd cattle], learn everything about *amakhaya* [rural areas]." He went on to talk quite openly about how Christianity promoted a closer nuclear family. "Traditionally," he said, men and women used to sleep apart, but he and his wife, both Christians, used to sleep in a single bed because "times had changed." Being civilized was now more important, he said.

Love, Sex, and Money

To recap, young people's greater autonomy in courting and marriage became manifest in provider love (when young men saved to marry a woman) and romantic love (when partners valued marital choice and companionship). Yet both became largely contingent on wage labor. This new dependence on money was vividly displayed when ilobolo was increasingly given in cash and not cattle.

A lot has now been written about the extraordinary power of money to recast social relations and bodily experiences: as Karl Marx wrote to make this point, "I am ugly, but I can buy for myself the most beautiful of women. Therefore I am not *ugly*."[36] Men with wages attracted women in new ways, but did wage labor lead to penetrative or non-penetrative "sex" being exchanged for money among young people in South Africa? In the main, I argue no. The extent of the contemporary materiality of everyday sex is relatively new, as I will show later; to make this argument I need to look at sex exchanges that took place in the past and show that most were formed in relation to a more significant project of "building a home."

The historical records are certainly replete with examples of urban "prostitution" that involved men and women of all "races."[37] These show, on the one hand, the new ways that capitalism and colonialism enabled women to abandon the patriarchal home. Yet, as radical a departure as this was, most rural African women did not follow this path. A young woman's movement to an urban area could permanently scar her reputation and, consequently, single young women without children were probably the people least likely to migrate. On the whole (and there is great variation), migrant women in the early parts of the twentieth century were more likely to be abandoned or divorced women, those with "illegitimate" children, or those going to join husbands in town.[38]

Urban "prostitution," in short, was a growing but still minority occupation and while, as we shall see, women could engage in various kinds of material relations with men in urban areas, these relations did not prevent men from returning to rural areas. The vast majority of South Africans in this period married and built a home, and extramarital sex was just that, extramarital, rather than the sex in the virtual absence of marriage that takes place today.

If urban "prostitutes" were numerically quite rare, how can we understand accounts of penetrative sex being associated with gifts in rural areas quite distant from the formal labor market? Monica Wilson's 1936 ethnography of Mpondoland, an area adjacent to Natal, suggested that a group of women called *amadikazi*, though not explicitly trading sex, could benefit materially from sexual relations, including relations with married men. Wilson described these women, whom she believed predated colonialism, as the "artists of the community."[39] But even this example has to be understood in relation to the overwhelming emphasis on building a rural home. Wilson's rural amadikazi women were largely divorced or widowed women or single mothers, who were usually seen as ineligible for marriage as first wives, generally the most prized position for a young woman.[40]

Certainly, all the elderly people I spoke with suggested very strongly that, for most unmarried rural women, a male suitor's commitment to paying ilobolo and building a home were much more important than any immediate gifts he might make. Anthropologist Absolom Vilakazi also encountered great shock when he asked about courting gifts in the region in the 1960s: "To give

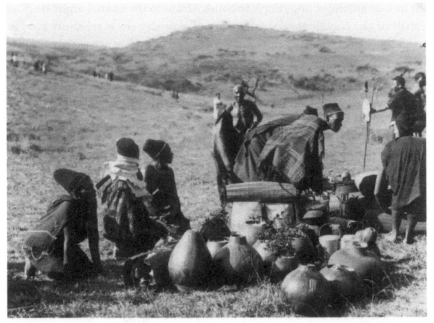

FIGURE 3.1. People on their way to a wedding ceremony in 1928, bearing gifts. The exchange of gifts between families was an integral part of African marriage, with ilobolo the most significant gift from the man's family to the woman's. Courtesy of Campbell Collections of the University of KwaZulu-Natal (d07–145).

gifts at this stage would be highly improper among the traditionalists, and the boy would be accused of trying to bribe the girl to love him."[41] While some of my informants said that gifts were given by boyfriends to girlfriends, they were adamant that a woman would not abandon a man if these gifts were not forthcoming. The very language employed to discuss courting gifts supports this view. Vilakazi uses the word *gwaza* (bribe) to suggest that gifts given to attract women would be seen as improper, even immoral, interventions. Similarly, some of my informants used the word *umkhonzo* to describe gifts given in rural areas. To *khonza* is to pay respects or send compliments (you *khonza* a chief to show that you are under his authority), which suggests that gifts were seen as a sign of commitment and trust.

Most gifts before marriage, therefore, were associated with ilobolo and went from family to family rather than directly to a woman. Yet once women were married, they could pursue gifts from men more explicitly. Indeed, it was sometimes accepted that a married woman living apart from her husband for long periods might have intimate relations with a "secondary" lover who could provide economic support. As noted in more detail in chapter 9, I refer to these as "secondary" rather than "casual" lovers because women's relationships with these boyfriends might endure for some time and be thought of with reference to a "primary" lover, here a husband. Certainly, many of my older female informants smiled wryly when relating how a secondary lover was dubbed an *isidikiselo* (the top of a pot), while the husband was an *ibhodwe* (a pot). Informants distinguished between this pot metaphor, which was related with some humor, and the more judgmental word for "secret" secondary lovers, *amashende* (the singular is *ishende*), associated with "loose" women.

Mrs. Mathonsi, in her fifties, explained the partial acceptance of secondary lovers in more detail to me. I had been asking her why it was that men in rural areas in the mid-century were allowed to be isoka (have multiple partners) and yet women were not allowed to have amashende. She quickly corrected me. Amashende were new, she said, and these were immoral extra partners. Past isidikiselo relationships, she noted, could be arranged by a husband's family:

> It wasn't ishende before, because when the father left to work in Jo'burg there would be a man who would look after his home, so that if something went wrong, maybe in the homestead, he would have to help. That man became isidikiselo. When the woman was pregnant she used to have to go to visit her husband in Jo'burg and sleep with him, so that when he returned he would find her pregnant with his child—and yet really the baby belonged to the isidikiselo who was looking after the family.

These types of isidikiselo relations, like the *bonyatsi* relations (extramarital relations) described by Spiegel for Lesotho, were one important route through which migrants' earnings were diffused within rural communities.[42] But they operated in an ambiguous moral space. On the one hand, a married woman was expected to remain faithful and could be divorced for infidelity; on the other, her husband's absence for long periods justified her having a secondary lover to meet her intimate and monetary needs. This arrangement could, in fact, be seen as congruent with the maintenance of a homestead's integrity.

Love, Ilobolo, and Violence

A lot has been written about how ilobolo represents a form of male domination because it constitutes men's exchange of women. I have tried to complicate this history by showing how ilobolo became attached to ideas of commitment and love. In fact, both positions are compatible: to the extent that ilobolo both indicated a man's love for a woman and justified male domination in the form of violence, love and violence have never been opposites.

It is certainly the case that men's payment of ilobolo could work to insti-tutionalize male violence. Tholakale recalled how during her courtship with her future husband he used his leverage over marriage in the most intimate moments. Following Tholakale's qoma-ing of the man, who at that stage had another girlfriend, the couple began to engage in ukusoma ("thigh sex"). Soon, however, Tholakale's boyfriend began asking to have penetrative sex. One time he tried to force her, as she remembers:

MH: When he tried to persuade you, what did you say?

INT: I said, no, the law doesn't allow . . .

MH: Did he try and physically force you?

INT: Yes, we were fighting and I pushed him. . . . My husband said, if you are refusing like this, I wonder whether you can marry me or not.

After marriage, women might also experience a certain level of domes-tic violence. Yet this violence cannot be seen as deriving from a static Zulu culture, as violence is often portrayed today. Indeed, it was white male Native Commissioners who sometimes had the last word in deciding whether African men's violence was justified. If a woman deserted her husband and the Native Commissioner deemed her action justified, her husband could lose some or all of the ilobolo cattle he might receive upon their divorce—although such penalties appear not to have been common.[43] The transfer of ilobolo then both justified, and to a lesser degree imposed limits on, a husband's violence.

The Making of the Isoka Masculinity

I have emphasized thus far how social forces engendered by colonialism reworked traditions of courting in important ways. It is important to remem-ber also that the very idea of "tradition" is socially produced and thus mutable. Both points are important: even when AIDS interventions have attempted to be culturally sensitive by recognizing different "sexual cultures," the tendency has been to present these as quite static (and geographically bounded). Thus it is often said that Zulu men are aggressive or violent; or, in a more sophisticated way, that longstanding Zulu masculinities place a high value on violence or on men's acquiring multiple partners. Tradition, from this perspective, can be modified, but rarely are its historical-geographical foundations and the reasons for its resonance questioned. Yet the court I had sat in was part of a dynamic set of processes that made tradition as well as interpreting it; traditions, including Zuluness, and indeed the very idea of traditions, never stood still. To create a sense of the historical dynamism that I believe should be more emphasized in AIDS work, I look at the philandering figure of the isoka and argue that the masculinity he represents was never static.

During the course of my research I became fascinated with the term "isoka," which broadly speaking means a man with many girlfriends, although it can also simply mean a boyfriend. Many informants told me that the idea that men can have multiple partners and women cannot (what we might call an "isoka masculinity") was simply inherited from the custom of polygamy, which granted men the sole right to have multiple wives. Isoka bore many similarities to dominant images of masculine men I grew up with in the UK—images that celebrated as "studs" men who attracted multiple women and, relatedly, chastised as "sluts" supposedly "loose" women. And isoka's reach extends to the upper echelons of politics: when President Jacob Zuma defended himself from rape charges by declaring that he was not *isishimane*, a man unable to find a girlfriend, he evoked the naturalness of the isoka, a man who could. This masculinity, he said, was part of his culture, and so why would he rape a woman?

But is it the case that isiZulu-speaking men have always celebrated having multiple partners and, relatedly, that women have been denied this entitlement? I believe not, at least not in the way portrayed today. My evidence for this is somewhat limited by the sources, but they paint a consistent picture. I begin with language, which is both an important and difficult window into social change: isiZulu itself only became a written language when missionaries wrote Bibles, dictionaries, and other texts.[44] Dictionaries certainly do not simply reflect the meanings of words in society; they also help to produce them. But successive dictionaries can provide some clues to the changing meanings of words over time.

One possible root of the word "isoka" is *ukusoka* (to be circumcised). Shaka abolished the lengthy ritual of circumcision to gain greater control over his army, though it had served as a formal rite of passage for those leaving boyhood. The first dedicated isiZulu dictionary, compiled by the missionary John Colenso in 1861, defined ukusoka in these terms and then went on to define the noun isoka as an "unmarried man; handsome young man; sweetheart; accepted lover; a young man liked by the girls."[45] Although there are several meanings contained in the definition of isoka, including a man popular with women, seen alongside its association with circumcision, "isoka" signified a young man who had begun to court as a first step toward marriage.

Masculinities and femininities are always forged in relation to one another, and today isoka defends not only a man's entitlement to have multiple lovers but his exclusive right to do so. Yet the scale of this gendered differentiation appears to be new: numerous records from the nineteenth and early twentieth century suggest that young women were, in fact, able to ukusoma with several lovers.[46] In an era when fertility faced the greatest restrictions, elders appear to have been less concerned with the practice of ukusoma than with matters unequivocally related to pregnancy. Of course, ukusoma always stood a chance of leading to impregnation.[47] But what seemed to be of paramount importance was the need to prevent pregnancy by an unknown man. Ndukwana's description in 1900 of ukusoma captures these points well: "A girl is not penetrated. She crosses her legs and tightens them as she feels the man is about to spend, and the man spends on the girl's thigh. . . . It was a common thing for a woman to have three lovers . . . one lover one month, another the next month, and so on. . . . When a girl was made pregnant, one could easily find out what lover she was with on the month preceding that in which her courses stopped."[48]

Evidence of a growing gap between the acceptable courting behavior of men and women can be found in Doke and Vilakazi's 1948 dictionary, which differentiates between an "original meaning" of "isoka," which is "one old enough to commence courting," and later meanings that include a "young man popular among girls."[49] Speaking of this later meaning, anthropologist Absolom Vilakazi describes in powerful terms the masculine status of the isoka in the mid-twentieth century: "Courting behaviour among traditional young men is a very important part of their education; for a young man must achieve the distinction of being an *isoka*, i.e. a Don Juan or a Casanova."[50] Celebrations of isoka circulated in stories, songs, praises, and new media such as newspapers.[51] An isoka, many old men and women told me, used his charisma to shela women.

My discussions with elderly informants who recalled the mid-twentieth century also support the view that something of a "sexual double standard" became more pronounced in the early twentieth century: they did not recall an earlier era of women's relative freedom and instead noted harsh consequences for a woman and her peer group if she had multiple ukusoma partners. Any woman with more than one boyfriend (overlapping or close together) risked being labeled *isifebe* (a loose woman), and this could greatly hinder her future marriage prospects.[52] The significance of the insult "isifebe" is vividly seen in the defamation cases pursued by women branded by this name.[53]

Although we must be cautious about drawing firm conclusions from the available evidence, it appears that masculinities and femininities were reshaped such that young men's entitlement to have multiple intimate partners increased relative to women's in the early twentieth century. I am, of course, only considering one aspect of intimate relations. A fuller review would emphasize changing practices within marriage and the rapidly rising number of women in urban areas: from 98,000 in 1911 to 357,000 in 1936 to 904,000 in 1951.[54] The relative anonymity of town life, as we shall see, could grant women some new intimate freedoms, including the ability to have more than one lover. But all of my informants said that by the early to mid-twentieth century in rural areas, an isoka was celebrated for having multiple partners, whereas a young unmarried woman who had more than one partner was derided as isifebe.

Yet an isoka was by no means given free rein to seduce women. Notably, a man found it difficult to secure even one girlfriend if he did not work. Vilakazi wrote in 1962, "Throughout my stay among the Nyuswa, I did not meet a single young man who was not at work but who was courting a girl or expecting to be qonywa'd [chosen by a girl]."[55] Similarly, despite the bravado image of the isoka, many elderly men told me that they had had only one or two concurrent girlfriends when they were young.

An isoka also faced restrictions precisely because other paths to manhood were ultimately more valued. In the mid-twentieth century many expressions of masculinity overlapped: from prowess in stick-fighting, to knowledge about cattle, to literacy. Yet to become a truly respected man a young man had to marry and build a homestead (becoming umnumzana, a head of household). The phrase isoka lamanyala could be employed to rebuke men with too many girlfriends; amanyala means "dirt" or "a disgraceful act," and the phrase signified an unseemly masculinity, a masculinity gone too far. Though some men did recall a certain status associated with being isoka lamanyala, for most it was a reproach.

Indeed, parents with a heavy stake in their daughter's future ilobolo could call a philandering man to account, asking if he intended to marry all of his girlfriends. Underlining the importance of the expectation of marriage, Mr. Buthelezi from Isithebe, seventy-four, compared the isoka lamanyala to the isoka: "An isoka lamanyala is a person with a lot of girlfriends, a person who takes from every place; he is qonywa'd here and qonywa'd there and he will never get married." He contrasted this figure to an isoka, who eventually marries his favored girlfriend and therefore "doesn't destroy people's children."

Preachers too, especially those from Western churches, were generally virulent in their opposition to isoka, preferring Zulu men to espouse respectable monogamous values. They looked with distaste not only at "heathens" but at members of African initiated churches who could retain African customs, including polygamy (Shembe, mentioned later, is one example of such a church).[56] Moreover, in contrast to customary marriages, Western Christian marriages allowed a woman to divorce her husband for adultery. Indeed, while reifying women's purity, churches also introduced certain ideas of equality in intimate relations; perhaps for these reasons, they attracted more women worshipers than men. And, in other embodied ways, the physical dangers of "immorality" seemed increasingly obvious: the rise of STIs, especially syphilis, also challenged the isoka to temper his behavior.[57]

Another reason why isoka was not a static or uncontested figure is the existence of same-sex erotic relations. The isoka celebrated and thus natural-ized a man's pursuit of women. But in the many mining compounds where men lived for months at a time it was quite common for residents to engage in ukusoma (ukmetsha in isiXhosa) relations with one another in "mine mar-riages" that typically crossed large age differences.[58] These same-sex intimate relations challenged isoka's claims that men had a natural need to pursue multiple women.

Dunbar Moodie argued that men engaged in these forms of intimacy partly as a way to resist proletarianization: distant from their rural wives and girlfriends, men wanted to avoid penetrative sex with urban women, which might waste money and expose them to disease. Their overarching aim was to maintain investment in a rural marital homestead. Over the years, this thesis has faced criticism for not stressing the pleasure in these relationships: Marc Epprecht's detailed history shows that same-sex relationships preceded the mining industry and that anal penetration also took place.[59] What Moodie did do, however, was show how male-male relations at the mines did not exist in a binary opposite to masculinities centered on a man and a woman building a rural home; indeed the two could mutually reinforce one another.

But this example also reminds us that we must apply caution when using any social category relating to intimacy. Only with a great deal of qualification can we say that these miners were MSM or "men who have sex with men" (to use a phrase now common in the AIDS world). Moreover, to talk of "male-male relations" is really only to report, in a quite unspecific way, eroticism between two male-bodied persons. Rather than participants seeing these simply through sex-centric terms (homosexual, male-male, or same-sex relations), these social arrangements, which also incorporated domestic labor and material support, appear to have been understood partly as temporary marriages between "men" and "boys." In the face of strong claims today by some African leaders that homosexuality is new to Africa, it is of course crucial to recognize the existence of same-sex intimacy in the past. At the same time, consideration must be given to the danger of reading "homosexuality" back into history, as though the meanings of same-sex relations did not change over time.[60]

How did the "isoka masculinity" come to celebrate men having multiple partners but criticize women doing the same? What is the history of this stud / slut dichotomy in South Africa? It is difficult to draw firm conclusions, given the lack of available evidence. But there are three changes, all critical to the region's history, which are certainly consistent with this redefining of gendered norms in the early twentieth century. The first, already described, is that men moved into wage labor. A young wage-earning man had new powers to choose a wife. The second is that the isoka masculinity, and related femininities, emerged as colonial authorities actively promoted male-led "traditional" institutions. The third is that Christianity promoted a clearer moral domain of "sex" that attached ideas of morality to women's bodies in new ways.

Historian Shula Marks's work provides probably the best example of how these forces could converge on and redefine gendered bodies. She notes panicked attempts in the early twentieth century to prevent women leaving rural areas for towns. On the one hand these efforts show the new spaces that women could enter in the twentieth century. But Marks also demonstrated how in Natal in the 1920s and 1930s a coalition of forces—white missionaries, Zulu nationalists, African Christians, and the Department of Native Affairs— railed against the disintegration of "tribal discipline" evidenced by the increasing "immorality" of single women in urban and rural areas. According to Marks, "It was in the position of African women that the forces of conservatism found a natural focus."[61] Key contours of masculinities in the early twentieth century similarly emerged at this juncture.

COLONIALISM: AN ACCOMMODATION OF PATRIARCHS

Why does "tradition" resonate so loudly and in such a gendered way in South Africa? If moralistic calls on the past are heard all over the world in various guises, the form of colonialism pioneered in Natal bestowed on "tradition" a particular institutional inertia that is still palpable today. Let me explain.

In the 1840s, when Natal became a British colony, its white settlers faced a daunting challenge: they were heavily outnumbered by Africans and yet received little material support from Britain.[62] Over time, Theophilus Shepstone, the secretary for native affairs, developed a system of "indirect rule" to address this quagmire. Central to this system was the state's devolution of certain powers to chiefs, who then ruled over their subjects in rural "locations" (later called "reserves"). Overseen by white administrators, chiefs had to administer the system whereby African subjects effectively funded their own domination through paying a hut tax.

On the one hand, this system stripped male chiefs and *abanumzana* of authority and made them answerable to white settlers. But Shepstone's strategy also rested on what historian Jeff Guy calls an "accommodation of patriarchs," a coming together of settler and African men.[63] A main tool for this alliance was the application of customary law, a legal framework overseen by white government officials but administered at lower levels by chiefs. While this legal system allowed some women to go over the heads of fathers and chiefs, in general it became infamous for positioning African women as "minors" and therefore always subject to the authority of a man.[64]

The Natal Marriage Act of 1869 is a good example of how indirect rule both modified and, at times, fixed gendered customs. One of the Act's main aims was to ensure that a bride explicitly state at her marriage ceremony that she was marrying freely. This reveals how Shepstone defended his strategy by modernizing certain unpalatable "traditions"—in this case to effect a limitation on male authority. But to ensure that all men had the ability to marry and thus become patriarchs, the law also set a maximum payment for ilobolo at ten cattle (not including the single animal given to the bride's mother). The justification for this intervention was that rich men were inflating the value of ilobolo and making it difficult for young men to marry.[65]

Over time isiZulu speakers came to think of eleven cattle as the standard rather than maximum ilobolo payment. Moreover, as officials codified ilobolo and other practices in a written document (the Natal Code of Native Law), the very idea of tradition became institutionalized in powerful ways. Today very few isiZulu speakers are aware that it was a settler law that established the standard ilobolo payment, which is now one of the most sacrosanct Zulu traditions. Nor are they aware that payments of *imvulamlomo* (literally, open the mouth to commence ilobolo negotiations) and *izibizo* (a set of additional presents for the bride's family) were instigated by isiZulu-speaking men as a way to circumvent these new rules.[66] If no tradition can be simply invented, neither is it possible to find present-day practices that are untainted by history.

Importantly, Natal's system of indirect rule came to heavily influence state policy after the modern South African state was formed in 1910. The racial contours of this new state were complicated, but in many respects they rested on continued land dispossession and the devolution of restricted responsibilities to male chiefs.[67] Famously, the Union of South Africa's first major piece of legislation was the 1913 Land Act that granted Africans only 8 percent of the country's land (extended to 13 percent in 1932). The post-1948 apartheid era, in turn, oversaw massive forced removals as Africans, especially, were relocated from towns and freehold land.[68] The sustained devolution of power to chiefs was also brought to a head during apartheid when ten ethnic homelands were created and encouraged to embrace "independence." But this later period is for another chapter. What is important for the argument here is that neo-traditionalism tended to extend certain controls on rural women, and this extension was consistent with the hardening of the isoka/isifebe (stud/slut) dichotomy in the early twentieth century.

CHRISTIANITY: PRUDE BODIES AND SEXUAL GUILT

Powerful modern forces forged new symbolic divisions within society: between amakholwa (believers, Christians) and amaqaba (heathen) or being phucukile (civilized) and following *amasiko* (customs). And "sex" became formative of, as well as viewed through, this new register. According to missionaries, to be civilized required rejecting "lewd" practices of "sex" and embracing Christian virtues of self-restraint and sexual prudery. "The body is the temple of God," I was told many times by informants relaying to me the guilt-ridden Christian view of sex.

Yet it is important not to take these boundaries too literally. What came to be called "modern" and "traditional" were in fact a shifting set of practices that were mutually constituted; both were expressed not in stable beliefs but through a fluid set of habits and practices, signaled by dress, speech, diet, and other aspects of everyday life.[69] Indeed, Inkatha, the Zulu nationalist movement set up in the 1920s, was propelled by not only King Solomon kaDinuzulu but also members of the Christian educated elite, revealing the extent to which these worlds overlapped in the political sphere.[70]

Moreover, despite Christian efforts at promoting sexual morality, penetrative sex became increasingly practiced before marriage.[71] This draws attention to a great irony: missionaries had huge influence in associating sex with sin, but they almost completely failed to prevent its enjoyment. Indeed, certain Christian teachings actually encouraged penetrative sex. By introducing modern ideas of intimacy—symbolized by lovers' right to choose their own partners—missionaries promoted love as a matter between two individuals. Partly as a result, though the practice of ukusoma persisted, penetrative sex became increasingly associated with modernity and manhood. As Vusumuzi, an eighty-year-old man, told me, "Boys used to talk to one another and say, we don't want to ukuhlobonga [soma]." Someone who engaged in ukusoma, he said, might be derided as isishimane, not a true man. Other informants told me that ukusoma began to be thought of as "old-fashioned" (tellingly, they usually used the English phrase).

Indeed, men seemed to increasingly conceive of premarital penetrative sex as a domain of pleasure and an expression of masculinity. And this is certainly also consistent with the reduced importance of fertility to society.

Discussing the Eastern Cape in the 1940s and 1950s, Anne Mager links rising sexual violence to the erosion of labor-intensive rural agriculture. The lesser value of rural labor, she argues, devalued the connections between women's bodies and fertility, since children were no longer such an asset. Consequently, men "were individually concerned with sex as an experience of the flesh."[72]

Yet while Christians could construct men's "sexual" actions as immoral, male indiscretions could still be resolved through the payment of compensation; this was called by several names, including *inhlawulo* (the term is widely translated today as "fine" or "damages"). Revealing the growing acceptance of premarital sex, however, by the mid-century inhlawulo was moving from being a payment required for taking a woman's virginity to a payment incurred for rendering a woman pregnant. Reasons for this include the decline in the practice of virginity testing and men's greater mobility, which made it difficult to hold them accountable.[73]

One reason why women faced more censure than men for premarital sex is that pregnancy—increasingly seen less as a mistake and more as a deliberate act of "sex"—could reduce a woman's chance of marriage. But, as we have seen, women also had a lesser ability to ukusoma with more than one man, even though this non-penetrative form of intimacy typically did not lead to childbirth. Important to greater restrictions on ukusoma, we might surmise, was how this practice became increasingly coded as a form of "sex" ("thigh sex") in ways that offended a new emphasis on sexual purity.

Christian notions of "sex" also transformed meanings around hlonipha (respect) that gendered the body in new ways. Today, hlonipha is usually seen as a "traditional" form of respect—a set of practices that reflect the very essence of being Zulu. Yet, importantly, Christianity engendered strong new associations between sexual guilt and hlonipha: modern ideas of sex as a sin became steadfastly entangled with feelings about and perceptions of hlonipha. Practices associated with hlonipha therefore helped to mediate the embodiment of "sexual" purity, especially for women. This never happened in a mechanistic way, and we shall see later how some women moved to urban areas and gained new opportunities for intimate relations. Nevertheless, it happened in rural areas in ways that—while complex—are certainly consistent with the emergence of a more pronounced isoka/isifebe dichotomy that pressured women not to have multiple partners.

In nineteenth-century South Africa, what came to be translated as "marriage" was a pivotal—the pivotal—institution that structured material flows, moral obligations, lived geographies, power relations, and pleasures and pains.

However, in the early part of the twentieth century wedlock became dependent on wage labor. From this time, emotional and material commitments, understood as a form of love, became attached to men's working and paying ilobolo. These were radical shifts—by no means easy to document—and represent a very different scenario from dominant accounts of "modernity causing family breakdown" or "love coming to Africa."

What is also clear is that masculinities like isoka were produced in numerous realms, and key to their production was the convergence of Christian prudery, neo-traditionalism, and migrant labor. A formidable force—comprising white missionaries, Zulu nationalists, African Christians, and the state—coalesced in ways that probably further restricted rural women's courting behavior. The early twentieth century, however, cannot be seen as a time when colonialism simply led to the greater oppression of women. Christianity, as we have seen, resulted in certain notions of intimate equality; moreover, capitalism led to urban spaces to which women could move, abandoning rural lives. And making things even more complicated was the fact that not everybody was talking about the same thing in talking about "sex." Indeed, the word ukusoma today reveals overlapping, sometimes contradictory, meanings: its translation as "thigh sex" suggests that it became increasingly sexualized; yet the laughter it caused in the court I visited, and the ease with which old people still discuss it, speaks to a time when "sex" was not a distinct domain central to defining the self. As we shall see, the association between "sex," penetrative intercourse, and individual and group identities was to become increasingly strong over the course of the twentieth century.

FOUR

Urban Respectability:
Sundumbili Township, 1964–94

Mr. Nkosi's home, completed in 1964, is small and rectangular in shape, one of the thousands of "matchbox houses" built in South Africa's townships during the apartheid era. Its main entrance opens directly into a small lounge, off which open a kitchen, two small bedrooms, and a tiny bathroom. Paint now peels from the house's inside walls and the absence of ceiling boards means you can see right up into the corroding asbestos roof. Privacy is virtually impossible in this tiny structure.

When I interviewed Mr. Nkosi he brought out a large collection of photographs. He particularly wanted to show me two: one that commemorates his twenty years of work at the SAPPI paper mill and another that marks his twenty-fifth year of service. In the first he is wearing a smart suit and tie and shaking hands with a white manager, dropping his left shoulder and bending his knees as a sign of respect. In the second he is wearing only a "traditional" *ibheshu* (loincloth) and is looking at the same manager, who is handing him a commemorative plaque.

A few weeks later it was my turn to take some photos to give to Mr. Nkosi, as one way of thanking him for his time. On this occasion, he and his daughters wore traditional dress, consisting of animal skins, and posed in their small front yard next to a dilapidated isibaya (cattle kraal). Placed as it was in a township, the isibaya struck me, and many residents I knew, as a rather out-of-place symbol of rural life. Thefts had forced him to sell off his livestock, and the structure looked somewhat sorry in its current empty state.

This brief vignette invites a number of interpretations. Mr. Nkosi's long employment at SAPPI was consistent with the economy's expansion from mining into secondary industry, a move that required a more stable labor force. His failure to establish a viable isibaya signified urban residents' gradual severing of ties to their rural homes. And Mr. Nkosi's insistence that his daughters dress "traditionally" signals the valorization of women's purity in the time of AIDS.

In my mind, however, what resonates the most in my encounter with Mr. Nkosi, and in similar encounters with many men of this era, is the figure of umnumzana, a respectable patriarch, which overlays all of these interpretations. A word long used to denote a rural homestead head, umnumzana quickly came in urban areas to mean "gentleman" or "mister." It signaled a man of worth and status and was a flexible symbol, as the two work photographs demonstrate. Versions of umnumzana could encompass men who lived in rural areas, those who moved to urban areas permanently, and those who straddled the two. The figure of umnumzana, the head of a household, provided a kind of masculine moral compass that allowed men to navigate many economic and social settings but retain the authority and material benefits of being a household head.

Urban Legends?

Many past accounts of South Africa's urban areas emphasize "family breakdown," and in doing so they neglect the respectable urban umnumzana figure. In 1959 anthropologist Laura Longmore published an influential urban ethnography called *The Dispossessed*. Subtitled *A Study of the Sex-Life of Bantu Women in and around Johannesburg,* the book graphically documented the "disintegration of family life" in an African township and warned, "It may well be that the new urban African generation is dispensing with marriage in its old forms."[1] Longmore's rich account of illegitimacy and extramarital affairs reinforced the findings of earlier groundbreaking urban ethnographers such as Eileen Krige, Ray Phillips, and Ellen Hellman.[2] In turn, these authors' close links to influential liberal institutions helped to determine the way that urban areas were perceived and apartheid criticized in subsequent years.[3] Urban "promiscuity" became a prominent symbol of the deleterious effects of racial segregation on the African family.[4]

Social historians have now overturned the idea that apartheid constituted an unfolding of a "grand plan."[5] Yet the theory that apartheid caused a straightforward and linear decline in family relations—or, relatedly, that the rise of "industrial men" fueled the collapse of families—has remained much less directly challenged.[6] Indeed, if anything, it was reinvigorated when AIDS came to the fore in the 1990s—and it is precisely for this reason that it must be confronted. I showed earlier how an "accommodation of [white and black] patriarchs" upheld the umnumzana figure in rural areas; here I emphasize how urban policy too promoted this figure, albeit in contradictory ways.

The reasons for the increasing number of abanumzana in urban areas lie in contradictory trends: while the early apartheid era witnessed horrifying new restrictions on Africans' access to urban areas, the rising demand for stable African labor meant that it was also the period when urban townships grew the fastest. In the twenty years after the National Party won power in 1948 under the banner of apartheid, many of the enormous townships that are well known today—Soweto, KwaMashu, and Umlazi, to name but a few— were built or greatly extended.[7] And at the center of planners' designs at this time were four-room "matchbox" family houses, allocated overwhelmingly to working men with wives.

This chapter covers much ground, but I think it is important to explain the tremendous changes in Sundumbili township over only a thirty-year period— and in a way that emphasizes its connections to other places. In addition to showing how the early apartheid township era engendered powerful meanings of, and physical structures devoted to, the patriarchal family, I address two further themes. First, I consider the gendered nature of the homeland/ bantustan project whereby the apartheid state devolved certain powers to ethnically constituted regions, especially in the 1960s and 1970s. Most accounts of Inkatha, the Zulu nationalist group which ran the KwaZulu homeland, stress its championship of an aggressive Zulu masculinity. There is much truth to this, especially in the period of political violence between Inkatha and the ANC that encompassed the 1980s and early 1990s.[8] Yet Inkatha has another important side: in its early years the organization in Sundumbili was run by "respectable" family men and the KwaZulu homeland itself spearheaded moves to grant women certain rights, including to own property.

If apartheid, including the homeland project, did not simply cause the family to "degenerate," a more robust periodization is necessary—my second theme. As I show here and develop in the next chapter, the 1980s were the key period when rising unemployment and housing shortages prevented younger men from accessing work and family housing. By 1994, as young people won political freedom, townships' ability to foster a patriarchal form of "welfare paternalism" had abruptly ended, and a women-led alternative had not become entrenched.[9] If we are to understand the palpable sense of conflict between men and women today we need to better understand the production of, and then the virtual ending of, a "patriarchal bargain" based, in urban areas, on male work and male-led housing. To make these arguments I draw from oral histories as well as archival sources.[10]

Sundumbili: A Model Ethnic Township

"SAPPI built the township." I must have heard this statement a hundred times when conducting research. Yet it is not strictly true—it was the national government that approved and financed the township. Still, the falsehood tells an accurate story about the importance of work and housing to residents' sense of place. The origin of Sundumbili, as the maxim suggests, was in the need to stabilize the SAPPI paper mill's African workforce after the plant opened in 1954. This factory, dependent on the water from the Thukela River, had chosen its location because of the abundance of labor in the adjacent rural "reserve."

The opening of Sundumbili township in 1964 was part of an emerging racial geography whose boundaries became hardened in the post-1948 apartheid era. The 1950 Group Areas Act instigated the removal of tens of thousands of people—mostly Indians, Africans, and coloureds but some whites—who had lived in racially mixed urban areas.[11] The apartheid state also strengthened influx controls that restricted Africans' access to urban areas, including by tightening laws that forced them to carry "passes."

Located relatively far from a large city, the SAPPI paper mill oversaw the construction of what amounted to two company towns. Mandini was built for its white employees; company directors gave their names to the town's first streets. Sundumbili was built for its larger but considerably lower-paid African workforce. SAPPI also established fifty-three Indian family houses next to the plant.[12] At this time, most Indians in the area lived in or near Tugela and were involved in market gardening or sugar cane production.[13] Job segregation meant that they were employed at SAPPI in semi-skilled work such as pipefitting and plumbing. Africans, at first, were overwhelmingly employed in work designated unskilled.

Race is a fundamental but not sufficient lens through which to understand urban planning at this time. Certainly, as they grew in numbers, African townships became a powerful symbol of apartheid racial planning. In the interest of state control, most were located far from "white" urban areas, and their roads were wide to allow police vehicles to patrol.[14]

At the same time, modernist American and British planning styles influenced the planning of these racialized spaces in wide-ranging ways.[15] Prior to the establishment of Sundumbili, the majority of SAPPI's male employees—typically hailing from northern KwaZulu-Natal—were migrants who lived in a single-sex compound on the paper mill's grounds. The move toward township family houses, planners hoped, would stabilize this labor force. Considering the township's image today as a place of violence and crime, it is remarkable that early plans included a swimming pool, a tennis court, a hotel, crèches, schools, businesses "with large open spaces, a sports centre, car parking lots and a reservoir."[16] Indeed, across the country, planners conceived of townships as spaces that created modern communities, including through promoting distinct social "neighborhoods."[17]

Urban planning also sought to divide Africans along ethnic lines. Johannesburg's Soweto, populated by residents from all over the country, was divided into discrete ethnic sections. And the state took this ethnic segregation to shocking new heights in the late 1960s: it halted altogether the construction of townships in large towns like Johannesburg and built them only in the ten ethnic homelands/bantustans to which most Africans were consigned. Sundumbili's location in what came to be called the KwaZulu homeland in the 1970s is consistent with this shift in urban policy.[18] Giving a sense of the prevailing narrative of ethnic modernism, one local paper described Sundumbili as "an important step forward in the development of the Zulu people."[19]

Sundumbili was built in roughly four phases. In 1964, 860 four-room family houses were constructed. These formed the first three sections, called by residents Thokoza (Be Happy), Skhalambazo (the name is said to derive from *imbazo*, "axe," because of the fighting that took place in this area), and Bhidla (said to have been derived from *ukubhidliza*, "to demolish," because of the removal of shacks to make space for this section). The area built in the second phase, in 1977, gained the name Dark City because it initially had no street lights. Sections built in the third phase, completed in 1980, were called Redhill (comprising red-brick houses on a hill) and Island (because at first it was surrounded by open space). Phases two and three added only around 1,000 houses. The final phase, opened in 1990, added roughly another 950 houses; these were the first houses built for private purchase and not rent and were financed by the KwaZulu Finance Corporation, the development wing of the KwaZulu government. This section was called Chappies, the name of the construction company that built the houses.

Making Modern Families in a Homeland Township

Mr. Ngcobo is a quiet man who lives in the Skhalambazo section of Sundumbili. Born in 1942, he attended a mission school until Standard 6; this gave him eight years of schooling in total, a quite high level for this period. Today, young and old residents speak of him, as of most of SAPPI's early employees, as a man of status—one of the founding fathers of the township.

Growing up not far from Mandeni, he took his first job at a sugar mill just south of Mandeni at Darnall, where he lived in the company's all-male compound. He recalls leaving the sugar mill after disliking the Indian supervisors' treatment of him.[20] In 1963, he moved to Durban to look for work. Not having Section 10 (residency) status did not stop him from securing several informal jobs, including construction work at the Toyota factory completed in that year.[21]

In 1966, escaping the constant harassment of "blackjacks" (Durban's influx control police) Mr. Ngcobo moved to Mandeni and found work at the SAPPI paper mill. In 1968, he finally married his childhood girlfriend, after four years of ilobolo payments, and they moved into a four-room township house that is still their home. Although wages rose after a strike in 1973, he says he left SAPPI in 1978 because of apartheid (white) foremen who "would kick like donkeys." He started a panel-beating business in the township and also worked for a while at the fast-growing factory complex at the nearby Isithebe Industrial Park.

Today, Mr. Ngcobo appears reasonably comfortable materially. Like many older residents, he purchased his house cheaply in the 1980s—in his case for only R1680 (US$210). He now pays it off at R35 (US$4.40) a month, and shares it with his wife and two children. Like many residents of his age, in the 1960s he supported the banned ANC and then joined Inkatha in 1977, soon after it was established.

Mr. Ngcobo's wife, when addressing me, referred to him respectfully as "ubaba walayikhaya" (the father of the house). Men's urban status became inscribed in the spatialized routines of everyday life that visits to houses such as Mr. Ngcobo's quickly revealed. The aura surrounding the isihlalo sikababa (father's chair), the most comfortable chair in the house, was easy to detect. I often witnessed mischievous grandchildren scampering from it when ubaba (father) entered the room.

As my research assistant and I sat down to talk, Mr. Ngcobo's wife and children quickly offered us drinks, a sign of respect to us but also to him. The small size of township houses made it difficult to uphold spatial divisions, but some hlonipha (respect) practices could be maintained; for instance, a child or woman might guqa (kneel) while serving food or drink to a man or older person. Underlining the household head's power was the fact that township houses were, at first, granted only to working men. And no better witness than Nelson Mandela describes the masculine feeling of moving into a township house (in his case, in Orlando in the 1940s): "It was the first true home of my own and I was mightily proud. A man is not a man until he has a house of his own."[22]

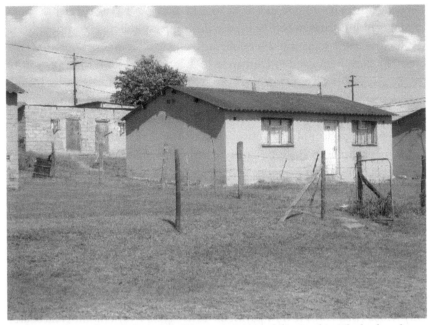

FIGURE 4.1. An early 51/9 "matchbox" house in Sundumbili township. The backyard contains *imijondolo* rented by the house's owner. Photograph by Mark Hunter.

Mr. Ngcobo was one of many Christian men who settled in towns. Missionaries actively promoted smaller nuclear families, and urban areas provided a modern geography for them. Since Christianity and schooling were closely associated, an urban abanumzana could gain status not simply as a household head but as an educated "gentleman." English took a relatively long time to master, but even a few years of schooling could enable a man to read the first isiZulu newspaper, *Ilanga laseNatal*, founded by John Dube in 1903.

Taught by Western missionaries but denied the benefits of liberalism, educated Africans—of whom John Dube himself was one of the most famous—were located in a kind of "ambiguity of dependence" on settler society.[23] And the difficult task of navigating manhood in the context of the political and cultural authority of whites is instanced by a 1950 clothing advertisement in *Ilanga* that displayed a sophisticated white man next to isiZulu text stating, "Banumzana!!" (figure 4.2). In addition to showing how being civilized (phucukile) was forged in relation to whiteness, the ad also demonstrates the salience of the term "umnumzana," a respectable urban man.

Yet African men's aspiration to urban "respectability" also served as a reminder of the flimsy justifications for racism; as Homi Bhabha noted, "mimicry" of the colonial master could be disruptive of colonial authority.[24] The *Ilanga* ad therefore indicates that South Africa's form of racial capitalism not only produced a rigid racial division of labor, about which much has been written, but also facilitated the reworking of identities in other arenas, including consumption. Like work, consumption was a domain of social struggle.

The physical structures anchoring urban life for Mr. Nkosi and Mr. Ngcobo were four-room "matchbox" houses. Virtually all township houses built in the apartheid era, including those in Sundumbili, were designed according to the NE 51/9 style ("NE 51" means the style was designed for non-Europeans in 1951). With an inside toilet, a kitchen, a living room, and two bedrooms, providing occupants with a living space of 51.2 square meters in all, a house of this design was seen as "capable of becoming a home that promotes family life and the nurture of children."[25] Such houses were typically granted to employed married men. Indeed, although the state manifested widely divergent views on whether to "stabilize" urban Africans, "there was never any disagreement about the centrality of the institution of marriage."[26]

Not only the prevailing housing design but also the philosophy of racial control drew on the symbolism of the nuclear family. Early white male township superintendents across South Africa saw themselves as "fathers" who "knew their natives" and were able to administer unpleasant laws in a relatively gentle way.[27] Sundumbili was slightly different in this regard because the nearby SAPPI plant itself played a significant role in township life. Tellingly, paper mill managers held quarterly meetings to discuss Sundumbili with "Bantu Affairs" personnel in Eshowe, the district's capital town. And SAPPI's influence extended well beyond housing: in 1971 it showed its workers—after having gained permission from the Eshowe Bantu Affairs Commissioner— films that included *The Three Musketeers, Cabin in the Sky,* and *Laurel and Hardy's Laughing '20s.*[28]

Apartheid's "matchbox" houses, then, gave a generation of men a foothold in urban areas. In contrast, new state controls constrained African women: in the 1950s, amid great protests, women joined men in being required to carry "passes" that limited their access to urban areas. Instead of building an urban shack and making a living through informal activities, as women had done for decades, by the 1960s they were allowed to stay in urban areas only "as units of labor or as shackled dependants of men."[29] These rules were never completely enforced, and woman-headed households existed in Sundumbili, as in other townships, being established, for instance, upon a husband's death (in these cases the house could be registered in a son's name). In white areas

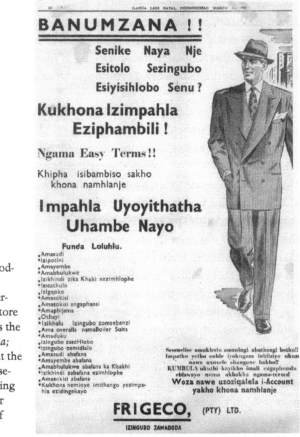

FIGURE 4.2. Selling the modern *umnumzana* in *Ilanga*, March 11, 1950. The advertisement is for a clothes store in Durban. *Abanumzana* is the plural form of *umnumzana;* the word originally meant the male head of a rural household, but in an urban setting came to mean "mister" or "gentleman." Courtesy of *Ilanga laseNatal*, Durban.

like Mandini, domestic work also provided a significant number of women with urban accommodation. Nevertheless, virtually all early township houses were rented to men.

Deeply patriarchal, this housing policy was also heteronormative, which placed it at odds with expressions of same-sex desire that had long existed in the country.[30] This point is well illustrated by the violent destruction of uMkhumbane (Cato Manor) informal settlement in 1959 as Durban enforced racial zoning. Many married Africans from the settlement were relocated to the new KwaMashu township and allocated family housing. Yet uMkhumbane's destruction undermined a vibrant and well-documented culture of same-sex intimacy, especially in the informal settlement's eSinyameni section. Here, men held ceremonies known as *imigidi wezitabane* (cultural performances of men who have boyfriends) as well as same-sex marriage ceremonies.[31] So well known was this area that one story in *Ilanga* in 1970, over a decade later, evoked the same-sex culture of eSinyameni to describe a marriage ceremony between two men in Durban that involved bridesmaids and the drinking of champagne.[32] Although they were by no means approved of by all South Africans, same-sex relationships existed, and they ran starkly counter to the state's post-1950s family housing projects.

All townships thus promoted a heteronormative model of family life. But Sundumbili differed from many others in that its location in an African reserve (later homeland) meant that residents did not have to have Section 10 urban residency status. Not being subjected to these controls, residents probably had more stability in Sundumbili than in many other townships in South Africa. Nevertheless, even townships located near larger white towns and thus subject to influx laws saw the growth of a quite stable population: a recent study of Soweto, Johannesburg, found that many of its residents had lived in this township for several decades.[33]

WOMEN AND THE NUCLEAR FAMILY

In a sure sign of domesticity, Mrs. Mthembu wore a neat pinafore (a sleeveless garment similar to an apron) when I met her in 2003. On her lounge wall she had hung three large photos of her children graduating from tertiary education and one of her late husband. This Christian lady was born in 1940 in Endulinde, some ten kilometers north of central Mandeni. After marrying in 1965, she moved into her husband's rural home. Mr. Mthembu, also an educated Christian, had secured a job with SAPPI and shortly afterward was invited to rent a four-room township house in Sundumbili. In such circumstances, a number of men whom I interviewed said that they preferred to live with a concubine while their wife looked after the rural homestead. Christian men, however, were by far the most likely to live with their wives in the township. Mrs. Mthembu also pushed for such a relocation: "When you marry your husband," she said, "you must go with him to the town."

She recalled that rural-born Christian women actively drew on ideals of romantic love to make the case to their husbands that they should move together to an urban area. In teasing out the prevailing narratives, it is difficult to separate the secular influences of ideas of romantic love from Christian beliefs about the virtues of the nuclear family. Images of romantic love promoting companionate marriage circulated widely in the media—yet these images were most accessible to those educated in mission schools. Moreover, with roads, electric lighting, and family housing, urban areas provided a modern geography for both secular ideas of romantic love and the realization of the Christian nuclear family.

In Sundumbili, as elsewhere in South Africa, *umanyano*, women's church organizations, were one institution that could promote a modern version of domesticated femininity.[34] Mrs. Mthembu remembers how members of these organizations baked and sewed together and visited ill residents. Christian women from these groups also struck up links with white-run Women's Institutes that were active in townships in the 1960s and 1970s. The Mandini Women's Institute was founded in 1952 and, even before the township was built, organized activities directed toward improving the health of Africans, for instance running a childcare clinic and providing subsidized milk.[35]

Though race shaped women's lives in profound ways, one issue that affected all women was contraception. In 1967 a family planning clinic was set up at SAPPI, and it came to treat white, African, Indian, and coloured women.[36] This initiative predated the massive family planning program aimed at Africans from the 1970s which led to the promotion of contraception (mostly Depo-Provera) in the township's clinic.[37]

In very different ways, then, white and black women were rethinking their own femininity at this time. Urban Christian African women still emphasized motherhood, but families rarely had more than two or three children; indeed, the tiny homes almost demanded this restriction. Township women's relatively good education also meant that some entered professions such as teaching and nursing. In these relatively rare cases the household had a dual income.

As has been widely noted, the apartheid period was marked by hugely oppressive laws: in addition to promoting urban segregation and rural home-lands, new legislation ended high-quality mission schooling, segregated ame-nities, and outlawed mixed-race marriages and sex. Yet the economic boom of the 1960s generally raised standards of living in Sundumbili. Producers of consumer goods in particular sought to capitalize on "the emergence of the African woman as a potent economic force."[38] In Sundumbili's houses, a sofa and coffee table were the most important furniture in the front room, and a "room divider" with bookshelves and a display cabinet was also prized. Some houses I visited had tiles on the floor and a ceiling board that hid the asbestos roofing. When electricity was introduced in the 1980s, stoves and T.V.s became popular.

Located on the other side of the SAPPI paper mill, white women liv-ing in Mandini enjoyed a higher standard of living and better work oppor-tunities. One 1963 newspaper article noted that "some girls choose a career . . . and finally become doctors, educationalists, artists, actresses or the like." But it went on to say that "all of them, including the career girls, have their secret hopes, to marry a handsome and competent young man, to make a beautiful home, to become a gracious housewife."[39] The white women active in the Women's Institute could perhaps find a temporary foothold for their own shifting identities in the active promotion of African domesticity. All white women of reasonable economic standing, after all, had an African "girl" as a maid.

MORAL AND IMMORAL GEOGRAPHIES

We can find in Sundumbili's early history examples of more "casual" relations, ones well documented by urban ethnographers such as Laura Longmore. Non-marital and extramarital relationships, in fact, preceded the building of the township. Longtime residents of the area remember a group of women living in one- and two-room shacks made from flimsy paper, cardboard, and wood in the early 1950s, when the SAPPI factory itself was being constructed. The shacks were called *imikhukhu* (*khukhu* is an idiom for washing away) and *izindlwana* (literally, "small houses"); the word *umjondolo* was not widely used until roughly the 1980s. The women typically sold homemade beer, meat, and other products.[40]

Once the township was built in 1964, both "marriages of convenience" and informal forms of cohabitation were relatively common.[41] Marriage was the easiest way for a man to gain access to family housing, although he could also register a house in his parents' name. When he had ties to both a township and a rural home, a man's income typically had to be divided; consequently, concubines often brewed and sold sorghum beer as a means to supplement the urban household. "Shebeen queens" also constructed tin shacks alongside the "matchbox" houses of the township for this purpose.[42]

Before the establishment of a government-run beer hall in the township in the 1970s, women's informal brewing provided men with their only access to alcohol. Yet Sundumbili's lively informal alcohol trade stoked sharp tensions within an increasingly differentiated population. In 1970 an outraged Mandini Bantu Women's Institute (named after the white-run version) wrote to Sundumbili's township manager and complained about the illegal sale of alcohol and men who lived with concubines.[43]

The presence of concubine unions became symbolic of an anything-goes attitude in urban life across South Africa, including in Sundumbili. Indeed, the expediency of cohabitation is reflected in the verb *ukukipita* (literally, "to keep it"). But temporary urban relationships also reveal that many early male township residents maintained close connections with wives in rural areas, to whom they sent remittances. Following anthropologist Philip Mayer, I argue that it is wrong, therefore, for observers to conceptualize non-marital urban relationships as simply immoral; what could appear immoral in the context of urban areas alone could be quite moral if we consider that many men's lives were stretched between urban and rural areas.[44] To the men who practiced them, these non-marital concubine relations represented not the "degeneration" of the family but a commitment to supporting it while away.

Reflecting these views, Mr. Dlamini, who lived in the SAPPI compound in the 1960s, recalls his colleagues' anger when he moved into a township house. There was a feeling, he said, that "once we take these houses we are going to neglect our [rural] families." People who took houses, he remembered, were seen as being "like Indians," visitors to the country, not belonging anywhere (in this racialization of space, whites were seen as oppressors but still geographically rooted in South Africa).[45] In making these points Mr. Dlamini used the scornful verb *ukubhunguka*, to abandon a home, which derided men's abandonment of a rural umuzi, including its amadlozi (ancestors). Men who did this were counterposed to the *amagoduka*, those who returned home. Men's moral stances were therefore highly contested: was a married man who lived with an urban concubine immoral because he lived "in sin" (a typical Christian interpretation) or moral because he lived in this temporary arrangement in order *not* to settle permanently and ukubhunguka?

Links between Sundumbili and rural areas persisted into the 1980s: Ardington's 1983 study found that 65 percent of the township residents claimed to have another home. But the study also reveals a weakening of these links: only 25 percent of respondents indicated they would leave the Mandeni area upon the termination of their employment.[46] Many men like Mr. Nkosi—whose story began this chapter—appeared to have initially anticipated a return to their rural homes, but subsequently became disillusioned by the pace of rural decline and accustomed to the better schools and services in urban areas.

Unlike men, women could not legitimately combine a rural-based marriage and temporary urban living. Women's often precarious urban existence is well illustrated by Mrs. Mngadi, whom I interviewed in her house in March 2003. Born in 1955 in Mtubatuba, in northern KwaZulu-Natal, she left this rural area to search for work after her father bhunguka'd (abandoned the rural home). Bhidla section was her home from around 1970, when she lived temporarily with her sister, who was in a *kipita* (cohabiting) relationship with a SAPPI man.

In the early 1970s, Mrs. Mngadi started a love affair with Siyanda, a man from Northern KwaZulu who worked for a firm of building contractors. They kipita'd and he supported her; Mrs. Mngadi used Depo-Provera to prevent pregnancy. However, she soon discovered that her boyfriend had a wife in the rural area whence he hailed. He offered to make her his second wife, but she refused and left him.

Forced to find a way to survive, Mrs. Mngadi found work at Isithebe Industrial Park and also, she says, had many boyfriends—especially men who worked at SAPPI who had left their wives in the rural areas. Eventually she found Christianity, and this helped her to turn her life around. In the 1990s, she fell in love with and married a man who worked at the state's electricity company, Eskom. However, after several years this man left her for another woman. She now lives in the house that he bought, hoping that he will not claim it for himself.

Mrs. Mngadi is both a victim of bhunguka (her father abandoned her home) and a potential cause of it herself (through her relationships with married SAPPI men). Looking back at why she did not marry her first lover, who already had a wife, she said that she "grew up saying I don't want a man who has polygamy (isithembu)." Such a relationship, she declared, would give her jealousy (isikhwele); in other words, the kind of love she favored (monogamous) resulted in, and from, bodily emotions over which she had little control. Influenced by schooling and Christianity, Mrs. Mngadi endorsed a more modern idea of love.

Yet, as her circumstances worsened, Mrs. Mngadi came to lament not marrying her first suitor: "Really, I regret it, I wish that I had carried on with Siyanda, the one I was in love with, because he said he was going to build me a home." Here she appears to turn away from romantic love and laud the virtues of a provider love that rested on a man lobola-ing and supporting a woman.

1974–84: The KwaZulu Homeland, Self-Help, and "Rights with Hlonipha"

During Sundumbili's second decade, from roughly the mid-1970s to the mid-1980s, the paternalism of the first era was recast as the administration of the township moved to Ulundi, the capital of the KwaZulu homeland. Building on more than a century of devolution of power to African authorities, the state in the 1960s and 1970s established ten ethnic homelands/bantustans, and in the four that became independent, it stripped millions of Africans of their South African citizenship.[47]

In the homeland of KwaZulu the chief minister of the KwaZulu Legislative Assembly was Chief Mangosuthu Buthelezi. A charismatic leader, Buthelezi refused full independence from South Africa but took the homeland to "self-governing" status in 1977. In 1975 he buttressed the homeland's ethnic vision by establishing Inkatha Yenkululeko Yesiswe (the National Cultural Liberation Movement), a revived version of the Zulu nationalist organization established in the 1920s. Although Inkatha subsequently became known as a violent organization, this was not how it was thought of in the 1970s. With the African National Congress banned and leaders like Mandela jailed, most residents of Sundumbili saw Inkatha as a legitimate means of political expression. The ANC, in fact, supported its establishment and saw it as an ally until around 1980.

In Sundumbili Inkatha was led by a group of respectable SAPPI men, most of whom lived in the township's four-room houses. One prominent local member was Prince Nhlanhla Zulu, a member of the Zulu royal house who found work in the 1960s in the SAPPI laboratory and eventually became an Inkatha Freedom Party (IFP) member of parliament in Cape Town. Capturing the flavor of this period, Buthelezi described Zulu after his death in 2007 as "a man of our time who relished progress and the beauty of tradition in equal measure."[48]

Another Inkatha member and prominent figure of this era was Rev. Mzoneli, who returned to KwaZulu-Natal in 1974 after studying for a degree in social work at Ohio University. Prior to leaving South Africa, he had been one of a large number of Christian activists in the Black Consciousness movement.[49] On his return to the country Mzoneli became the pastor of Sundumbili's Lutheran church.

Consistent with the Black Consciousness movement's promotion of self-help groups, Mzoneli founded Siwasivuka ("We fall, we rise"), otherwise known as the Sundumbili Community Development Association. The names of Siwasivuka's standing committees—health and nutrition, education and literacy, crafts and industries, agriculture, physical improvement, and cultural activities—give a flavor of the modernist ethos that pervaded the organization. Mr. Mzoneli told me in 2003 that he had sought to "inculcate in Sundumbili a spirit of home."[50]

Although Inkatha was a male-led organization that harked back to a glorious Zulu past, many women supported its project of ethnic uplift. By 1985, Inkatha's Women's Brigade numbered nearly 400,000—more than a third of Inkatha's total membership.[51] One important reason for the growth in the number of female Inkatha members was the rapid expansion of health and educational institutions. Schooling in particular not only raised women's expectations but brought them directly into employment: by 1979 there were 16,000 teachers in KwaZulu.[52]

Yet the steadily increasing numbers of women in industry and the professions conflicted sharply with customary laws that positioned Zulu women as "minors." In legal terms Zulu women were probably the most marginalized group in South Africa.[53] Responding to this dilemma, in 1974 the new KwaZulu Legislative Assembly established, as one of its first acts, a select committee on the "disabilities of Zulu women." Noting that urban women were influenced by work opportunities and "women of other cultures," the committee gave particular attention to the injustice of denying female teachers and nurses the right to own property.[54] The KwaZulu authority therefore sought to balance the middle-class aspirations of some women in KwaZulu and Inkatha's public image as promoting "traditional" Zulu institutions such as chiefs.

In 1981, building on this momentum, the KwaZulu Legislative Assembly reformed customary law so that women could be legally recognized as heads of households and could own property.[55] Around the same time, across South Africa, women gained increasing rights to access township housing in their own name.[56] Now any woman with means could apply for a township house, although township managers still often presumed that men were the rightful heads of households. One lady in her fifties, Mrs. Khuzwayo, who lives in a house in Chappies with her sisters, remembers hearing Buthelezi on the radio delivering pro-women messages. She told me, "Buthelezi realized that women knew how to develop the country." Indeed, the very institutions at which aspiring middle-class women were working—schools and hospitals— were precisely the ones that legitimized the KwaZulu homeland structure.

According to Mrs. Khuzwayo, Buthelezi explicitly spoke of granting women amalungelo (rights). Yet if Inkatha granted women certain rights, they were *not* rights premised on equality between men and women and the young and old (as "rights" have been presented after democracy). Rather than being granted an individual right to gender equality, Mrs. Khuzwayo told me, a woman was still encouraged to hlonipha (respect) traditional customs: Buthelezi proposed what we might call "rights with hlonipha." Essentially, women gained property rights and membership in an ethnic community, but not full equality with men or voting rights within South Africa.

Indeed, Inkatha's women leaders could combine support for women's legal "emancipation" with a neo-traditionalist embrace of purity, for instance through the annual reed ceremony for virgins held at the Zulu king's kraal.[57] This apparently contradictory approach to gender has to be seen as part of the homeland's broader culture, which combined both "modernity" and "traditions" in a way that kept white men at the apex of social hierarchies but created important other divisions along lines of ethnicity, class, and status.

Polyvalent understandings of rights evolved too from men's informal associations. In 1977 a survey of township residents sponsored by the University of Zululand found crime to be considered the main problem, followed by dusty roads, drunkenness, and uncontrolled youth.[58] The nearest police station, although it was only seven kilometers away in Nyoni, had little concern for crime affecting black South Africans.

To address this, a group of mostly SAPPI men began engaging in vigilante activities, calling themselves *oqonda* or *abelungisi;* Mr. Manqele, a member of the Inkatha-aligned town council, led the organization. These men drew on another aspect of "rights"; abelungisi took their name from the verb ukulunga, "to be right," and the men's aim was to right moral wrongs (similarly, *uku-qonda* means "to be straight"). In the early 1980s, groups of oqonda sprouted in many parts of urban KwaZulu-Natal. Armed with traditional weapons, such as sjamboks and knobkerries, oqonda would patrol the township and, according to one informant, *qondisa isigwegwe* (straighten the moral crooked-ness) of people.

As well as rising crime, the appearance of oqonda also signaled height-ened gendered conflicts as men's grip on work and housing began to come to an end. As it did in other KwaZulu townships, the reach of oqonda in Sundumbili extended deep into domestic politics.[59] It was not only criminals but also wayward women whom oqonda "straightened," including women who acted without respect by wearing trousers—clothes meant for men. One seventy-year-old man, Mr. Ncube, remembered their attitude toward trouser-wearers: "You have to show that you are a woman, you mustn't come as a man." Another supporter of oqonda from the area was quoted in 1982 as saying, "Most people were happy with *mbutho* ["regiment," another name for oqonda] . . . except the youth because it stopped the ladies wearing trousers or schoolchildren lying with their boyfriends outside."[60]

Some women were indeed acting like men at this time. One trend, described more fully in the next chapter, was the large number of rural migrants, including women, who were arriving to work in the factory com-plex established at Isithebe in 1971. By 1982, Isithebe Industrial Park employed 4,239 men and 3,207 women.[61] Concerned residents called a meeting at the township manager's office to discuss the shortage of accommodation for the large number of unmarried "girls."[62] A coalition of groups—the coun-cil, women's groups, and Inkatha—pushed for the establishment of a hostel for single women. These plans were never realized, and many single women continued to live in imijondolo (by now a more common term for shacks) in Isithebe and the surrounding Sundumbili.

An even stronger affront to a man's rightful position as a head of house-hold, however, came when a few women accessed township housing in their own right. In the early 1980s, a number of women bought plots in the new Island section of the township on which to build their own houses, sometimes room by room. What's more, all women now had the unequivocal right to take over the couple's four-room "matchbox" house upon the death of their husband. Women's ascendancy to the head of households—which overturned the social basis of umnumzana—resulted in a stinging letter of criticism sent from "the community" to the KwaZulu administration complaining that women were now favored in housing matters (its lead author was a man, Mr. Khumalo).[63]

Fast Love? Coming of Age in the 1970s

I have thus far briefly described the lives of the township's first residents. But what kind of intimate relations did their children engage in during the 1970s and 1980s? Despite the graphic warnings of early urban ethnographers like Laura Longmore, urban men and women overwhelmingly continued to marry: in the Mandeni area 67 percent of men over twenty-five were married in 1983.[64] Although certain traditions were looked down on as uncouth in urban areas, one that persisted was ilobolo.[65] Fathers had a material interest in securing ilobolo payments, but most daughters, too, strongly defended the custom: how else would a woman know that a man was serious about her and would be able to support her? Cash had to be earned, and this required commitment, sacrifice, and dedication to the project of "building a home"—all signs of a good man.

Conceptions of "sex" were also changing in this period, influenced by multiple factors. Drum magazine, which came to symbolize a new cosmopolitan urban culture, ran a famous series of articles on sex in 1972: "Everything You Ever Wanted to Know about Sex."[66] In the 1970s the growing availability of contraception was also a profound change. If Christians had long portrayed "sex" as a separate realm, contraception allowed the detachment of sex altogether from pregnancy. Ukusoma (penis-thigh intimacy), a practice long seen as "old-fashioned" in urban areas, was increasingly discarded during this period; in startling evidence of collective forgetting, some young township residents I spoke with in the early 2000s had never heard of it, although it was usually familiar in rural areas.

In this milieu, penetrative sex and love became interwoven and contested in new ways. Did sex before marriage signify love between two individuals or its opposite, lust? Morality or immorality? The answer was not always clear, and this ambiguity warns against taking illegitimacy rates as a sign of immorality, as early urban ethnographers typically did. Urban ethnographers who fixated on technical definitions of "illegitimacy" missed the fact that couples who parented children would often subsequently marry.[67]

In growing urban areas, to what extent could penetrative sex be exchanged for gifts? There are longstanding accounts, from across the continent, of rural-born women moving to overwhelmingly male-populated urban areas and living by exchanging sex for money in various kinds of arrangements.[68] In countries that gained independence, better-educated women were often reported to be engaging in relationships with older middle-class men.[69] Yet my interviews in Sundumbili suggest that until around the 1980s, gifts from men to women linked to sex were not common among unmarried young people in Sundumbili. This is not to say that such exchanges never took place, but those that did primarily involved women who were seen as less eligible for marriage, for instance widows and women who had borne children.[70]

As in rural areas, marriageable women who accepted gifts in exchange for sex risked being portrayed as izifebe (loose women). And in any case, many women would wonder why a man was giving her gifts and not paying ilobolo for her, if he truly loved her? These were, of course, values aspired to and not always kept. Hinting at a growing materiality around relationships and rising social inequalities (themes developed in later chapters), residents told me that the term "sugar daddy" began to be used in the 1980s to signify a man who supported a much younger girlfriend. Revealingly, however, an older and more common term, umathandezincane (a man who likes young women) was used to describe a man who had intimate relations with a young woman and might even, unlike a sugar daddy, marry her.

Mid-1980s Onward:
Political Conflict, Housing, and the Unemployment Crisis

Sundumbili's first two decades were marked by differing forms of paternalism within an overall violent racist system. The township's social structure rested on the male wage earner, but some women accessed housing as wives or concubines, and eventually in their own right. Although rapid economic growth marked this period, from the mid-1970s the economy began to stutter under the combined forces of a global economic downturn, increased oil prices, and the mounting strength of black trade unions and the anti-apartheid movement. Per capita growth drifted into negative numbers, and unemployment and inequalities expanded rapidly. By the 1980s, young people in most parts of South Africa had a slimmer chance of finding a job than their parents. This general picture was slightly complicated in Mandeni because of the growing number of factories established in nearby Isithebe Industrial Park.

However, thousands of in-migrants competed for jobs and this meant that, as in other parts of South Africa, unemployment increased.

Escalating unemployment coincided across South Africa with the state's inability to fund housing. By the beginning of the 1980s economic and political crisis meant that administration boards—the agents who took over the running of townships from local authorities—were in financial disarray, and urban township houses became harder to secure, more expensive, and of worse quality.[71] In Sundumbili in the early 1980s, the Port Natal administration board built the Redhill and Island sections, but the rent of the new houses was nearly three times the amount paid by those living in houses built in the 1960s.[72] By the late 1980s there existed in effect a nationwide freeze on government-funded township housing. The private sector was charged with picking up the slack, and in Sundumbili only better-off residents were able to get loans to buy new houses in the Chappies section. As a consequence of these housing shortages—and this point bears emphasizing—the ratio of residents to formal Sundumbili houses rose from roughly four in 1969 to seven in 1983 and twelve in 1991.[73]

Yet colossal political developments drew attention away from these changes. On June 16, 1976, Soweto township youth began the "Soweto uprising." The protests, violently quashed by police, centered on the state's attempt to introduce Afrikaans as a medium for instruction in schools. Although Sundumbili residents do not remember their township as being particularly politicized at this time, protests spread across the country. And the protesting youth opposed not only apartheid but their parents' apparent acquiescence to racial rule.

In the 1980s, as struggles against apartheid intensified, the benefits of state paternalism seemed even scantier, especially as unemployment escalated. Moreover, rising education levels came together with bleak economic prospects. Established in 1953, "Bantu Education" worsened the standard of education—effectively closing the mission schools, which had offered a high-quality education at least to an elite—but also significantly expanded schooling's scope, and with it young people's expectations. In Sundumbili by 1983 five schools hosted three thousand students and provided education up to Standard 10 (graduation from secondary school).[74]

In an example of the politicizing effect of increasing literacy, journalist Fred Khumalo recalls in his autobiography reading *Pace* in Mpumalanga township, close to Durban, and being struck by stories of successful black Americans such as Booker T. Washington, Martin Luther King, Marcus Garvey, and Malcolm X. When electricity was brought to township homes in the 1980s, Khumalo recalls, American pop culture on television "bombarded us."[75] Of course, America's political and cultural influence goes back decades, but the arrival of T.V. helped to bring the two worlds into more direct contact.[76] It made change seem imminent by depicting the political and economic power of post–civil rights African-Americans.

Another shift in the 1980s that was dwarfed by political developments was the rise of class inequalities closely tied to age.[77] Despite brutal state violence, some of SAPPI's first male employees grew more prosperous during this time. Seeking to create a buffer between the militant masses and the white elite, the apartheid government actively promoted the economic development of African-owned businesses. Moreover, a series of deeper shifts accentuated this trend. In the 1970s, labor shortages, rising trade union membership, and a relaxation of job segregation increased African wages among a core group.[78]

In Sundumbili, these new divisions are reflected in the emergence of a class of entrepreneurs, usually SAPPI workers with township houses, who invested their wages in lucrative businesses. The growth of factories in Isithebe in the 1980s created a massive demand for taxis; men with capital could procure a vehicle (usually a Toyota Hiaca, which can carry sixteen people), and by 1983 taxis were the most profitable small business activity in the area.[79] Building and renting imijondolo in the backyards of four-room township houses or in rural areas was also increasingly lucrative. Ironically, the much maligned four-room "matchbox" house became the springboard for accumulation. Increasingly purchased at knock-down prices from the authorities in the 1980s, some became barely recognizable as new rooms, garages, porches, and elaborate courtyards were added.

No history of Mandeni can ignore the terrible period of political violence that peaked in the early 1990s. Even though Chief Buthelezi did not accept "independence" for KwaZulu, by the early 1980s ANC supporters increasingly saw Inkatha (after 1990 the Inkatha Freedom Party) as an apartheid collaborator because of its complicity with the homeland project. For "comrades" exhibiting "struggle masculinities," Inkatha had sold out the liberation movement instead of joining forces with them to overthrow the state.[80]

Across KwaZulu-Natal and in the hostels that housed temporary (often Zulu) workers around Johannesburg, tensions rose between supporters of Inkatha and those of the ANC and the powerful union federation COSATU (Congress of South African Trade Unions). In Mandeni the social cocktail was particularly explosive. Tribal authorities and other structures linked to the KwaZulu homeland were firmly entrenched, and yet COSATU-affiliated workers rapidly organized in Isithebe's mushrooming factories to foster a new culture of resistance.

As battle lines became more firmly drawn, Inkatha transformed itself from a Zulu nationalist "development" organization run by respected elders into an authoritarian and violent organization heavily influenced by warlords. Spurred on by an increasingly confrontational Buthelezi, the organization positioned itself as the heir of Zulu masculinities and argued that Zulus had the right to self-determination in a homeland: it labeled Zulus aligned with the ANC feminine and "agents of the Xhosas."[81]

Anticipating this shift, in the early 1980s some Inkatha members, such as Rev. Mzoneli, left Inkatha or took a back seat in the organization. In turn, a number of oqonda took a more active and violent role in Inkatha. They were joined by some local chiefs who had a vested interest in homeland institutions. One COSATU activist told me that in the 1980s Chief Mathonsi worked in a metal factory and was a staunch union supporter, but repudiated this role to take over the local Mathonsi chiefship and become a feared Inkatha supporter.[82] Inkatha was also backed by businessmen like Sundumbili's Major Gcaleka, the owner of Sundumbili's largest store, who depended on trading licenses obtained from KwaZulu authorities.

Much of the South African and international media described the political violence as "black on black," but this deflected attention from its underlying causes. One of these was the "Third Force," the involvement of some elements of the apartheid state in political violence, including through supporting Inkatha. The "Caprivi trainees"—Inkatha members trained by the South African army in Namibia in 1986—became one of the most visible signs of this support.[83] The IFP-aligned KwaZulu police, notorious for their bias, were another group feared by ANC supporters.[84] Factory managers further stoked violence by employing Inkatha-aligned workers in preference to more militant COSATU-aligned workers.

The worst period of political violence occurred in the years between Mandela's release in 1990 and the 1994 elections. After a series of bloody skirmishes the township became geographically divided: Redhill and most of Skhalambazo were IFP areas while Bhidla, Chappies, and most parts of Island were ANC. In turn, Sundumbili's division into ANC and IFP zones facilitated new forms of sexual control; people were not allowed to court those from "enemy" areas. This coincided with, and shaped, an apparent increase in sexual violence. According to the master's dissertation of one former ANC comrade who lived in Sundumbili, IFP youth would "abduct couples and gang rape a girlfriend in front of her boyfriend before killing them. This culture of gang raping was also employed by the ANC youth."[85] Similarly, women "on the same [political] side" were pressured into providing sexual services to ANC comrades or Inkatha supporters.[86]

Yet sexual violence was also connected to rising male unemployment and shifting household structures, a link not often made at the time but one I stress later.[87] One manifestation of heightened gender conflict was gang rape, which seemed to become more frequent around this time, partly independently of political violence. Fred Khumalo describes the violent punishing of a "loose" woman in the early 1980s, before political violence had taken hold, in the form of "streamlining," the gang rape of a man's girlfriend to punish her for talking to another man. "It wasn't considered rape. Rape was associated with physical violence and force. Streamlining was about control." Khumalo's shocking account is also important because it shows the lingering presence of ideas of respectability, even in these violent moments. Reflecting the tensions in men's actions, Khumalo says that although the practice restored men's manhood, "Streamlining went against the values instilled in me. My father respected my mother and women in general."[88]

The IFP-ANC political violence described here was mainly concentrated in present-day KwaZulu-Natal and, to a lesser extent, in townships near Johannesburg, but it has to be seen as very much a part of broader urban struggle in the dying years of apartheid. All ANC-aligned township protests opposed the apartheid state or its "puppets" and demanded that they be overthrown. Young people, increasingly unemployed, unmarried, and unable to gain access to houses, were the foot soldiers of uprisings everywhere. This contrasted sharply with the earlier period of paternalism, symbolized by men being granted four-room houses. Sociologist Belinda Bozzoli writes that the pro-ANC "young lions" in Johannesburg saw their activism as being in opposition to "patriarchal and age-based authority inimical to the young." Young people, she argues, "rejected both paternalism and liberalism—and in doing so they rejected their own parents—upon whom the earlier hierarchy of control had depended, and whom they perceived as having failed."[89] Certainly, the model of "welfare paternalism" that underpinned early townships had by the late 1980s been displaced by political activism. But rumbling underneath this, too, was an emerging crisis in housing and employment whose full force, as we shall see, was felt after 1994.

———————

Sundumbili's history takes us through the racial paternalism of the 1960s and the respectable ethnic nationalism of the 1970s to the terrible violence of the 1990s. The anti-apartheid struggles in townships are perhaps the most discussed parts of this urban history. But the fostering of masculine values of urban respectability, ones that rested on work and housing, refutes ideas that urban areas were characterized only by sexual "degeneration." Certainly the majority of people, rural or urban, who came of age in the 1960s and 1970s did marry and "build a home," even if divorce and concubine relationships were not uncommon.

What ensued later in the 1980s and early 1990s, somewhat offstage, was a rapid transformation from the township's early period of "welfare paternalism." Male unemployment increased and women moved in large numbers into industrial work. The housing crisis intensified and, as we will see in the next chapter, shacks began to multiply in and around the township.

By 1994, the earlier life path of working and marrying had become less likely in either a rural or an urban setting, and even in a way of living that combined both types of place. Yet the younger generation was better educated than their parents, and massive optimism about political change drove violence, especially from 1990 to 1994—between Mandela's release and the country's first democratic election. Would men and women realize their urban dreams after apartheid? How would respectability, embodied in the figure of umnumzana, become reworked after apartheid? Before considering these questions, we must explore the growth of imijondolo, in which many women made a home in the 1980s and 1990s.

FIVE

Shacks in the Cracks of Apartheid: Industrial Women and the Changing Political Economy and Geography of Intimacy

It is an unusually wet fall even for the north coast of KwaZulu-Natal. The year is 2000 and I am moving into Isithebe's informal/jondolo settlement from the nearby farm where I have been staying for a few weeks. The contrast couldn't be more striking. At the farm, the rain nourishes the neatly ordered sugar cane fields that stretch comfortably across the hills above Isithebe; the small white farming community celebrates the heavy rains. Yet in the flat land of Isithebe, residents whose ancestors used to farm this land tie plastic bags around their shoes to navigate the muddy tracks. In the mornings, many walk precariously toward Isithebe Industrial Park, a large collection of factories that overshadow the settlement. When they return, they will find the roofs and walls of their imijondolo leaking water, and rain dripping with infuriating regularity on the floor; the puddles in turn breed mosquitoes that will feed enthusiastically on residents in the coming summer months.

The family I am staying with in the jondolo settlement own a shop, and I volunteer my help in it occasionally. Working as a shop assistant places me, an *umlungu* (white), in a situation where I can act with some deference and humility and slowly get to know residents. My body adapts to fit this new setting: I learn to place my right hand under my open left palm when receiving money and adjust to speaking mainly in isiZulu, since few residents speak English. One day, after I have interviewed a group of women in a room adjacent to the shop, one lady lags behind. She is in her late forties and has a strong presence, looking at me with a weathered smile. This lady is called Dudu Mabuza, and over the next five years I get to know her quite well. I visit Dudu from time to time at her two-room mud, stick, and stone home and also see her regularly at the shop. One day I ask if she will talk with me about her life.

Dudu was born in 1954 and spent her early years in Nongoma, a rural area around one hundred and fifty kilometers north of Isithebe. A mission school afforded her education up to Standard 5, a high level (seven years) for an African woman in the 1960s. Dudu's mother was also educated at a mission school and worked as a teacher until she married and stopped work to look after her marital home. When her marriage broke down she moved to Matikulu, a sugar mill town close to Mandeni, and worked as a cleaner in the local country club; employers preferred domestic workers who spoke English. Her boss—or, as Dudu puts it, her "mother's umlungu" (mother's white)—also employed Dudu to help clean the country club.

In 1972, Dudu worked as a domestic worker for a family in Mandini, the white company town established by the SAPPI paper mill: "It was 'my girl do this and this,'" she explained. Shortly afterward, she left this job for what was then the more lucrative work of buying vegetables from Indian traders based at Tugela and selling them to residents in African areas. In the late 1970s, Dudu changed occupation again, finding work in one of Isithebe's new garment factories. By 1982, this income had allowed her to "buy" a plot of land in Isithebe for R500 (US$63) from an *isakhamuzi* (original resident, pl. *izakhamizi*). Her purchase of land (or, more accurately, land use), though technically unlawful, was consistent with reforms to customary law at this time, which granted women certain property rights. Since she "owned" a plot, her two-room structure was called an *indlu* (house), to differentiate it from the growing number of smaller rented imijondolo that housed migrants from rural areas.

As Isithebe's one-room imijondolo grew in numbers during the 1980s, the area became one of many unplanned informal settlements emerging in the political and social cracks of apartheid—and in turn deepening these cracks. The two most widely cited reasons why these spaces mushroomed are the chronic shortage of formal housing and the urbanization resulting from the languishing of rural homelands. These pressures are typically said to have exploded when the state abolished the hated pass laws in 1986, thus allowing for the free movement of all South Africans into towns regardless of race.

Pointing to the tremendous rise of shacks in many poor countries, Mike Davis recently coined the term "planet of slums."[1] However, like many people setting out to explain the mushrooming of shacks in South Africa, Davis largely ignores the gendered shifts that these physical constructions also manifest. Importantly, women like Dudu who lived in South African informal settlements disturbed two apartheid fantasies: that most African women should live in rural areas and that all women should be subjected to men's authority in the patriarchal marital home. If apartheid partly sustained itself through promoting the patriarchal home, the unraveling of both apartheid and the male-led family were inextricably linked.

When Dudu came to Mandeni in the 1970s, there must have been an air of optimism among migrant women: not only was informal trading quite lucrative, but factories were also opening up quickly after the establishment of Isithebe Industrial Park in 1971. If "industrial men" moved to the area from the 1950s, "industrial women" were joining them two decades later. By the 1990s, however, employment opportunities had diminished considerably and many of the women who followed in Dudu's steps viewed Isithebe as a place not of potential economic independence but of dependence on lovers. Few "bought" land; most lived in rented imijondolo.

Wide-reaching gendered shifts drove women's continued movement into urban shacks despite declining employment opportunities. As men had greater difficulty finding work from the late 1970s, only a small number of rural-born women remained permanently in rural areas. The agrarian economy was languishing and women had less expectation of marrying and being supported by a husband. Important new connections between rising unemployment, declining marriage rates, and increasing female mobility became apparent, and the growing number of one- or two-occupant imijondolo were a geographical manifestation of this story.

Put another way, the 1980s reconfigured expectations, emotions, dreams, and intimate relations that for generations had been profoundly shaped by the joint but contested project of *ukwakha umuzi* (to build a home). Living in an umjondolo came to symbolize precarious economic circumstances and life without marriage—and this was true in townships where backyard shacks mushroomed as much as in informal settlements themselves. These shifts are what I refer to as the changing political economy and geography of intimacy. And they coincided with the introduction of the deadly HIV virus in the 1980s, which would come to be disproportionately found in informal settlements.

Some caveats are in order before proceeding. "The changing political economy and geography of intimacy" is a broad term, and like all analytical abstractions is quite crude: intimacy and geography are always changing and the growth of shacks today is best thought of as a recurrence —only the onset of apartheid halted the explosion of shacks in the first half of the twentieth century. The rhythm and effects of the changes I describe also differ widely across South Africa. The 1980s were a terrible period of rising unemployment, but Isithebe's burst of growth at this time shows that jobs were unevenly distributed across the country. Moreover, although I give attention to the role of men's unemployment in increasing the mobility of women in the 1980s, in the 1970s scholars were already noting an increase of woman-headed households despite apartheid restrictions.[2]

More broadly, a myriad of household types and attendant geographies exist in South Africa, a country long seen as exhibiting "domestic fluidity."[3]

Some urban shack dwellers, for instance, moved not from rural homelands but from white-owned farms to which they had no intention of returning. And, despite the common stereotype, many people living in informal settlements did not, in fact, come to cities from rural areas of any kind.[4] Townships, as we have seen in the case of Sundumbili, were overflowing with residents because of the chronic shortage of housing. Still, despite these qualifications, the general themes that I describe are widespread and came together from roughly the 1980s: unemployment rose in all regions and fewer men supported women in marital relations; women's movement increased significantly; and shacks mushroomed in many places. These changes demand greater attention in AIDS policy and I use the somewhat crude term "changing political economy and geography of intimacy" to make this point (see also table 2.1).

Isithebe Industrial Park: Industrial Decentralization, the Gendered Division of Labor, and Unionization

Red Street, Blue Street, Yellow Street, Pink Street—the names of Isithebe Industrial Park's roads betray planners' dreams of creating an ordered space as they sought to propel the area into the modern industrial age. The location of this huge factory complex in Mandeni resulted from a national strategy of "industrial decentralization." According to this state initiative, factories received generous subsidies if they moved to predominantly rural parts of South Africa, including ethnic "homelands" established in the 1960s and 1970s.

After its opening in 1971, Isithebe Industrial Park grew quickly, especially in the 1980s as state subsidies were cranked up.[5] It attracted a diverse spread of businesses: in 1991, clothing and textiles accounted for 33 percent of employment, metal for 25 percent, plastic for 12 percent, machinery and appliances for 8 percent, paper for 7 percent, and other types of industries for 15 percent.[6] Investment in the park came mostly from South African firms, but Taiwanese companies played an increasing role, reflecting the diplomatic isolation of both countries.[7] By 1990, at its peak, Isithebe Industrial Park was the most successful of the more than forty industrial decentralization areas in the country, employing approximately 23,000 workers, around half women, in more than 180 plants.[8]

Some economists argued at the time that the decentralization of South African industry was driven not only by the state's generous subsidies but also by capital's wish to reduce costs at a time of recession.[9] Certainly, industries' movement to rural areas, where more women than men lived, was consistent with a wider feminization of the workforce. The percentage of industrial

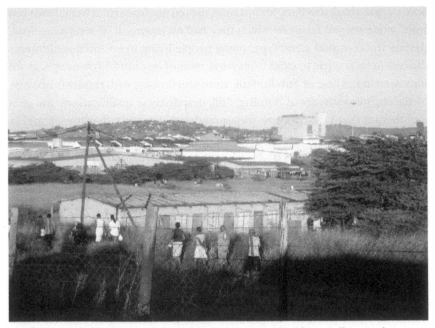

FIGURE 5.1. Isithebe *jondolo* or informal settlement, 2006. Residents walk to work, or to look for work, past a row of twenty-two one-room *imijondolo,* eleven on each side. In the background are a soccer pitch and the factories of Isithebe Industrial Park. Photograph by Mark Hunter.

employees who were African women rose significantly in the post–World War II period: from 1.8 percent in 1946 to 4.1 percent in 1960 and 6.2 percent in 1970.[10] Then a recession hit the country, and the number of black wage-earning women increased by 52 percent between 1973 and 1981: working-class women, sociologist Jacklyn Cock noted, were the "shock absorbers of the current crisis."[11]

In the Mandeni area, industrialization provided particularly secure jobs for white men: many lived in Mandini where they could enjoy a comfortable suburban lifestyle, including a nine-hole golf course. Earning lower wages, some African men who found work at Isithebe moved into Sundumbili township, where they joined SAPPI workers as patrons of four-room family houses. In Isithebe's factories, these men were disproportionately concentrated in the higher-skilled metal industry or worked as supervisors in factories employing mostly women. In contrast, "industrial women" typically toiled for up to twelve hours a day on sewing or textile machines. By the mid-1980s pay in the garment sector was between R18 and R38 a week, about a third of men's average salary.[12]

These conditions grew gradually better as unions gained strength in the 1980s, first within the predominantly male metal sector but by the late 1980s in the garment sector too. Men secured the largest pay raises, organizing under the rallying cry of the right to a "family wage." Some women supported these calls: as wives or potential wives, they still felt that they had a stake, if a floundering and contested one, in defending men's role as breadwinners. One female factory worker told researchers in 1984 that she "can't believe that a man can be paid only R30 a week like women because they know that a man is the breadwinner."[13] On the other hand, many women, like Dudu, had an independent and sometimes militant outlook; her mother's life was proof of the unreliability of men and the relative economic autonomy possible without a husband.

The independent spirit of some early industrial women was described by a social worker interviewed in 1984: "But now, a lot of women are choosing not to get married because they cease to be themselves once they are married. You just become something that doesn't exist. You have no opinions of your own."[14] Women's economic autonomy, and the need for solidarity to challenge white privilege on the shop floor and in society more generally, encouraged many to join unions. As Dudu told me, "Around 1985, an organizer [a man] came from Empangeni and told us that the whites were playing with us. We went to APEX [a large metal firm that was unionized by that time] and made a union committee. We were told how to make a union and be a comrade."

The making of Isithebe Jondolo Settlement

> Q. [to a member of the Skwatta Kamp hip hop band]:
> Where did the name "Skwatta Kamp" come from?
>
> Sello [band member]: We sort of compared ourselves with the people who come from the informal settlements—in the music industry hip hop is kinda looked at from a rather low angle. So we took our situation and we compared it to the people of the squatter camps and thought, OK . . . they are also looked at as a kinda nuisance, you know, put on the outskirts of the towns and nobody cares about them. So we felt we were on that type of trip as well so that's how the name came about.[15]

A few young residents of Isithebe jondolo settlement today call the area a *skwatta kamp*, a phrase made popular by the contemporary South African hip hop band of that name. Yet, unlike many informal settlements in large towns, Isithebe jondolo settlement has never had a squatter population, people who neither own land nor pay rent. The main reason for this is that the settlement grew on KwaZulu land that was under the authority of an inkosi (chief) and therefore had long-established land-use patterns. As factories grew in number in the 1970s, it was longstanding residents who began to "sell" land to workers like Dudu who needed a place to stay. While the chief told outsiders that no payment was given to him when land changed hands, residents are adamant that both the chief and izinduna (the chief's officials) took a cut from each transaction.[16] By the early 1980s, many longstanding residents (izakhamizi) had begun to divide and sell their land, and migrants typically built structures with several rooms on these plots.

It was in the late 1980s and 1990s, as the population mushroomed, that most of the thousands of rented one-room imijondolo that now define the informal settlement were constructed. They were built and rented out primarily by the families that had lived there for many years and those who had, in turn, bought smaller plots from this group (these people could also come to be called izakhamizi over time). The family with whom I stayed were members of this latter group; they had fled to Mandeni in the 1980s to escape IFP-ANC violence in a notoriously tense part of KwaZulu. The male household head bought a plot of land from an isakhamuzi at a relatively cheap price and eventually built about fifty imijondolo, a shop, and his own family's house.

The "selling" of land wedded together inkosi, izinduna, izakhamizi, and tenants in quite robust ways.[17] While I have heard of occasions when residents contested land boundaries and even resorted to threats of violence, on the whole land disputes were minimal.

Local chiefs, however, faced a particular—but not irreconcilable—dilemma in land sales. On the one hand, every sale eroded chiefs' control over their only real social asset—land. But chiefs have long been aware of the money economy's ability to buttress their "traditional" authority. Hence, in the 1970s, when Mcatshangelwa Mathonsi agreed to allow a portion of Isithebe to be used for the industrial park, the government gave the tribal authority a *bakkie* (pickup truck) and, to sway the general population, promised the tribal authority a new school (which was named Tshwana, after the chief).[18] Two decades later—now well into the industrial era—Mcatshangelwa's grandson used gifts gained from land sales to promote his economic status and therefore retain authority in the area.

The explosion of imijondolo in Isithebe from the 1980s, while certainly facilitated by the area's distance from a large white population, was consistent with the expansion of informal settlements across South Africa at this time. Present-day KwaZulu-Natal became particularly well known for its large number of imijondolo, many of which were already appearing in the late 1970s. Patterns of land allocation stemming from the colonial period meant that KwaZulu was the most fragmented of all the homelands.[19] And the rural fingers of the KwaZulu homeland extended deep into the areas surrounding central Durban. Consequently, many shacks were located on peri-urban land controlled by chiefs.[20] A contrasting pattern was illegal squatting on government or privately owned land; this model was evident in KwaZulu-Natal but became the typical means by which shacks grew in other provinces.

A pivotal moment in the growth of shacks, especially in South Africa's large towns, came in 1986. At that time, after a series of failed urban reforms, the state scrapped the hated pass laws that prevented most Africans from living in urban areas.[21] "Not content to wait for the millennium," Mabin wrote, capturing the flavor of growing shack dwellings in South Africa in 1989, "the inhabitants of the Bantustans and evictees from the farms built new informal 'urban' environments which gave them as much access to the benefits of an urban life as they could achieve."[22] By 1995 nearly 18 percent of KwaZulu-Natal's population eked out a living in these informal settlements.[23] And these growing informal settlements were, as the Skwatta Kamp member said, home to a marginalized class who lived near cities but in the most makeshift accommodation and sought work just at the time when the country witnessed a massive increase in unemployment. The entry of thousands of unemployed people from surrounding countries into South Africa, especially after 1994, fueled further shack growth.

Yet just as shacks came to house thousands of poor urban dwellers, expanding supermarket chains weakened the profitability of trading, the bulwark of the informal sector for women. Located north of SAPPI, Renckens, a family-run shop, took advantage of the explosion of the industrial population in the 1980s and became the biggest franchise of the SPAR grocery store chain in Africa. Renckens managers I spoke with put the company's success down to its Scandinavian missionary roots that gave it an intimate knowledge of local tastes: it concentrated on selling cheap and popular staple foods in a warehouse-like store (oil, rice, flour, corn meal, sugar beans, and sugar). But the company's achievements also reflected racialized biases in state support of businesses, not least of which was the restriction of Indian traders, who had long sold household goods, to land south of the Thukela River.

This circumstance of a rising number of shacks and growing social differentiation can be visualized in Isithebe through a mapping exercise I carried out in 2006 with the help of an Isithebe resident (see figure 5.2). Using his discussions with elderly residents, we reconstructed the boundaries of the izakhamizi's *imizi* (homesteads) before land began to be widely sold; each one would have consisted of several huts and an isibaya (cattle kraal). Figure 5.2 illustrates the old boundaries of imizi (in roughly the 1970s) and the present-day boundaries of the plots bought by people like Dudu in the 1980s. These new owners, in turn, built thousands of imijondolo for rent mostly to migrants. At the apex of the social scale are the original residents; in the middle are owners of subdivided plots, who tend to have bought their land in the 1980s; and at the bottom are the tenants of imijondolo who moved into the area from the 1980s onward.

The Changing Political Economy and Geography of Intimacy

I use the term "changing political economy and geography of intimacy" to refer to a group of interconnected trends, including rising unemployment and social inequality, diminishing marriage rates, and increasing female mobility. These trends, embodied in attitudes, institutions, and habits, and especially manifest from the 1980s, rest on both sharp changes and historical continuities. Dudu's story speaks directly to this point. When Dudu moved to Mandeni in the early 1970s, she was one of a minority of women who left the rural areas of the KwaZulu homeland. As well as being constrained by apartheid-related restrictions on movement, most women still had a strong, if waning, commitment to rural areas.

Yet more and more women like Dudu moved to urban areas over time. And women's greater economic independence overlapped with, and helped to produce, changing meanings of "work." As outlined earlier, rural men tended to be attracted to women who were khuthele (diligent); at the core of the concept of diligence was women's ability to nurture children and help build a rural umuzi. But another vision of diligence appeared in interviews I conducted with migrant women like Dudu, one that emphasized the ability to survive independently. And the bodily practices that signified a good, self-sufficient woman were resourcefulness and independence, in contrast to the deference and inhlonipho (respect) expected of a rural wife.

What gave added force to these shifts was the rapid rise in unemployment from the mid-1970s that birthed a new class of rural-born men who had never been formally employed. Men's growing unemployment—from the perspective of women, their increasing unreliability—yielded a greater expectation that a rural woman should migrate and seek work. Isithebe holds a rather

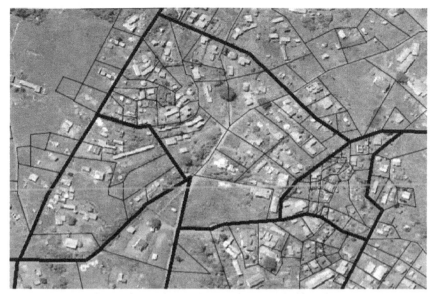

FIGURE 5.2. Boundaries of *imizi* (home plots) in the 1970s (bold) and in 2006 (light). By 2006 most plots had been subdivided and portions sold. By this time, thousands of residents lived in rented *imijondolo*, the rectangular buildings identifiable in the photo.

exceptional place in this overall story because, hosting more than 180 factories, it served as a powerful magnet to pull women from northern KwaZulu-Natal into industrial work in the 1980s.[24] In larger towns formal work opportunities were harder to find and residents of shacks could maintain weaker links to the more distant rural hinterland. But what is vital to grasp is that by the 1980s women born in rural areas had a vastly reduced expectation that they would marry, and virtually no belief that rural areas could provide them with a meaningful life-path. Three spheres—marriage, mobility, and intimacy—became interconnected in important ways.

DECLINING MARRIAGE RATES

Although data are far from perfect, it is clear that marriage rates in South Africa plummeted from the 1960s. In 1951, census data showed that 54 percent of Africans over the age of fifteen were married; in 1960, 57 percent; in 1970, 49 percent; in 1980, 42 percent; in 1991, 38 percent; and in 2001, only 30 percent.[25] This is a staggering reduction, among the sharpest for any country for which I have seen figures. It is reflected today in the virtual absence of weddings on weekends in Mandeni, in contrast to the steady flow of AIDS-related funerals. Study after study today reveals extremely low marriage rates among Africans.[26]

Why did marriage rates drop so starkly? The initial decline from the 1960s can be largely attributed to three forces: domestic instability caused by male migrant labor, women's increased work prospects, and the growing economic failure of rural areas. Particularly from the late 1970s, however, when unemployment rose sharply, men's inability to pay ilobolo and become dependable "providers" also became a factor. And falling marriage rates and women's growing mobility became mutually reinforcing trends: why would women stay in a languishing rural area when their chances of finding a man to marry and support them were so obviously diminishing? Better, some thought, to join women like Dudu in informal settlements known for allowing cohabiting relations.

MOBILE WOMEN:
FROM MIGRANT MEN TO MOVING WOMEN

In the mid-twentieth century, rural areas were predominantly occupied by children, women of all ages, and older men. There were always women who moved to urban areas, of course, but these were a minority. The classic pattern of STI infection was a man moving to an urban area, becoming infected there, and returning to infect his wife. Today, in contrast, it is often a rural-based woman who can infect her partner with HIV.[27] And, signaling equally dramatic shifts, almost as many men as women now live in rural areas: only 5 percent more women than men reside in rural Hlabisa, an area 120 kilometers northeast of Mandeni where I conducted research.[28]

The contours of this shift are difficult to capture through most migration statistics. Census data show a rise in women's migration from the 1970s but indicate that men still migrate more often than women.[29] More recent household survey data, however, reveals significant recent increases in women's movement and provides possible reasons for this trend. Showing the importance of marital status to movement, Dorrit Posel was able to determine that considerably more female migrants were unmarried than married.[30] The presence of an employed man in a household also deterred migration. These findings support the view that women's migration is connected to declines in marriage and the spatial reorganization of households.

More intensively researched but geographically smaller demographic studies provide important additional details. The Africa Centre for Population and Health Studies, based in rural Hlabisa, visits each household twice a year in a geographical site it calls the Demographic Surveillance Area (DSA). It is

therefore able to document in some detail the lives of the area's 85,000 inhabitants and better able than census data to capture shorter-term movement.

I use here the term "movement" to emphasize that women's changes
in geographical location are often quite different from men's. The classic
"migration" pattern is men's spending long periods in distant mines; that
national statistics best capture this trend reflects their gender bias. Rural-born
women today, however, tend to move shorter distances for shorter periods—
especially women who leave children in rural areas, who return for visits more
frequently than men. Able to record these patterns, the Africa Centre found
that gross movement rates (in- and out-migration taken together) were nearly
the same for women as for men.[31] Put simply—and signaling a quite dramatic
social transformation over the latter parts of the twentieth century—a gender-
sensitive account of movement shows that rural women are now moving as
much as men.

LOOKING BACK FROM RURAL KWAZULU-NATAL

By now it is clear that Mandeni must be understood through its connections to other places, and foremost among these is rural KwaZulu-Natal.
Affiliated with the Africa Centre in Mtubatuba, Thembeka Mngomezulu and
I probed these links by visiting twenty-eight rural homesteads in the Hlabisa
district of KwaZulu-Natal in late 2003; I stayed with a rural-based family while
conducting this research.[32] A chance encounter during our travel around the
area gave a sense of some of the meanings ascribed to rural-urban movements.
I was with two employees of the Africa Centre. Slightly lost, we stopped at
a rural school to ask for directions and began chatting with the teachers, all
women, who wanted to know about my study; in turn I used the opportunity
to ask about the movement of people between this rural area and Mandeni.
The conversation, undertaken in isiZulu, went like this:

> MH: Why do women leave here and go to Mandeni?
>
> INT: They want the fat of men [*Bafuna amafutha amadoda*].
>
> [*Great laughter.*]
>
> MH: What is the fat of men?
>
> INT: Sperms [*Amasperms;* the plural prefix *ama* is often used when
> mixing English with Zulu].
>
> [*Laughter.*]
>
> MH: There are no sperms here?
>
> INT: There is no work, there is no money.

The metaphor of men being without sperm illustrates graphically how unemployment undermined rural men's role as breadwinners, and thereby the basis for their provider masculinity. The very make-up of rural households today reveals fundamental challenges to men's authority. Strikingly, most rural households no longer revolve around a male umnumzana (head of household): the majority we visited were three- or four-generation households where most family members, especially younger ones, were unmarried. In effect, this meant that *ogogo* (grannies) or *omkhulu* (granddads) lived with their adult children, grandchildren, and even great-grandchildren. This household structure suggests that only a minority of the generation coming of age in the 1980s married, formed their own households, and then took in the elderly; in fact, a granny's pension (women typically live longer than men) often replaced a migrant man's salary as a dependable source of income around which a household became organized.

Interviews we conducted in rural Hlabisa supported my findings in Mandeni that marriage was an institution for the better off: of the few families we visited where a recent marriage had been reported, all were comparatively wealthy. Approaching one such rural umuzi, we were struck by its neat wire fencing. We entered through a brightly painted gate to find a large round hut and, to its side, four square ones of various sizes; the *igceke* (courtyard) was neat and well swept. This house's wealth came from the earnings of a man who had recently died; he had been in his sixties. Thulile had worked in Durban for Spoornet, South Africa's rail operator, for many years. Until recently the household had consisted of this umnumzana, his wife, his daughter, his two sons and their wives, and fourteen grandchildren. At one point Thulile was said to have owned around sixty cattle; he gave some of these to his sons to enable them to marry.

This senior man's provision of ilobolo cattle demands discussion. At first glance, it echoes the situation before migrant labor, when a father financed his son's marriage. But the dynamic process of building an umuzi was stunted: the father had ensured that his sons could marry, but these young men were not working and had been unable to accumulate cash or cattle in order to move out of their father's home and build their own.

Households therefore became dramatically altered by the reduction in marriage and the waning of the male-provider model. Marriage revealed itself, in the eyes of many women especially, to be a rather rigid and undesirable institution. What emerged was a shift toward more flexible intimate alliances and geographies spanning multiple connected households. One of the best examples of this is households run by siblings rather than a married couple, such as those Isak Niehaus described in 1994.[33]

Over the 1990s, the need for more flexible forms of cooperation within and between households increased even further as unemployment continued to rise. In another Hlabisa household we visited, Gezekile, then fifty-two, had separated several decades ago from her husband and returned to live with her widowed mother. In the early 1980s, she found work in one of Isithebe's clothing factories and used the money to support the rural household while the eldest daughter looked after her young siblings. Then Gezekile's son, Dumisani, was fortunate enough to find work in Mandeni and left his children in the family umuzi. By 2003 her younger daughter was looking for work in Mandeni while her mother stayed in Hlabisa, looking after her and her brother's young children.

This household therefore tells a story of ongoing cooperation between mother, son, and daughter and continuous but varied movement between rural Hlabisa and Mandeni. The valuable point that Niehaus made is that this type of cooperation and flexibility would be harder if a man headed the umuzi (that is, if the umuzi had an umnumzana, a male head of household). Among the poorest South Africans especially, wedlock became exposed as a decidedly inflexible institution through which to organize social alliances and the flow of resources. Gezekile was, in fact, deeply suspicious of men: "If you get a man he will want to eat your money and you will end up not giving your children anything."

As young men failed to work and marry, yawning new gaps between employed and unemployed men reconfigured intimate relations in rural areas.[34] One consequence was that migrant men could distribute their wages through sexual networks, such as by returning to a rural area and entering into a relationship with a woman, perhaps even a married woman.[35] These gaps between men's ability to attract women were not unprecedented, as we have seen, but became more pronounced in circumstances where a smaller number of men had access to disposable incomes.

Just as significant for the future, however, were sexual relations in the absence of (rather than simply outside of) marital relations. Let me illustrate this point further through the case of Fikile. Twenty-six at the time she gave this account, Fikile had grown up in northern KwaZulu-Natal, not far from Hlabisa. After moving to Isithebe she could only find work washing and ironing one day a week, for R50. Two employed boyfriends provided her with support. Her main boyfriend gave her food and money, some of which she sent home. The other, an *umakhwapheni* (secret lover, literally "under the armpit"), gave her R50 or R100 irregularly. Her main boyfriend, she said, did not want to use condoms, and she said that she trusted him but used condoms with the other.

Fikile's story bears similarities to those of many women in the early twentieth century who moved from rural to urban areas. But it differs from older accounts because she maintains strong links with her rural home. Also, she was expected to migrate rather than waiting to marry. Showing how women's movements can now, like men's, link rural and urban areas through intimate relationships, Fikile said that she also slept with a boyfriend from her rural home. They didn't use condoms, she said, because he claimed to be *indoda yami ngempela ngempela* (my man, for real, for real).

Imijondolo Meanings: Cohabitation and Partial Independence

As a result of these transformations, today many people's geographical experience of everyday life is not a family homestead but unmarried life in an umjondolo. What meanings are caught up with this geography? Imijondolo are testimony, on the one hand, to the growth, from the 1980s, of a generally marginalized population who found steady work and formal housing difficult to secure. But, importantly, they are also a geographical manifestation of a set of deeply gendered processes of movement and migration. In 2001, more than 54 percent of Isithebe's residents were women, a figure that would be higher were it not for the large number of AIDS deaths among women and if we were able to distinguish people living in imijondolo from those living in other types of homes on the rural land surveyed in the census.[36] The gendering of informal settlements, however, involves much more than simply numbers; indeed, many men do live in informal settlements. One reason why these spaces are profoundly gendered is that most residents live outside of marriage or a family home.

The very word "umjondolo" indicates the ambiguous social position of the unmarried women who often live in these structures. Although the etymology of the word is unclear, it appears to have been coined around the 1970s.[37] Several informants told me that it may have been derived from the word *umjendevu*, an old spinster; others with whom I spoke acknowledged that this sounded possible. One sixty-year-old man explained to me that an unmarried woman, an umjendevu, had "expired," just like the temporary building materials used to construct imijondolo.[38] Although we cannot be certain of the word's origin, this explanation captures the way unmarried women living in imijondolo were perceived as engaging in a form of gendered transgression because they were not living with a male guardian, be it a father or a husband. This was certainly the feeling in the 1940s, before apartheid removals, when thousands of women lived in urban shacks—and yet the sheer numbers of imijondolo from the 1980s gave them a new pertinence.

Most imijondolo in Isithebe are rented, and this is not uncommon on former KwaZulu rural land where homestead boundaries prevail. Thousands of other imijondolo, however, are located on government-owned land, and these are more likely to house "squatters." One such shack settlement in which I conducted research during 2009 was situated next to a railway station in south Durban. Here, the imijondolo were nestled in a dense forest area bordering a former white suburb. They were constructed from wood planks, plywood, plastic, tarpaulins, and reeds, all materials collected free in the area. Residents had previously been living in a diverse group of places: rural areas, hostels, other shack settlements that had been destroyed by the government, and townships (where the monthly rent for an umjondolo adjacent to a family home could be R400). Most residents sold scrap metal or sought temporary work in nearby factories or *ejalidini*, suburban homes. The gendered nature of informal settlements was evident in this place's very name, *Emantombazaneni* (Place of Women). Indeed, instead of referring to the area's founding fathers, figures that loom large in townships, the name commemorated its first settlers, five women.

Imijondolo, however, imply not only gendered but generational transgression. One of the first words Dudu used in describing Isithebe to me was "ukukipita" (to cohabit); she uttered it in a kind of mischievous tone, telling me it was against amasiko (traditions). "Ukukipita" and similar terms, such as *ukuhlalisana* (to stay together), have long been used in South Africa's towns to describe cohabitation. The subtly derogatory connotations of all these words result from the fact that men and women are said to be rebelling against kin and traditions by not marrying. Some residents say that this rebellion brings bad luck, because it upsets the amadlozi (ancestors), the spirits of the dead who reside in a family imizi.

Yet the changes in household structure marked by imijondolo must be thought of not simply as a "breakdown of marriage" but as a reconfiguration of material resources, emotions, and geographies. Signs of quite positive meanings appeared one warm summer night during my stay in Isithebe. I was dozing in my umjondolo, exhausted after a day of interviews, and noticed that the music playing outside was quite different from the usual tunes I heard from the Ukhozi FM isiZulu radio station. It was ballroom music. Curious, I walked out of my umjondolo and saw unmarried women and men locked together in intricate dance moves in the moonlight. South African urbanites have long engaged in ballroom dancing, but such public expressions of intimacy would not have been tolerated in most of the rural areas whence migrants hailed. To this day, men and women in rural areas are usually not able to cohabit without the man paying at least some ilobolo (bridewealth). In contrast, at Isithebe, while the threat of violence restricts women's (and, to a lesser extent, men's) movements at night, the appearance of a group of "industrial women" living in imijondolo in the 1980s helped to give new meaning to these spaces.

That meanings are not fixed and are deeply gendered can be seen in an ongoing debate in Isithebe about whether I lived in an umjondolo. My one-room structure, slightly to the side of my host family's main house, was identical to many imijondolo typically built in long rows (and dubbed by residents *isitimela*, "train"). Each measured around 10 X 15 ft (3 X 4.5 m), was built of 150 X 450 mm M150 hollow concrete blocks, and had a corrugated iron roof and a single door and window. A few residents (and often the landlords) called these structures not imijondolo but *amakotishi* (cottages) to differentiate them from the less-desired mud, wood, and stone structures that are also rented in the area. Another reason why the term "umjondolo" might be regarded as inappropriate in my case was that the structure was situated within the umuzi (homestead or property) of the family with which I was staying. This meant it could also be positioned as an indlu (house), drawing on the image of a rural umuzi (homestead) that could contain several izindlu (houses). Hence, new acquaintances often asked, *Uyaqasha?* (Are you renting?), trying to get a better sense of my arrangements. If I was renting, I was living in an umjondolo; but if I was staying with the family, I was living in an indlu constructed like an umjondolo.

Who owns an imijondolo, where it is located, and how it is constructed are thus the structure's most important defining features. In Isithebe, the cheapest imijondolo for rent are made from mud, sticks, stones, and paper and are sometimes called imikhukhu, meaning flimsy shacks. These are the most fragile structures in the area: water perpetually leaks through their walls and ceilings, they are very vulnerable to break-ins, and a strong storm can completely destroy them. The solid concrete-block structures therefore have considerable advantages, reducing the chances of rain or wind damage and deterring break-ins—but they have their own cost. The outside air cools in the late afternoon, but the hollow blocks retain the day's warmth and radiate it until the early hours of the morning. I awoke many nights saturated in sweat in what seemed like a slow-cooking oven.

And water always seemed to come in extremes in Isithebe, especially in the summer: if the settlement wasn't knee deep in mud, there was a shortage. In the hot months from November to March, the draining heat was temporarily disrupted only when the prevailing northeast wind switched to a cold southwest one on the arrival of a cold front. Within minutes, the settlement reverberated with the sound of doors slamming and residents rushing to collect washing from the line. Downpours could quickly flood the settlement. Yet clean water was in frustratingly limited supply, making cooking and bathing difficult. Residents (including myself) regularly got boils, skin infections that start as lumps under the skin and then erupt into a painful bloody mess.

The English words for imijondolo areas are no less contentious than the isiZulu ones. "Informal settlement" is a problematic term but one that I ultimately decided to use in this book to describe densely populated areas with informal housing and minimal services. The term became increasingly used in the 1980s as the state reformed urban apartheid and sought to differentiate between tolerated "informal settlements" and undesirable "squatter" settlements, which were to be removed.[39] Today, this term is favored by planners and, while it has a depoliticizing and homogenizing tone, residents of "informal settlements" do describe these areas as being without piped water, tarred roads, flush toilets, and other services found in "formal" settlements. Another common term is "shack settlement," but the problem with using this for Isithebe is that the area does not contain simply "shacks"; as I have described, imijondolo can also be sturdy concrete-block buildings. Finally, as we shall see later, the post-apartheid state's return to the language of "slums" to justify removing urban shacks is a vivid sign of how racialized labels can be employed in the name of "development."

A key tenet of urban apartheid was the violent destruction of informal settlements. As the political cracks in apartheid grew wider in the 1970s and 1980s, shacks reappeared. In Isithebe, the rhythm of the jondolo settlement's development was slightly different—it was a homeland area and not a large "white" city, and generous state incentives artificially promoted local industry and rapid population growth. African people, including women, could move here freely and settle, whereas they could not live legally in white South Africa until the collapse of influx controls in 1986.

But Isithebe serves as a very good illustration of a major theme of this chapter: that rising numbers of imijondolo are not only a sign of the shortage of urban housing but a geographical manifestation of unraveling gender dynamics. At the beginning of the century, only a relatively small number of women moved to urban shacks. From the 1980s, however, marriage itself was uncommon for all but the better off. Imijondolo, despite their poor construction, provided some kind of alternative to rural life.

The rise of imijondolo had important implications for the gendered nature of apartheid. Unemployment reduced the male umnumzana's authority, and it did so as women forged alternatives in the form of imijondolo and, in the case of women like Dudu, even accessed forms of informal housing akin to houses. We should not, therefore, look back with nostalgia at the period when abanumzana ruled households. Nor, in turn, should we see the recent period as one of "marital breakdown." Rather, in it women themselves have charted alternatives to the male-led home. As the next chapter shows, when women's unemployment rose in Isithebe, this alternative to the male provider model based on women's economic independence became increasingly unfeasible.

PART 2

Intimacy after
Democracy, 1994–

SIX

Postcolonial Geographies:
Being "Left Behind" in the New South Africa

In the last chapter we met Dudu, an "industrial woman" who found employment as a garment worker in Isithebe's factories in the 1970s. With a regular income, however small, women like Dudu often shunned marriage to men—who, in turn, had become progressively less able to afford it. Yet in the 1990s, despite the joy of being able to vote for the first time in her life, Dudu faced declining personal, economic, and health fortunes, and her troubles were representative of the harsher circumstances women in the jondolo settlement faced.

In 1999, Jonathan, Dudu's longstanding boyfriend who lived in her two-room home, was laid off from a large metal-industry firm. He cut a sad picture of an unemployed man battered by his inability to work. As is common with alcoholics, it was impossible to determine when he was drunk: his eyes were always bloodshot, his speech slurred, and his stare never fully engaged. Jonathan died in 2004.

In April 2006 I returned after a year away to find that Dudu herself had passed away and their son, in his early teens, was living alone. As was common in the area, rumors of AIDS followed the death of two lovers one after another.

The last years of Dudu's life were spent complaining bitterly about "factories leaving the area," her perception of abandonment occasioned by the closure of some of Isithebe Industrial Park's firms. But Dudu fared better than most local women. Clothing factories often employed her for brief stints in preference to newer arrivals because of her long experience working with industrial sewing machines. Owning her own plot meant that Dudu didn't pay rent, and she also made some extra money through running a shebeen (an informal tavern in a home). Especially when she was not working in a factory, she could often be seen rolling a beer-filled wheelbarrow through the jondolo settlement.

In contrast, newer migrants to Isithebe found it more difficult to find work and were forced to come up with rent payments for imijondolo. Yet, notably, this younger generation also arrived with high hopes of surpassing the social position of women like Dudu. Most, after all, had more years of schooling than she did, and had been young when apartheid was abolished.

This dream of a better life was perhaps even stronger in the formally built Sundumbili township, several miles away. The younger generation wanted to surpass the steady paternalism that characterized their parents' generation: an era when four-room "matchbox" houses were the best available housing and their price was racial humiliation in the workplace and society at large. Young people had gained their rights, and now was the time to reap the benefits.

In this chapter I sketch out how the social and geographical contours of South Africa were modified, but not fundamentally redrawn, after democratic elections in 1994. Areas denoted as black under apartheid remained sites of the most extreme poverty. As both a cause and a consequence of this, social mobility typically required a new form of geographical mobility: a move out of a poor area to a richer one. Yet, in tension with these new geographies of inequality, the onset of democracy brought with it powerful new ideas of citizenship and rights for all.

Political Freedom in the Era of Unemployment

The 1980s was a decade of intense anti-apartheid struggles and brutal state oppression. Full-scale civil war seemed imminent. Then, somewhat unexpectedly, in February 1990 President F. W. De Klerk released Nelson Mandela and other political prisoners and unbanned the ANC. Massive pressure exerted from inside and outside the country had produced the beginning of the end of apartheid.

With democracy in sight, the ANC and its allies in the unions and civil society got to work drafting the Reconstruction and Development Programme (RDP), an ambitious plan to reduce poverty, improve housing, and create jobs. But this emphasis on promoting growth through redistribution did not last. By the time the ANC was elected in 1994, with a 66 percent majority, it was already watering down its commitment to social equality. One early casualty was job creation: the ANC effectively sidelined a 1993 Keynesian macroeconomic plan produced by its ally MERG (the Macroeconomic Research Group).[1]

The reasons for the ANC's rejection of a more radical economic strategy are disputed.[2] Communism's collapse in the Soviet Union ended the party's patron-client relationship with this formerly mighty power; this was undoubtedly a paramount factor. So too were deep divisions within the ANC. The redistributive RDP, drafted by activists, reflected only one side of the ANC's thinking: throughout the 1980s the exiled Thabo Mbeki had championed talks with big business that centered on preserving a market economy while installing democracy.

Yet, whatever the reasons, the ANC's embrace of the market strengthened even further in the early years of democracy. In 1996, amid rumors of Mandela's ill health, the currency plummeted and, wishing to placate the markets and attract foreign investors, the ANC quickly rolled out a policy called GEAR (Growth, Employment and Redistribution). This broadly neo-liberal macro-economic plan promoted foreign investment, export-oriented growth, fiscal discipline, and privatization. COSATU, the main trade union federation, and the South African Communist Party threatened to abandon their alliance with the ANC, but GEAR remained in place.[3]

The foreign investment on which the ANC pinned its hopes largely failed to arrive. It was only in the 2000s, as the strategy's inability to address poverty became ever more apparent, that the ANC reintroduced the language of the "developmental state."[4] Jacob Zuma's ousting of Mbeki from the helm of the ANC in December 2007 and his election as president of the country in 2009 seemed to take this impulse further—although it is unclear how it will materialize in major policy changes, especially in the midst of a global recession.

In business circles, the ANC's economic record was largely celebrated as a success. Economic growth rose steadily, inflation came under control, and the currency maintained some stability, at least before the 2008 financial crisis pushed the country into recession.[5] However, unemployment continued its painful rise from the late 1970s. The 2003 United Nations Development Programme report painted a depressing picture: the Human Development Index for South Africa declined from 0.72 in 1990 to 0.67 in 2003.[6]

One especial point of controversy was trade liberalization that exposed South Africa's inward-looking economy to furious competition. The new government, keen to establish its credibility as a supporter of free-market "globalization," went even further than World Trade Organization rules demanded, swiftly lifting trade tariffs to reduce local industry's protection. To cut costs and evade new labor regulations in this more competitive environment, employers casualized labor, especially through subcontracting out key parts of their businesses.[7]

A sphere that did attract sustained government spending was social payments for the poor. In truth, this was more by accident than by design; the means-tested payments were a way to address the failure of the growth strategy to create jobs rather than a planned intervention. Payments had been made to more than a quarter of the South African population by 2007, and more women had received them than men.[8] The state pension was significantly increased, and a child support grant was introduced that at first subsidized children under seven years old and was later extended to children under fifteen years old.[9] By 2009, a child's guardian was eligible to a R240 (US$30) monthly grant, and pensioners saw their payments rise to R1,010 (US$125).[10] This weak form of social citizenship became vital in ensuring the ANC's continued support at the ballot box despite rising unemployment, and indeed the ANC achieved impressive national election victories in 1999, 2004, and 2009.

The new government pointed to these social grants and to programs of house building, electrification, and water provision as evidence of its "delivery"; others noted that fiscal constraints limited these programs.[11] On both sides, however, "development" became largely measured by discrete programmatic interventions.[12] Of course, programs have an ability to alter the race, class, and gender inequalities in society. Yet the deep-seated structural shifts that I have noted—rising unemployment and inequality, greater population movement, and falling marriage rates—continued unabated in the post-apartheid period.

One dramatic sign of women's increased movement, especially from rural areas, is their growing participation in the labor force (i.e., seeking work as well as performing both formal and informal labor). Between 1995 and 2005, the number of women in the labor force increased by 59 percent, whereas for men the increase was 35 percent; much of this growth was both a cause and a consequence of a ballooning informal sector. More women than men found formal employment during this period, and new labor legislation helped to increase women's average wages more than men's.[13] Yet a saturated informal sector offered very low remuneration for hundreds of thousands of other women.[14] Moreover, the sheer number of women entering the labor force increased female unemployment in the first ten years of democracy, from 40 percent to 47 percent, while male unemployment rose from 24 percent to 31 percent.[15]

Another shocking trend in the democratic era was the rapid increase in unemployment among young people: from 1995 to 2005 unemployment rose among 15–24-year-old women by 12 percentage points, to 72 percent, and among men of the same age by 11 percentage points, to 58 percent.[16] Thousands of young people failed to find work and remained dependent on others, including kin—and, as we shall see later, lovers. More widely, while the increase in the state pension and the introduction of the child support grant provided some important new stability to households, other ongoing processes linked to the employment crisis made households more precarious. The thousands of AIDS deaths also occasioned enormous economic stress on families who had to pay for expensive burials and meet new dependents' needs.[17]

By 2000, Habib and Padayachee were arguing that "the ANC's implementation of neo-liberal economic policies has meant disaster for the vast majority of South Africa's poor."[18] A group largely cut off from formal employment opportunities became consolidated in the dying days of apartheid, and their poverty was accentuated after 1994.[19] At the same time, stark new riches became apparent in the country: in 2005 South Africa had the fourth biggest jump in the number of dollar millionaires of any country in the world.[20] The most successful beneficiaries of Black Economic Empowerment (BEE) were "comrades in business," a small but high-profile group with close links to the ANC.[21] More inclusively, by 2007 Black South Africans came to fill around a third of professional and middle-management positions.[22] As a result, some young black South Africans could for the first time hope to get a good education, a white-collar job, and eventually a senior management position, a life path that had been open to middle-class whites for years.

Postcolonial Geographies: Social Reproduction on a Shoestring

Confining the black majority to poverty-stricken places, the apartheid era violently brought together race, class, and space in profound—if never completely impenetrable—ways. Seeking to reform this racial geography, legislators after 1994 redrew political boundaries at the provincial and municipal levels to enable cross-subsidies from richer (formerly white) to poorer (formerly black) areas. To address racist land laws that had granted Africans only 13 percent of the land, the state embarked on land reform and restitution programs, if at a painfully slow pace.

Yet it was market forces that occasioned some of the most spectacular reforms to apartheid's geography, most notably in residential patterns. Middle-class Africans, Indians, and coloureds were quick to move out of apartheid-designated spaces in search of better schools and a safer environment. This reversed the "class compression" engendered by apartheid.[23] Today, former white suburbs are home to a multi-racial middle class, and former coloured and Indian areas now host some Africans. However, although most African townships have growing middle-class sections, they remain, like informal settlements and rural areas, populated almost entirely by Africans.[24]

One spatial strategy that did attract considerable government attention was housing. The ANC made it clear that building thousands of low-cost houses would be a key priority, and this commitment is reflected in the colloquialism "RDP houses," named after the ANC's flagship Reconstruction and Development Programme. Driving through South Africa today, one cannot fail to be struck by the new housing developments scattered across the country.

However, with few exceptions, housing projects worked through apartheid's geography rather than providing a basis for its transformation. In the apartheid era, townships for Africans were usually built long distances from central urban areas, cementing the tie between racial and spatial inequality. Today, the market mechanism for delivering RDP houses means that many are also built on the outskirts of towns, where land is cheaper—a new house, yes, but extremely poor access to the urban labor market.[25] "There has been no attempt to intersperse them in the former white areas," says Cosmas Desmond. "This means apartheid has not died: it has had a makeover and bought some new clothes."[26]

Revealing too is the fact that housing policy lacked any coherent gender strategy. If apartheid's modernist housing rested on the figure of "industrial man," gender rarely received any attention in post-apartheid housing policy, at least until a 2006 government document on the topic.[27] The post-apartheid state's vision of "development" was technocratic and did not aim at integrating the domestic and economic spheres. Symbolic of this, RDP houses are typically two-room residences, unlike the four-room family houses built under apartheid. And whereas the "matchbox" township houses provided a minimum of 51.2 square meters of living space, in an era of fiscal austerity the minimum living space in RDP houses is considerably less, only 30 square meters. Housing policy did benefit more women than men, since single people could acquire an RDP house only if they had dependents, such as children. But this fact, although of great significance, seems almost incidental to policy and is qualified by the fact that many RDP houses are tiny structures built on the outskirts of towns.

Free RDP houses, which were certainly popular among many recipients, were therefore overwhelmingly cast in a technocratic mold. Housing debates concentrated on the number of houses built and the number of shacks destroyed rather than on wider questions of urban inequalities. Tellingly, official language tended to position the shacks of informal settlements as simply a "legacy of apartheid" or a "backlog," not as social geographies driven by dynamic and active processes and inequalities.

Certainly, despite many new housing projects, shacks refused to disappear. From 1994 to 2003 the state funded the building of one million RDP houses, only to see the number of informal/shack dwellings rise by 688,000 from 1996 to 2003.[28] Housing provision accelerated in the 2000s, and by 2007 two million low-cost houses had been built—yet two million households still lived in informal dwellings.[29]

How can informal housing still be so prevalent when the state has built so many houses? And why did the state not link housing, gender, and economic policy more closely with its efforts to stem the AIDS pandemic? If the apartheid state could develop a social engineering program that, however draconian, succeeded in building thousands of homes with a particular model of patriarchy, why could the post-apartheid state not better embrace housing's ability to transform urban poverty, gender, and race and class segregation in more far-reaching ways? The consequences of this failure are not clear, but we can legitimately ask if burgeoning informal settlements would have the country's highest AIDS rates if these policy links had been made.

To better assess the connections between housing and AIDS, we must foreground the gendered social forces driving shack growth. Notwithstanding the housing shortages apartheid bequeathed the democratic state, the persistent growth of shacks must be understood through what I call the changing political economy and geography of intimacy. By this I mean a series of interconnected shifts that include rising unemployment and inequalities, reduced marriage rates, and the greater mobility of women.

Seen through this lens, housing planners are dealing with not a "backlog" but a moving target: households are stretching, splitting, and therefore proliferating. From 1995 to 2002 average household size fell from 4.3 to 3.8 and single-person households rose from 12.6 percent to 21 percent of all households.[30] Put simply, as the state built RDP houses, thousands of new, overwhelmingly poor, households mushroomed—a reality speaking to the dynamic nature of movements, space, and the household. Shacks are not simply a "legacy" to be overcome through technocratic "development."

Of course housing policy, like all spheres of government, is not monolithic, and considerable variation exists between provinces and municipalities. Moreover, national policy makers did shift in 2004 toward recognizing the demands of many shack dwellers that informal settlements be upgraded rather than residents relocated to houses distant from work opportunities.[31] Yet, as we shall see later, in the late 2000s hawks in the KwaZulu-Natal government demanded an aggressive new drive for "slum elimination."

Industrial Decline in Mandeni

With a substantial industrial base and a large shack population, Mandeni experienced these social-spatial changes in a distinct but not exceptional way. We begin with the economic heart of the area, Isithebe Industrial Park. Here,

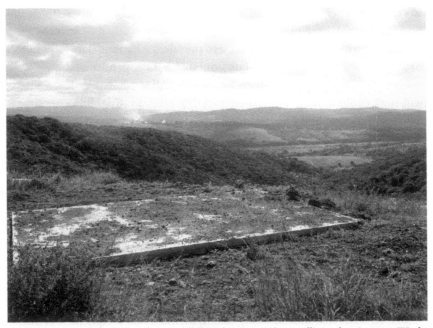

FIGURE 6.1. The foundations for a small RDP house at Hlomendlini, taken in 2006. Work opportunities are distant—across the Thukela River in the background is the fuming SAPPI paper mill. Photograph by Mark Hunter.

business boomed until the early 1990s. At that time, two waves of economic change affected the area. The first was rooted in the general economic malaise that had been felt much earlier elsewhere in South Africa but which Isithebe had been partly spared because of state subsidies for industry. The second was the industrial restructuring caused by post-apartheid trade liberalization.

In the 1990s Isithebe's firms laid off many men. Capital-intensive factories, especially in the prominent metal industry, argued that without government subsidies there was little incentive to remain in the industrial park—1,400 jobs alone were lost at the prominent manufacturer of shipping containers at which Dudu's partner Jonathan had worked. This shrunk the number of "industrial men" in the area. Yet men lucky enough to still be employed had relatively stable pay and solidly unionized workplaces. Moreover, even men who lost their jobs secured comparatively large layoff packages that could be used to start *spazas* (small informal shops) or taxi businesses, or build imijondolo to rent out.

Industrial restructuring in the female-dominated garment industry connected Isithebe to new international nodes of investment and consumption, but in doing so worsened pay and conditions at first. After trade liberalization, South Africa's national clothing retailers greatly increased the proportion of garments they sourced from overseas, especially from China. Consequently, most of the ten or so large unionized South African–owned clothing firms in Isithebe closed or relocated.[32] Women in Isithebe came to depend on the growing number of smaller Taiwanese-owned clothing and textile firms that had begun to invest in the industrial park in the 1980s; these were at first rarely unionized. Although also shaken by rising competition, these firms' longer experience exporting garments meant that they drew immediate benefit from a favorable U.S.-Africa trade agreement reached in 2000.[33] Low wages also increased their profitability: workers in these firms told me in 2000 that some earned as little as R65 per week, although a more common salary was R100. These salaries were less than half those paid by the shrinking number of South African–owned factories that had become unionized in the late 1980s.

Worse still, many new garment factories circumvented labor laws by subcontracting labor out to brokers who employed workers as "individual contractors."[34] I gained a sense of the power of these employers in 2001 when I visited a Taiwanese-owned firm with a union official. The meeting was cordial until the official mentioned new labor laws on minimum wages and the manager said, "Look, if you are going to talk about that I will relocate to Swaziland."

The resulting changes meant that by 2001 total employment in Isithebe Industrial Park was relatively steady at around 15,000, a decline from the peak of 23,000 in 1990 but a much smaller one than most other artificially created industrial parks in "decentralized" areas had seen.[35] The greater proportion of garment manufacturers in the park meant that women came to constitute around 65 percent of the workforce. These figures, however, hide the turmoil (and the sense of factories' abandonment) created by the closure of dozens of unionized South African–owned garment factories and the opening of smaller, non-union Taiwanese ones. And these shifts also increased the gender wage gap. In 2000, when I conducted most of my interviews with workers, men could earn R1,000 a week at one of the remaining metal firms or at the SAPPI paper mill, more than ten times the earnings of some female factory workers.

The bulk of my research was conducted in the first half of the 2000s, but in the second half of the decade the story was slightly different. During this period, wages increased in the garment industry but employment dropped rapidly. Although employers still found ways to evade labor laws, the minimum wage for garment workers rose to almost R400 a week by 2009. Yet, jolted not only by wage increases but by the global recession, many companies shifted production to lower-wage locations, especially Lesotho. Consequently, garment industry employment dropped dramatically, to only around 3,500 workers, less then half the figure in the early 1990s.[36]

Furthermore, women who lost their jobs were often in a perilous economic position. Whereas men who were laid off might receive significant severance payments, women received tiny amounts or nothing at all. And the gendered nature of the informal sector meant that women moved into largely saturated and unprofitable areas—a difficulty seen in women's jostling for position on the sides of roads to sell fruits and vegetables.

In shifting ways, then, global networks of production and state policy reworked gender inequalities in the 1990s and 2000s. Crucially for the sexual economy, as we shall see, a smaller group of men maintained, even enhanced, their superior economic position compared to most women—especially compared to the large number of women who continued to arrive in the area but failed to find work.

In this already economically volatile environment, one might have thought that an AIDS crisis, with roughly half of the workforce likely to be HIV positive, would have further threatened the industrial park's viability. But AIDS was little more than an inconvenient blip on the radar screens of most employers in the area. Especially in low-wage sectors such as clothing, hundreds of people stood at the factory gates ready to replace sick workers; cynically, we might surmise that employers preferred some labor turnover to discourage unionization. Unlike the large unionized factories, such as SAPPI's, that were predominantly staffed by men, garment companies had never had an ideology of paternalism: a worker's health (and other aspects of social reproduction) was her own problem.

Consequently, the main employer-led initiatives against AIDS in the area have come from "high-skill" companies that predominantly employ men. Nationally, a similar picture prevails, with large mining companies investing most heavily in AIDS prevention and treatment. In August 2000, one white manager described to me the blasé attitude of employers toward their overwhelmingly black work forces: "AIDS is not seen as a real business problem like stock flow. Put it this way: it is not something that managers talk about on the golf course."

The incomes of rich and poor moved farther apart, and so did the difference between their working conditions. In 1997 I witnessed the consequences of intensified competition in low-wage sectors. I conducted interviews in a firm in Isithebe that assembled harnesses (bundles of wires) for automotives and employed mostly women. Although the firm had introduced an array of fashionable new "post-Fordist" interventions, such as quality circles and participation schemes, workers complained that increases in productivity had been primarily driven by management taking away their chairs and implementing other speed-up mechanisms. The net effect, workers complained, was that many could not even find time to use the toilet.[37] The conditions in the smaller, less unionized garment factories were by all accounts worse.

Mandeni's Social Geography after Apartheid

As table 6.1 shows, after apartheid there are stark differences in the employment levels, incomes, and marriage rates of the four racial groups. Yet, as revealing as they are, these figures fail to capture growing divisions within racial groups. Understanding both tendencies requires a sense of how geography and power became reconfigured after apartheid.

In the democratic era, Mandeni's residents faced and shaped four principal changes to the area's social geography. The first was the amalgamation of formerly racially segregated spaces (coloured, white, Indian, and African) into a new municipality. This municipality, called Mandini in 1995, was renamed Mandeni in 2000 when local government boundaries were extended to encompass rural areas. The second was the quite dramatic movement of middle-class black South Africans into the former suburbs previously reserved for whites and, to a lesser extent, Indians. Even when whole families have not relocated, many children have been sent to schools in these areas. The tremendous growth of imijondolo both in the township and in nearby informal settlements was a third significant change. The fourth was the development of new RDP low-income housing projects, the biggest of which is at Hlomendlini, south of the Thukela River.

One revealing feature of recent transformations in Mandeni is that the area's most privileged elite has been able to partially insulate itself geographically from the consequences of apartheid's demise. The highly paid factory managers who work at Isithebe, mostly white and male, tend to live in the picturesque, and still overwhelmingly white, seaside resorts such as Zinkwazi or Ballito, thirty or forty minutes' drive away. Yet almost all other groups have experienced significant change. Mandini—the town built for white SAPPI employees—was, as some whites put it, "going black." Black and white residents now share this urban space not only as mistress and maid, or master and garden boy—though these relations are still common—but as equals in income and as fellow workers in occupations like teaching or skilled industrial work.

If Mandini changed forever from its roots as a white company town, Tugela, the former Indian area, is now somewhat similar to what it was in the

TABLE 6.1.

Demographics and Employment in Mandeni Municipality, 2001

	AFRICAN	INDIAN	WHITE	COLOURED
Total Population	122,595	3,126	2,340	611
Married	14%	43%	54%	28%
Employed (15–65)	30%	47%	58%	46%
Employed men earning less than R800 a month	49%	12%	2%	26%
Employed women earning less than R800 a month	74%	25%	5%	29%

It should be noted that the data in this table is derived from the census; labor force data drawing from dedicated labor surveys is outlined elsewhere in this chapter.

SOURCE: Statistics South Africa, "Interactive and Electronic Products," *Census 2001*, http://www.statssa.gov.za/census01/html/C2001Interactive.asp.

pre-apartheid period. In the 1970s, the ideology of racial purity had required the removal of Africans from proximate areas like Hlomendlini. The growth of the Renckens supermarket near to Sundumbili then eroded the retail trade that had hitherto centered on Tugela. Yet in the early 1990s, Africans began to return to Hlomendlini, led first by ANC comrades who fled the terrible political violence rife in central Mandeni. Then in 2006, following a land restitution settlement, the municipality built a thousand two-room houses at Hlomendlini (figure 6.1). Like many housing projects, the Hlomendlini houses were located some distance from the main employment areas, in this case nearly ten kilometers away from Isithebe (a smaller number of RDP houses were subsequently built near Sundumbili township). The Tugela area gained a further economic boost from African parents sending their children to the former Indian school there. This school charges lower fees then the former white "Model C" school in Mandini, but still gives students the chance to learn from teachers whose home language is English.

Tugela's partial return to a more racially mixed and economically prosperous past struck me one day when I visited a shop run by Mr. Hassan, who has been trading there since the 1950s. Mr. Hassan traces his ancestry to

Muslim traders who arrived in Natal from India as passengers; they were not, therefore, indentured to sugar cane farms like most immigrants from India. I arrived with a former customer of Mr. Hassan's, an African shop owner who had eventually decided to stock his shop with goods bought from larger retailers.

I watched as the two men reminisced about the past, and at one point African teenagers who were enrolled in the local school came in and bantered with Mr. Hassan in isiZulu. It struck me that Mr. Hassan had sold basic household items in his shop for the last fifty years, and from this quiet vantage point had witnessed tremendous change north of the Thukela River: the massive growth of factories, the deadly IFP-ANC political violence, and the tremendous growth of the local population. Now, in contrast to Mandeni's general economic decline, his shop is experiencing something of a boom. Pointing to his business's rising prosperity, Mr. Hassan said that the small Muslim community had recently funded the building of a new mosque.

ISITHEBE AND THE RISE OF IMIJONDOLO

The flow of people into the former white and Indian areas like Mandini and Tugela was one-way—no one moved from these richer, well-serviced areas to poor ones, and consequently, Isithebe jondolo settlement and Sundumbili township continued to have only African residents. Yet the population of these mostly poor areas rose quickly. Isithebe, which I consider first, became saturated with imijondolo as rural migrants continued to arrive in the area despite job losses in the surrounding factories. In the two wards roughly comprising Isithebe's informal settlement, the population more than doubled between 1996 and 2001 alone; this tremendous population growth is captured in figure 6.2.[38] In the 2000s this trend slowed or halted, with many migrants still arriving in search of work but a roughly equal number leaving or dying. I would estimate that the number of imijondolo stayed roughly constant during the time of my research (2000–2009).

The rising demand for imijondolo drove up rents in the 1990s, further worsening the position of new migrants in the area. By the early 2000s, the cheapest rent for an umjondolo in the jondolo settlement was R20 per month for a mud and stick shack without electricity; a concrete-block one with electricity cost R80.[39] Moreover, the going price of a small plot rose from around R500 in the 1980s to R2,000 by the 2000s. As a result, the jondolo settlement was a hostile environment for recent migrants, a high proportion of whom were women. Some women undoubtedly found formal work, but many moved into informal work and, as we shall see, it also became common for women to depend on men for material support.

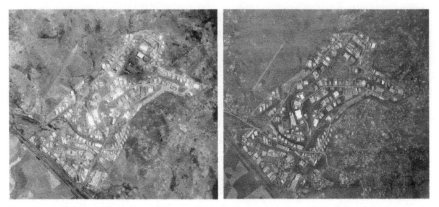

FIGURE 6.2A AND B. Isithebe, 1989 and 1999. In these ten years, the informal settlement surrounding the park grew tremendously, although the number of jobs in the industrial park fell from approximately 23,000 to 15,000. This growth highlights the continued agrarian decline, the high levels of movement by both men and women, reductions in marriage rates, and smaller household sizes.

Yet, as intimidating as this environment was, most migrants believed that remaining in a depressed rural area was an impossible long-term option. Whatever Isithebe's faults, it was a place of considerable economic activity. Moreover, because of longstanding movement patterns, most rural migrants could stay temporarily with a relative or friend. Indeed, unmarried rural migrants were in the majority in Isithebe: according to the 2001 census 75 percent of the population was unmarried and more than 50 percent of Isithebe's households consisted of only one or two people. As a result of its rural roots, the population is generally less well educated than that of the nearby Sundumbili township. In 2001, 20 percent of the residents over the age of twenty had had no schooling, and only 16 percent had passed the final year of high school.

SUNDUMBILI TOWNSHIP

Like Isithebe, Sundumbili grew substantially: from 1983 to 2001 the township saw its population double to around 24,000.[40] While some new residents were migrants, many were born in the township itself. Yet most of the new inhabitants were housed not in formal houses but in backyard imijondolo. In the early 1980s a typical Sundumbili resident lived in a four-room "matchbox" house, and this would have been home to around seven people.[41] Today, after the explosion of smaller rented rooms, median household size has dropped to between two and three.[42] In one typical part of the township, a section of Bhidla, my research assistant conducted a small survey and recorded 176 rented imijondolo in the backyards of 145 houses, more than one per house.

The rising cost of township housing was one reason for the expansion of imijondolo. One former township administrator told me that a "matchbox" house could be purchased in 1991 from local authorities for around R5,000, but by 2004 they were selling on the open market for between R35,000 and R50,000.[43] And this hugely unequal access to housing typically follows generational lines. It is common for a man employed by SAPPI to live in an extended four-room house and rent out a one-room umjondolo to a young man who is unemployed or employed in casual work, and this pattern demonstrates the strong connections between age and class.

Rights and Body Politics

How are these stark inequalities experienced in an era of democracy and citizenship? Importantly, social rights enshrined in the 1996 constitution allow citizens to hold the ANC accountable for its promises of a "better life for all"— its election slogan in 1994. Some social movements use this collective vision of rights to justify redistributive claims: groups have drawn on the constitution to fight for gender equality, access to AIDS drugs, and protection against shack evictions. I address AIDS activism in Mandeni later.[44]

At the same time, most young people I know, whether former ANC comrades or IFP stalwarts, profess apathy about what they call *ipolitiki*, a term that implies party politics. By shunning ipolitiki, residents say that they are reacting to the tragic history of IFP-ANC violence that still haunts the area. Engagement is also discouraged by the common belief that there is now little to fight over, because politicians are only interested in their own advancement.

Political realignments after apartheid are complex, but one point I'd like to stress is that many important contestations seem to have been re-scaled to the body and, in particular, work through notions of amalungelo (rights). I introduce this point here as a prelude to exploring the centrality of rights to gendered contestations in the next three chapters. Rights, according to many young people with whom I spoke, are gained through democracy and are a cornerstone of post-apartheid personhood. The publicity surrounding the constitution (in isiZulu called *umthetho sisekelo*, or "foundation of the law"), a document agreed in 1996, was especially apparent in the early years of my research (the early 2000s).

Colonialism, as we have seen, profoundly molded notions of "rights": it brought a vocabulary of liberalism to the country but restricted political rights to whites and devolved certain powers to "traditional" institutions that often upheld gender and generational hierarchies. Now that democracy has been achieved, one consequence of this binary logic is that rights can signal equality and be contrasted to a set of "traditional" practices justified through hlonipha (respect). Reflecting elders' distress at youths' apparent new power, one letter written to the newspaper *Isolezwe* abhors that "more rights have been given to children than parents" and argues that traditional forms of discipline, such as hitting a child, should not be seen as *ukuhlukumeza* (in this context meaning child abuse).[45] Moreover, as I show later, calls for women's rights tend to be interpreted in terms of equality between men and women in all respects, whereas in the homeland years the prevailing discourse propagated by homeland leaders like Buthelezi advocated what I called "rights with hlonipha"—the granting of some property rights to women, who still had an overarching duty to respect men.

This sense that individuals can challenge long-established hierarchies on the grounds of their rights is reflected in many statements I collected:

> [Rights] are to do whatever you want, any time. . . . No one can take them away from you. . . . Some are using them in the good way . . . some they don't use them good, because they just go anywhere without telling their parents; . . . when the parents ask, he says that it is my right to do that. (twenty-five-year-old man, Sundumbili)

> Rights started being practiced only after the black man came into power. (sixty-year-old woman, Sundumbili)

> It is hard to describe a right, it is like the foundation of the country. It is said that we are equal: a man cannot do anything, because she has the right to say no. (twenty-year-old woman, Sundumbili)

Yet while rights have an egalitarian flavor, the emerging middle class, as elsewhere in the world, is often able to shout the loudest, arguing that rights should be realized in a rise in its standards of living. "We want rights that were denied to us by apartheid, like access to elite schools," some parents say. The resulting class divisions are little noted in AIDS research, even if poverty is included in the analysis. But if we are to understand AIDS' structural and symbolic roots, we must attend to the juxtaposition of poverty and extremely rapid social mobility. In particular, both gendered identities and the failures of recent AIDS interventions cannot be understood without placing poverty and riches in the same analytical frame.

Uneven Rights: Schools for the Rich, Cell Phones for the Poor

South Africans have a constitutional right to education, but the educational system meant to provide it is highly skewed, and there are few work opportunities once schooling is completed. Professional work is now open to black South Africans, but new industrial jobs have virtually disappeared. This sharp division has particularly intensified competition for Model C schools, former white public schools that maintain high standards by charging fees.[46] Virtually all whites were educated in these schools in the apartheid era. Fully private schools still educate a smaller elite, but at a very high price.

In the Mandeni area, the most sought-after school is Mandini Academy, the previously all-white Model C school perched in the leafy and spacious surroundings of Mandini, the former white town. Parents' fees pay for extra teachers and other staff, in addition to those funded by the government. It is easily possible to commute to this school from the township, but students living in Mandini are more likely to get a place. Three out of four of Mandini Academy's students are now African and, signaling the sharpening of educational inequalities, one teacher told me that many of these students were actually the children of teachers working at cash-starved former African-only schools. This is in itself a vivid condemnation of "Bantu Education," under which only a quarter as much money was spent on black students as on white students.[47]

Even a casual visitor to Mandini Academy cannot fail to be struck by the large amount of racial mixing, with black and white students walking and talking openly together. A decade and a half after liberation, former Model C schools remain one of the few spaces in South Africa where race can be just one, rather than *the,* signifier of difference—the elite education gives all bright students a potential springboard into middle-class jobs.

In sharp contrast, in 2000 I visited a township school that had a flimsy roof, crumbling brick walls, and graffiti-filled rooms. The vast majority of children in Mandeni are educated in similar run-down schools in the township, rural area, or informal settlements. Above the considerable noise of children, the vice principal took the opportunity to complain to me about the poor learning conditions: there were 1,265 pupils (all African) in twenty-one classrooms, as many as four students had to share one desk, and others had to stand.

I kept in touch with Sipho, one of the students I interviewed that day, and four years later he provided me with information about his cohort: only four people out of his class of fifty-two had passed the final exam. By 2004, three had died (one in prison), three were still studying (including him), twelve were working (often part-time in the local factories), eight were untraceable, and the majority, twenty-four, were unemployed. By most accounts, schools in rural areas and informal settlements had even worse records.

In the apartheid era, white South Africans carved out a middle-class lifestyle that typically included a maid, private health care, and at least one annual vacation. Today, the new multi-racial middle class, as well as a growing number of international tourists, enjoy the country's golden beaches and rich game parks. *Isolezwe*, the popular Zulu newspaper aimed at urban residents, has a regular section called *Ukungcebeleka*, a verb meaning roughly "to go out," for instance to the beach, a restaurant, or the cinema. In general, consumption has exploded among the middle class, and rich South Africans, black and white, now flaunt luxury cars like BMWs.

This consumption boom is evident in poor areas and not only in expensive suburbs. Indeed, advertisers have become skilled at portraying consumption as one way to bring middle-class life to everyone's doorstep. Own the latest cell phone and you can live like the rich even if you are unemployed. Of course, advertisers have long promoted material goods as a sign of social distinction, from the clothes and soap that missionaries urged Africans to purchase to the automobiles that a few of the better-off could buy. But by tying consumption to freedom, post-apartheid advertisers deliberately reworked images of political struggle to convey the message that black South Africans have won the right to consume.[48] To consume is to be free—to be aware of one's rights and citizenship. The specific contours and experiences of this social distinction depend, of course, on different geographies, and I consider first Sundumbili township and then Isithebe jondolo settlement.

LOXION KULCHA: RIGHTS AND INEQUALITIES IN SUNDUMBILI TOWNSHIP

Townships, made famous by their anti-apartheid militancy, also fostered an aspiring middle class. The best-off residents of Sundumbili today are factory workers, teachers, clerks, and nurses, and some can afford to place a child in a Model C school in hopes that the child will attain a middle-class lifestyle. But for the majority of young township dwellers, who cannot enter on this path to middle-class prosperity, life seems to have stood still. Inhabitants use the verb *ukuhlala* (to stay) to describe, with resignation, how the unemployed just hang around the township.[49]

Sometimes sharp divisions open up within a single household. I knew one family in which the eldest son, thirty, had attended a township school and was unemployed, and constantly rued his inability to wed his girlfriend. Yet his sisters attended a Model C school and aspired to become actors or T.V. present-ers. Of course, the dreams of a middle-class life do not always come true; but they are certainly more likely to be realized if the dreamer was educated in a former Model C school rather than a township school. And even the small possibility of social mobility in townships can produce self-blame. I sensed that the thirty-year-old unemployed man was asking himself, "Why have I not made it? What is the difference between me and others who are successful?"

At the same time, it would be wrong to paint a picture of township youth, even the poorest, as simply disenchanted and depressed. Although they com-plained of boredom and were frustrated at the lack of jobs, I found that young people from Sundumbili could quickly steer conversation toward new local sites of fun. Kwaito music—a mixture of "bubblegum," rap, and house styles—exploded in townships after 1994, symbolizing the optimism and energy of the post-apartheid "Y generation."[50] In Sundumbili it is most famously enjoyed in an *ibheshi*, a late-night street party or "bash" whose organizers blast loud music and sell alcohol. Youth freedom and rights in the post-apartheid period are symbolized by all aspects of the event: alcohol, loud music, dancing, and its location in a site—the street—that had been reclaimed from political violence and apartheid oppression.[51]

Moreover, the new sense of freedom, cheek by jowl with great poverty, can inculcate not only self-blame but a sense of injustice among unemployed township dwellers who feel that they should not be facing such a painful dearth of opportunities. One way this is manifested is in the reluctance of township-born women to work in local garment factories. Although some women from Sundumbili do end up working in Isithebe's factories, many I knew told me that this kind of work was beneath them; they had not gone to school to earn a pittance sewing for twelve hours a day in a Taiwanese factory. This work is typically seen as more appropriate for rural migrants with poorer educations. Townships were where middle-class lives were to be launched—such status was their right.

Furthermore, the new divisions that arose after democracy can make townships feel like down-to-earth representatives of black South African cul-ture. At its birth in the 1960s, Sundumbili was coded as a modern space. Roads, water, and electricity serviced many of Sundumbili's brick houses, and these modern structures clearly distinguished the township from the surrounding informal and rural areas. Most township residents came to consider themselves phucukile (civilized), in comparison with the inhabitants of the nearby infor-mal settlements, areas they described as *amakhaya* or *amafamu* (rural homes or farms). Revealingly, however, residents today often favorably contrast the township, with its vibrant culture, to the modern but culturally dead former white suburbs to which some of the richest residents move. By celebrating *loxion kulcha* (township culture; significantly, Loxion Kulcha is also the name of a fashionable clothing brand), township youth across South Africa challenge the perceived arrogance of *amaModelC*, students who abandon township life for former white schools.

The sometimes derogatory label "amaModelC" is, in fact, a potent symbol of deep new cultural divisions after apartheid. It suggests that confident young students with posh accents look down on the uncouth styles of less well educated residents. Township schools today are supposed to be run in English; however, they are rarely staffed by native speakers and usually cannot bestow on students the fluency that employers typically desire. Indeed, South Africa's move from having two official languages under apartheid (English and Afrikaans) to eleven after it coincided with the gaining of English's status as "first among equals" in the sphere of work.

These class-based cultural divisions, as I show later, are significant because the largest AIDS program aimed at youth, loveLife, understood youth culture primarily in terms of the aspirations of English-speaking black South Africans. Indeed, AIDS messages have largely failed to take into account the profound effect of rising inequalities on South Africans' identities.

Of course, this social differentiation along divisions of education and language has long precedents in urban areas. In Cape Town's Langa township in the 1960s, anthropologists Monica Wilson and Archie Mafeje recorded strong signs of social differentiation, including the rather insulting term "ooscuse me" applied to well-to-do adults "accused of being aloof and conceited."[52] But today, it is the young amaModelC who are gaining vast new opportunities for social mobility, ones denied to nurses, clerks, and teachers—the most common high-status professions for Africans under apartheid.

The resentment of Model C schooling, in turn, grants high status to those who succeed after attending lesser schools. The most high-profile rags-to-riches figure today is, of course, Jacob Zuma, who is largely self-educated and became the country's president in 2009; his ousting of Thabo Mbeki as president of the ANC was, in part, connected to a popular rebellion against the perceived elitism of the well-spoken and well-educated former president.

Moreover, Zola (Bonginkosi Dlamini)—Kwaito star, actor, and T.V. presenter—has been described as "the second biggest brand in the country next to Nelson Mandela."[53] Film buffs outside South Africa will know him as the lead gangster in the Oscar-winning South African film *Tsotsi*. Zola's rough street slang contrasts with the smooth talk of the amaModelC T.V. presenters who dominate the national networks and who sometimes describe themselves as "coconuts" (black on the outside, white on the inside).[54] By naming himself after the notoriously violent part of Soweto township where he grew up (and which he promises never to leave), Zola indicates his pride in township life. He is popular because he not only demonstrates the stardom and success that are attainable after apartheid but also stands firmly in support of those "left behind."

I want to stress, however, that poorer township dwellers' sense of being "left behind" is always lived out in gendered ways. The paternalism upon which Sundumbili and other townships were founded rested on the provision of relatively cheap accommodation and a strong demand for male employment. As younger residents walk past the hundreds of "matchbox" houses— many now enlarged and extended—they are reminded daily of the period when "SAPPI built the township." And in doing so, the paper mill built meanings and expectations that centered on male work.

Certainly, there is no more potent symbol of employers' neglect of the area's welfare (and thus of social reproduction) than the changing role and status of the SAPPI paper mill. In the 1960s SAPPI helped establish the township and employed nearly two thousand African men, many of whom gained access to the township's family houses. Yet today the company, now part of a global-orientated business, employs around half the number of people that it did in the 1960s. Though SAPPI still supports a number of local charities and institutions, no longer does it play a pivotal role in Mandeni. The factory's toxic fumes still pollute the area, but it has now become an industrial island largely disconnected from residents' everyday lives.

AWUKHO UMSEBENZI KWASITHEBE: "NO WORK IN ISITHEBE"

Isithebe jondolo settlement is only two miles from Sundumbili, but it is a very different place. It is located literally in the shadow of Isithebe Industrial Park, and work, or the hope of work, dominates the lives of the mostly migrant residents. Whereas in the township unemployment is largely experienced as hlala-ing (staying or sitting around), Isithebe residents tend to be highly mobile and to maintain close links to rural areas. Moreover, every day unemployed residents walk miles around the factories to actively *ukufesa* (queue for work). In isiZulu, *ukufesa* is a relatively new verb, said to be derived from the English noun "face." It evokes the frustration of job seekers who press their faces against the gates of businesses in the hope of finding employment.

Unemployed residents in this jondolo settlement generally have only temporary support from family members, or perhaps lovers, and so finding employment or another form of subsistence is of paramount importance.

In 2000, a group of women in their twenties described for me the search for work: "You wake up in the morning, you go on the road, you arrive at the gate, maybe you hear rumors that they are hiring; you arrive, you wait until four, if they don't hire you go back to your place . . . every day. . . . There is no longer hiring [using the emotive term *akusekho ukuqashwa*]. . . . If you go to a firm, it depends on what work you know: if it is a clothing company there are operators and those that clean, the service workers." In addition, it is often necessary to bribe or have sex with the hiring manager: "He just comes out, then he points to the person that pays him," one woman told me.

Residents blame the ANC government and *amaShayina*, Taiwanese investors in the park, for their worsening employment prospects. The decline of "white" (South African–owned) firms and the rise of Taiwanese-owned factories roughly coincided with the end of apartheid. As a result, local people perceived the larger white firms, in which unions had won recognition and better working conditions, as leaving and being replaced by poorer-paying ama-Shayina. This makes people nostalgic for the past—though no one, of course, would want to return to the apartheid era. Certainly, when one Taiwanese manager was robbed and shot to death in 1998, Taiwanese investors believed the attack to have been racially motivated and threatened to leave Isithebe.

The wider political significance of job losses became clear in December 2000 when Inkatha unexpectedly defeated the ANC in the Mandeni local elections. Instead of campaigning on an ethnic Zulu platform, Inkatha maintained that it was the only party that could stop the factories from abandoning the area. This tactic garnered support among residents who were aware that Inkatha had long collected CVs from its supporters and delivered them to firms wishing to hire compliant non-union labor. However, in 2004 the ANC won back the municipality as Inkatha splintered into factions.

Nevertheless, despite changes in the council, life seemed to get worse in Isithebe jondolo settlement. Not a single house was built in the jondolo settlement (or in Sundumbili township either) in the first ten years of democracy. Early on in my stay, residents collected money to install a network of taps that they connected illegally to a water pipe that ran close to the settlement. In 2006, however, government officials removed these connections, and now standpipes are crowded with children and women waiting their turn to draw water.

Moreover, while most of the area became electrified in the 1990s, electricity cuts remain common. Residents are rudely reminded of their low social status when the settlement is plunged into darkness in the evenings when electricity is most demanded; as if inhabiting a different world, the nearby factories always remain floodlit. It took until 2007 for the first sign of *inthuthuko* (development) in the area to appear. In that year, every plot in Isithebe was given a free pit latrine toilet. But these are such tiny constructions that jokes abound about how the largest residents cannot even fit into them.

In Sundumbili township, social mobility for the young typically depends on studying at former white or Indian schools, but in the jondolo settlement ascent of the social ladder is still overwhelmingly achieved through owning land, renting imijondolo, and running taxis. And newer residents can rarely manage these, because the area became increasingly overpopulated in the 1990s. Indeed, the rural migrants who predominate in Isithebe have even less hope of reaching the middle class than township dwellers. The exceptions to this are the few richest residents, who send their children to former white or Indian schools. Yet, on the whole, the best the newest arrivals can hope for is some kind of casual work (*itoho*).

Many of Isithebe's residents leave their children in rural areas, but Isithebe does have children among its population. I first met Dingane in 2000, when he was thirteen years old. One of my more vivid memories is of seeing him one day standing outside a neighbor's house, peering longingly through the lounge window toward the television set. The well-to-do owners of the house, who owned a successful local business and rented out imijondolo, sent their children to Model C schools. While Dingane was welcome to play with the family's children in the yard, he was not allowed to enter the house. Captured in his awkward squints at the T.V. seemed to be the agonizing elusiveness of post-apartheid prosperity.

As the years went by, I watched Dingane's friends gain confidence through their privileged schooling and talk optimistically (in steadily improving English) about working in the media industry—a favorite dream of young, educated children. Dingane, however, slumped deeper into depression. One day he told me that he worked illegally for R5 a day in a bread factory, and another time I found him playing on his own and asked why he wasn't going to school. His mother, he said, couldn't afford the fees (his father had left them when he was young). I had previously interviewed her; she was trying to raise her four children on a small salary earned working at a factory that makes paper bags.

I paid his school fees so that he could attend the secondary school in the jondolo settlement, but after a year he complained about its poor quality. Over the course of my research, I had come to know the headmaster of a township school with a better reputation, and in 2003 I asked this man to enroll Dingane, which he did. Dingane told me he didn't want to imitate the womanizing and drinking that he saw men in the area doing. He dreamed of working at the SAPPI paper mill, the heart of the town and the symbol of "industrial man"—if only he could become educated.

However, when I returned to Mandeni in 2006 after a year's absence, Dingane was in prison, having been caught stealing cell phones from residents. He was nineteen by this time, and everyone said that he had changed; this was evident in his drinking and stealing. In 2009, my friends told me that he had acquired a gun and was involved in armed robberies in the area.

Dingane's case was not uncommon. In Isithebe, so banal is crime that it barely reaches the level of gossip unless it is particularly violent or involves a well-known person. During my stay in the area, one of my neighbors acciden-tally shot and killed his friend while they were playing cards. Another robbed a factory with an AK47 and fled the police. The shop attached to the house where I stayed was held up at gunpoint in 2005, and in 2007 a group of men and women attacked and killed a burglar trying to enter an umjondolo.

The most frightening incident I witnessed was the father of my adopted family firing a gun a few meters from my door at 3 AM to scare off an intruder. Indeed, it was at night when I most thought about violence. As a white person I figured that I signaled wealth and might attract attention from criminals. At the same time, I undoubtedly enjoyed certain privileges: I was not subjected to the same risk of sexual violence as a woman; moreover, because I was white, any violence directed at me would probably have demanded more immediate attention from the police.

From April 2005 to February 2006, seven murders, twenty-nine rapes, and seventy-four burglaries were reported to the local police station in Nyoni.[55] Left behind in the whirlwind of opportunity, many young men found that their only possible way up was through crime; for women, as we shall see, richer men provide a dangerous avenue for social mobility.

Political struggle had created great optimism for the future in Mandeni, and yet rising unemployment steadily undermined the possibility of marriage and housing for the young. In this chapter we have seen that this dream of prosperity eluded most South Africans but was realized dramatically by a few.

Today, townships still host inadequate schools and are still inhabited pri-marily by those designated African under apartheid. Informal settlements have continued to grow, despite the building of over two million RDP houses by 2007. Only a small proportion of black South Africans managed to move up the social scale, and doing so often necessitated families or at least school-children moving into former white or Indian suburbs. Moreover, just as HIV was introduced to the area, the social conditions that fueled its spread worsened: the gender income gap increased, women continued to move to the area despite job losses, and imijondolo multiplied rapidly.

Seen through a historical lens, both the state and employers played a more reactive than proactive role after 1994 in matters of everyday life and social reproduction. The increased scope and size of social grants, the state's most significant intervention to reduce poverty, were primarily responses to the failure of economic policy. Yet people's lives *were* transformed; for the first time they were citizens with rights, and changes were evident in everything from the rocking street parties to the quickening pace of consumerism. How did these changes come together to affect masculinities and femininities? How did economic changes became manifest in gender politics? What happens when consumption becomes the only way to increase social status in a climate saturated with both rights and inequalities?

SEVEN

Independent Women: Rights amid Wrongs, and Men's Broken Promises

In 2000, the U.S.-based band Destiny's Child released the song "Independent Women." The R'n'B track quickly became a hit in South Africa: the music of the African-American female band seemed to especially resonate with African women to whom democracy had brought new rights. The song demanded confidently, "All the women who are independent, throw your hands up at me."

But in the following year the South African male music stars Mandoza and Mdu released a strong musical response. Their hit song "50/50" deliberately mimicked the rhythm and tune of "Independent Women," but its chorus went "*Wonke umfazi oindependent,* let's go 50/50" (Every woman who is independent, let's go 50/50). The two male artists' lyrics warned women that if they want equality, then they must not rely on men financially—they must split all costs 50/50.

If the optimistic beat of "Independent Women" accorded with the new liberal democracy, Mandoza and Mdu's retort illustrates how notions of gender equality quickly became a heated point of contention. And it was "rights," as I show in this and the next chapter, that often became a lightning rod for these tensions. In the new era of freedom, all citizens had "rights," and it was often debated whether women had gained too few or too many.

Rights' authority is vested in their audacious claim that they are transhistorical and transgeographical—that they are the very essence of what it is to be human. Yet both the construction of this universal liberal human subject and the historical geographies that institutionalize rights in different settings must be probed. In 1996, two years after the end of apartheid, South Africa adopted one of the most liberal constitutions in the world, enshrining non-discrimination on the basis of gender as well as race and sexual orientation. The new democracy gave birth to a Commission for Gender Equality and new national legislation bolstering women's rights to maternity leave, the termination of pregnancy (abortion), and child maintenance.

Although these developments can be celebrated, the framing of gender in terms of rights also has other consequences. It could lead some to position rights as an uncomplicated modern alternative to backward traditions, and thus occlude the political-economic changes that mold gender inequality and intimacy today. And it could also downplay the creative way women themselves draw on and subvert notions of rights.

Certainly, despite rights' promises of equality, social and geographical divisions continued to sharpen after democracy. Moreover, unemployment's destabilizing of gendered expectations drove what can only be described as extreme levels of hostility between many men and women. Though we should be mindful of generalizations and of downplaying differences between women, it is clear that the longstanding "patriarchal bargain" based on marriage continued to buckle after apartheid: in a climate of chronic unemployment, it became less common for a man to work, earn enough to lobola a woman, and then provide for her as his wife. Furthermore, it also became more difficult for women to chart an alternative path economically independent of men.[1]

I am deliberately using the concept of rights both loosely and provocatively. My intention is not to evaluate the effectiveness of new institutions and laws aimed at promoting gender equality after apartheid. Instead, I want to place rights in a more historical context to think through some of the limitations of rights-based approaches. While gender rights are often spoken about with certitude, rights have never been hermetically sealed entities. As already noted, the verb "ukulunga," from which the noun "amalungelo" (rights) derives, means "to be right" or "to be in order," and it therefore has wider meanings than modern understandings of rights: it evokes historically embedded moral claims that do not rest on inalienable bodily traits. This chapter's central focus therefore is on a *cultural politics of rights*—how women deploy rights narratives to navigate intimate relations with men after apartheid.

Women in Mandeni tend to use rights in creative ways; typically they blend discourses of liberal rights with wider moral claims about what is "right." This chapter is organized around their key claims. I use four examples—women's right to "safe" sexual pleasure, to consume, to live alone, and to make decisions about their own children—to show how moral justifications (claims about what is right and wrong) are shifting through women's encounters with daily life after apartheid. They illustrate that liberal rights can never be completely estranged from the wider, historically and geographically constituted moral codes of "rights and wrongs" that have been sketched out in previous chapters. Hence, women do not have preexisting interests and identities on which modern liberal rights act; rather, rights help to construct their interests and identities, often in unanticipated ways. Put another way, rather than starting from the perspective that rights must be constantly increased in society to fuel a straightforward development of gender equality, this historical ethnography draws attention to multiple sites of struggle that always need to be historically situated.

Moral claims about what is "right," as each of the four examples show, are deeply contested. But these examples build up to a scenario that I think best captures the paradoxes of rights in post-apartheid society: some women employ rights to argue that, in a 50/50 world, they now have the right to have multiple partners, just like men. Women's assertion of an entitlement to multiple partners is, as we have seen, by no means new. Yet today it is framed in a language of absolute gender equality and universal rights—though at a time of unprecedented social inequalities and the rise of a deadly virus that causes AIDS. Of course, women's strategies and life paths are incredibly diverse, and many women do not fit neatly into the examples I choose to highlight. I end with some residents' attempts to adopt the identity of "a good woman," an effort that requires them to partially exchange the notion of rights for the more traditional virtues of hlonipha (respect).

The "It Girls": Rights with a Capital R

Before exploring shifting femininities in Mandeni, I begin with South Africa's "It girls." The term "It girls" is used worldwide to describe bold, sexy, and powerful women. Its use in South Africa demonstrates how transnational media links help to construct femininities today. But the It girls are also illuminating for two other reasons. First, all South African women's sense of themselves is formed in relation to the rising wealth of the middle class, which has now become multi-racial. Second, the It girls' modern, assertive, and individualistic femininity is precisely the model that is favored by some "gender and AIDS" narratives that circulate in international and national organizations.

Let's start with Nomakula (Kuli) Roberts, a prominent South African It girl. In 2004, Roberts—journalist, fashion icon, and former beauty queen—was featured on the front cover of South Africa's *Elle* magazine to advertise an article on the It girls. These women, *Elle* said, are "sexy, spunky, successful . . . having loads of sex appeal, being worshiped and envied in equal measure and, above all, possessing the kind of unstoppable self-confidence that requires validation from no-one else. . . . Almost every girl has fantasized about becoming an It girl."[2] It is certainly the case that the It girls' images are widely circulated in South Africa, especially in urban areas. They represent a new elite, entry into which is now dependent not on race but on class.

Indicating the importance of consumption to this world, Kuli Roberts was asked to present the T.V. fashion show *What Not to Wear.* In her opinion women should "not be scared to shop. . . . You work. You earn your own money. You've earned the right to go out and spend lots of it on yourself."[3] In line with President Mbeki's wish to realize an "African Renaissance," she sees consumption as affirming an Africanness that apartheid denigrated. Hence, in her *Elle* cover photo Roberts wears a large gold necklace that spells out *ubuntu*, a word denoting an African philosophy of humanness.

Roberts also writes a controversial column called "Bitch's Brew" in *Sunday World*, a popular newspaper with a predominantly African readership. In this forum, she bluntly argues that women should beat unfaithful men at their own game. Here is an excerpt from a 2004 piece entitled "Let's Three-Time Those Randy Dogs":

> A bunch of rather resourceful women have come to the conclusion that since their attached men are not always around to lie and tell them they love them, it makes no sense not to have three bastards all doing the same thing, at different times of course! Instead of dreaming about and pining for your man, you are constantly showered with attention from various flames. Think about the fact that you are always loved, amused, never lonely and always have an audience— and the advantage is that you do not have to bear him children, clean his skidmarks or cook for him. . . . The men will forget that you are doing exactly what they are up to, but because you're female you're expected to live by a different set of rules. . . . So I say to you, fine sister, have your cake and eat it three times.[4]

In a piece written five years later—the longevity of the column indicates its popularity—Roberts touches on interracial dating. Marriage and sex across racial divides were illegal under apartheid. Now that these laws have been repealed, Kuli Roberts makes it clear that, no matter who a woman sleeps with, her own sexual satisfaction must be her primary concern. Peppered with phrases like "dazzle you with his tongue," the article ends with the words "Look ladies, I say this to you all the time: men are men and unless they will go South and stay there, then they are not worth your while—white, black or green."[5]

Sometimes associated with "third-wave feminism," Roberts' sex-positive femininity is perhaps most famously symbolized by the enormously popular T.V. show *Sex and the City*, which is broadcast to South Africans. The program's four New York women gained iconic status for promoting a femininity that rests not on marriage but on women's economic independence, consumption, and sexual satisfaction. However, as one critic has noted, "With this focus on individualism, feminism becomes reduced to one issue: choice."[6]

There is more, however, to *Sex and the City* than just sex. As any fan knows, much of the program's appeal derives from the incessant tension between the stars' desire for sex and their yearning for true love. This interplay of love and sex is similarly reflected in popular magazines and newspapers in South Africa.

As marriage has become virtually a middle-class institution, a number of glossy new wedding magazines now promote ever more expensive weddings as a means of distinction. Large payments of ilobolo and extravagant weddings are big news for the media: in 2009 it was reported that businessman Mbongiseni Duma paid a whopping R1 million (US$125,000) in ilobolo to marry his business partner, the Zulu princess Ntombizosuthu (the ilobolo for the king's daughters has historically been very high).[7]

One popular woman's magazine is entitled *True Love* and speaks directly to this goal of a fairy-tale marriage. But in addition to love, the magazine also frequently discusses sexual pleasure outside marriage. Tellingly, one of its articles drew on a "sex expert" to portray the body as transcendental—and therefore severed from class, race, and other axes of inequality.

> Dr Eve feels that casual sex can be fun if it's a phase—not a lifestyle.
> *"This is a choice adults have a right to make,"* says Dr Eve, "but it carries the need to take responsibility for protecting your body and mind."[8]

Of course, many middle-class women will not identify with Dr. Eve's prescriptions or the bold sexuality of the It girls. Nevertheless, bodily rights are a framework lived very differently by poorer South Africans.

Right 1: The Right to Safe Sex and to Sexual Pleasure

I begin exploring "rights" in Mandeni through the issues of "safe sex" and sexual pleasure. I generally support, though with important qualifications, the prevailing view that rights provide women with an important tool to challenge certain aspects of men's control over women's bodies. Most of my discussions with young women and men do suggest that rights narratives can drive greater condom use and, to a degree, a new sense of equality between lovers.

Before considering these issues in depth, however, we have to take a step back and remind ourselves of what we mean by "sex." AIDS prevention narratives tend to assume that sex is a universal phenomenon to which rights can easily be attached. In contrast, as we have seen, sex's construction as a domain at the core of a person's identity has a long, uneven, and incomplete history in South Africa; it is entangled with shifts in the household, employment, migration, religion, healing, and fertility.

Yet, erasing this ambiguous history, since 1994 powerful narratives have portrayed sex as the cornerstone of life after apartheid. Here the English

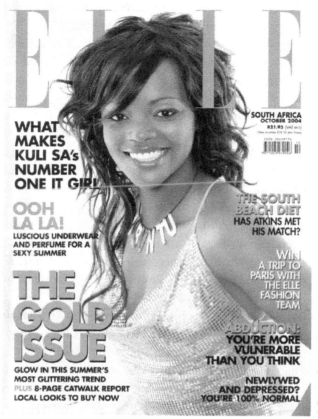

FIGURE 7.1. Nomakula Roberts, an "It girl." *Elle,* October, 2004. Courtesy of *Elle* Magazine South Africa, Avusa Publishing; photograph by Merwelene van der Merwe.

term "sex" (widely used by isiZulu speakers) serves to stand in for an array of genital pleasures, while simultaneously directing attention to penis-vagina penetration. Apartheid's censors were notoriously prudish and intolerant of pornography (and even banned television until 1976), but watch T.V. late at night today and you'll regularly find soft-core porn. The website Sondeza.com was established for sexual discussions and images under the motto "supplying what black South Africa is deprived of" (*sondeza* means "bring closer").[9] The impression that sexual freedom came with democracy was strengthened, therefore, by the proliferation of erotic images in the media after 1994.

One way to capture sex's changing construction over the course of the twentieth century is through the shifting vocabulary used to denote sexual anatomy. Elderly informants I interviewed typically used phrases like *inkomo* (cow) for a woman's genitalia. This reference to (*ilobolo*) cattle evokes the strong connection between women's bodies and kinship, since a woman with a baby would attract a lower ilobolo payment (similarly Zuma used the term "father's cattle kraal" for a woman's genitalia during his rape trial).

Today, a woman's genitalia may still be politely spoken of as *inkomo*, but young people are more likely to use the words *ikhekhe* (cake), *iGold*, or *iEighteen*—the latter is a reference to a soccer pitch's eighteen-yard box, and connotes scoring a goal.[10] Similarly, whereas sexual intercourse was denoted in the past through the verb *ukulala* (to sleep) or *ukuya ocansini* (to go to the grass mat), a word used today is *ukubhebha*, which is typically translated into English as "to fuck." These terms, which are used by women as well as men, indicate that sex is involved less with the bringing together of two families and more with a woman's sense of self—or a man's wish to gain pleasure from a woman's body.

Yet despite its widespread association with individual freedom, sex today holds an ambiguous position in the lives of many South Africans—it is a site of pleasure by right, a thing to exchange for necessities, and a site of intense gendered violence. I consider the two latter points in much greater detail in the following two chapters.

In line with the messages of AIDS campaigns, many women I knew insisted that they used rights in the now more distinct domain of sex to protect themselves from the risks of sex or to demand more sexual pleasure. Regarding the first of these, many young women said that in principle they had a right, especially in a time of AIDS, to use condoms, even if men often denied them this right. I was not therefore surprised to find that surveys subsequently reported rising condom usage over the 2000s. In 2003 my research assistant and I spoke with three women in their twenties in Sundumbili township; their words reflect a sense that the domain of sex is subject to new egalitarian discourses—if, as we shall see, this must always be qualified.

> Nonhlanhla (research assistant): Do you use condoms with your boyfriends, or only if you sleep with someone else besides your [main] boyfriend?
>
> Nelisiwe: I don't use condoms with the father of my baby, for I know what he does. With the others I am strict about using them.
>
> MH: If you compare people from the past and today, which generation used condoms the most?
>
> Nobantu: People today are used to the idea of wearing a condom. Even boys don't have that much problem anymore; they expect a girl to protect herself.

MH: Why is that?

Gugulethu: It's because they see how the situation around them is.
We listen to radio and hear that the rate [of AIDS] is high.

Statements such as these indicate a growing acceptance of condoms in
an era of high HIV prevalence and modern notions of gender equality. But
although they seem to suggest that a woman's right to protect her body from
potentially harmful secretions is being recognized, women can rarely do so on
their own terms. For instance, Nelisiwe's ability to use a condom with a "secondary" lover is strengthened by the fact that she does not use one with the
father of her child. She is therefore exerting not an abstract individual right,
but one formed in relation to moral obligations that she has to her primary
lover. The backdrop to these multiple sets of obligations, discussed at length
later, is that intimate relations can be both the site of pleasure and a critical
means of securing men's material support.

Turning to pleasure, sex today is not without "shame," as if Christian
ideas of the "body as the temple of God" have been forgotten. New discourses, including those of rights, can be employed to partially overcome
"shame." Young people I knew spoke fairly openly about how, in principle at
least, sex should be enjoyed by both men and women. Most saw this equality
as relatively new and linked it to the coming of democracy. As we saw earlier,
this is not true: until the early twentieth century both men and women might
have multiple partners with whom they engaged in "thigh sex" (ukusoma).
Moreover, the word *ukuromensa*, derived from the English term "romance,"
emerged in the twentieth century to mean "to engage in foreplay" (with penis-
vagina sex here the symbolic end act). Indeed, most elderly informants I spoke
with stressed that Christianity and literacy brought a sense of equality in certain spheres of intimate relations: an increase in mutual foreplay, I was told
many times, accompanied new romantic bonds that were symbolized by the
demise of polygamy.

But the allure of democracy can help to position equality in intimacy as
a post-apartheid phenomenon. Many young people I spoke with discussed
"new" practices such as oral sex (*ukumunca* is the verb used, meaning literally "to suck") and new sexual "styles," often said to be learnt from racy T.V.
programs. And most young people I know told me that women, as well as
men, demand sexual pleasure today. As one twenty-three-year-old woman
from the township put it, "I am not a cow; when I start, I do romance" (i.e.,
she and her partner engaged in mutual stimulation before intercourse). In the
jondolo settlement, I heard a group of women discussing the naturalness of

sexual desire, saying, "I just don't believe a woman who says she abstains." These women used the word *ushukela* (sugar) to refer to sex. Like sugar, sex is a pleasure, but it has the potential to rot the body. The idea that a woman who enjoys sex is "loose" (an isifebe) still exists—but it is countered by new narratives of intimate equality.

AIDS campaigners often say that it is taboo to talk about sex in African culture. Leaving aside questions of what exactly is meant by the word "sex," intimate bodily relations have often been discussed graphically in the past.[11] These discussions, however, tended to be limited to single-sex age groups (i.e., they did not cross gender or generational hierarchies). Today the language of rights and new forms of sex talk seem to have disturbed gendered and generational lines of authority denoted by the concept of hlonipha (respect).

As an example of this, one day I was sitting with a good friend, Bongi, then in her early thirties, and others in a shack in Isithebe. (I say much more about Bongi's life in chapter 7.) She turned to me and asked if it was true that whites had anal sex. As I tried to explain whites' exotic sexual practices, various other people came into the shack. One man in his fifties entered and overheard us using the words *ucansi* (penetrative sex, literally a grass sleeping mat) and *emuva* (behind). There is no simple word for anal sex in isiZulu and, not having heard Bongi begin the discussion by using the English term, he presumed we were talking about penetrative vaginal sex from behind. "Of course I know about that," he said, to the amused glances of three or four younger women and me. When he found out we were talking about anal sex, he screamed in disgust at white peoples' sexual antics.

Certainly, few people I know would doubt that more forthright sex talk has become common after apartheid. The following love letter from a twenty-four-year-old woman to her boyfriend of the same age, written in English, shows how the writer positions herself as a sexual subject who is deeply in love.[12] It also reveals that marriage, although rare, still plays a powerful role in romantic discussions that include sex. For her, sex is an expression of love—but this must not be taken for granted: the love that she embraces, and perhaps the womanhood she aspires to, depend on her boyfriend marrying her in the future.

> Dear Sweetheart,
>
> It's a pleasure to me to write this letter to you. I just want to let you know how much you mean to me baby. I love you like crazy since the first day I lay my eyes to you for better I love you, for worse I love you, in joy I love you, in sorrow I love you. I love you where you are. And about last night thank you I can't forget it you make me feel like a natural woman. Baby you do satisfy me especially in bed you like 'o'

I can't say it I can't describe it. But I love u for it and always when I'm not with you I keep missing you honey I wish to sleep next to you all the time. If I am a men I would ask you to marry me because I don't want to loose you sweety . . . you are the men of my dreams

Always love you !!!
Always miss you !!!
Please don't stop loving me
Take care
All my love

Right 2: The Right to Consume

Discussing popular culture after apartheid, Deborah Posel argues that there has been an explosion of discourses on sex, or a "politicization of sexuality." Consumption, she notes, is a key sphere for this: "Sex is consumed," she says, "at the same time as consumption is sexualized."[13] This association is not unprecedented. In the 1950s, sexy images of black women were widely used to promote beauty creams and other merchandise in magazines and newspapers aimed at black South Africans; actress Dolly Rathebe was "the country's most photographed, bikini-clad, black pin-up."[14]

Yet democracy unleashed a powerful new wave of sexualized advertising images connected to—indeed formative of—meanings of freedom. In Mandeni, this consumer impulse is most evident in Sundumbili township, which I consider here. In this space media connections, including to the It girls, are the most dense, and average incomes are higher than in the rural and informal areas. Young township women today frequently claim the "right to consume." Or, to put this "right" in a more textured way: historically rooted moral claims and modern notions of liberal "rights" intersect to give women a sense that they *should* benefit from consumer goods. But this intersection is thick with revealing contradictions and tensions.

In the 1960s, when the township was built, a husband's salary could purchase furniture and other items for a four-room house. From the 1970s, a wave of "industrial women" earned salaries in Isithebe's fast-multiplying factories. These factories engendered new ways of becoming a woman. They enabled women to move from their family homes and gain some control over the sphere of consumption.

Today, *uzendazamshiya* is an emotive term for a woman passed over by suitors, who remains unmarried in her family home (the verb *ukushiya* means "to leave behind").[15] Such women used to be a minority, an exception. But plummeting marriage rates and the high price of housing now mean that many township women in their twenties and thirties still live with family members. Being an uzendazamshiya is certainly more acceptable now than in the past—indeed a young woman's friends are rarely themselves married. But being left behind in a family home means that a woman becomes disappointed with her life because she so openly fails to traverse the path from girlhood to womanhood through either wedlock or working. And even if a woman does leave her township home, she is unlikely to do so to marry. She is more likely to live in a rented room in a house or in an umjondolo. Kipita-ing (cohabiting) is common today, although newspaper columns and letters can still portray the practice as a disgrace (*ihlazo*).[16]

One reason why being an uzendazamshiya is intensely painful is that intergenerational social mobility has historically been reflected in working women's buying things for their mothers. This dynamic was brought starkly home to me when I interviewed a mission-schooled grandmother who had been employed as a domestic worker for many years. Her daughter now works as a teacher, and her granddaughter became an executive of a large private company after attending a Model C (former white) school. Each reached a social peak in the racially and gender-stratified labor market of her day, and each was encouraged, especially by her mother, to progress to do better than her mother had. In turn, each helped to raise her mother's standard of living. This expectation of advancement means that a woman who fails to attract ilobolo or earn an income can feel herself to be a failure and be seen as a failure. Instead she is left behind as an uzendazamshiya, dependent on her family in a world of upside-down obligations.[17]

So how can we reconcile what appears to be a quickening beat of consumption across South Africa with the great poverty of much of its population? Exploring the site of consumption provides some starting points. The domestic femininity that characterized the township wives of SAPPI men in the 1960s is still reflected today in the pinafores this group can wear in the home and in the coffee tables, room dividers, kitchen products, television sets, and music systems that are commonly found in "matchbox" houses; in many cases, better-off families have even added several extra rooms or a garage to their house. This is not to say that consumption aimed at the body was not important to women in those years. Cosmetics and clothing have certainly long been markers of distinction. And yet, with high marriage rates in the township, a well-kept home became formative of a married woman's identity.

In contrast, young women today are virtually all unmarried. They typically live in an umjondolo or an overcrowded family house. Relatively uninvested in a project of home building, women can instead spend disposable money (whether acquired through work, through child support or other grants, or from boyfriends) on fashion items such as clothes or, in the words of Sarah Nutall, on "stylizing the self."[18] Women will invariably be expected to spend some of their disposable income on items such as food for the household. But this is usually seen as *maintaining* rather than *building* a home.

Thembi, a young woman from the Sundumbili area, described in 2000 the pressure to follow fashion in the public sphere: "You are nothing if you do not have fashion. I am scared to even leave the house; if you don't have something to wear people laugh at you, they point at you and say, 'Look what she is wearing.'" In the township, mocking fun is sometimes made of residents who shop at *emukrosini* (the crossroads), a market adjacent to the nearby Isithebe Industrial Park that is held on Fridays and sells cheap items, including second-hand clothes, mostly to the migrant employees of Isithebe's factories.

In a climate of wealth amid poverty, the body becomes both a focal point for consumption and a source of consumption, including from boyfriends. The story of twenty-three-year-old Thandi, who lived on the outskirts of Sundumbili township, illustrates how a sexualized femininity helps to refashion a woman's body and, in turn, how intimate relations can become a means to attain fashion items. Because her mother worked, Thandi had some income, unlike many women who migrated from rural areas to Mandeni. However, since her mother's salary was low (she was then employed in a poorly paying clothing firm that had just cut salaries) Thandi's sexual partners, attracted by her sense of style, served both to support the household and to provide consumption goods. She spoke in 2001 of having three boyfriends who gave her money, clothes, and groceries and emphasized that she had multiple partners because she had many needs: "To dress, I don't work, a cell-phone . . . doing my hair so that I am beautiful for my boyfriends, they won't love an ugly person."

Fashion items modify the body, but alcohol consumption, which has been rising among young women, can alter it in more immediate ways. Indeed, alcohol captures particularly well how rights, the body, and intimacy have become connected in new ways after apartheid—and the dangerous consequences of this linkage. In the early period of the township, the 1960s and 1970s, shebeens (illegal drinking places usually run by women in houses or shacks) and a beer hall (a public drinking space established by the state) generally catered to working men. The small number of female patrons gained a quick reputation as izifebe (loose women, or prostitutes). Today, a new breed of shebeens aimed at youth have emerged across Sundumbili. And these "joints" stock an array of drinks aggressively marketed to women, such as

Redd's cider. Almost as many women as men visit these new youth shebeens; women now have the "right" to celebrate freedom and enjoy loud music and new dance styles—and equally to drown life's stresses in alcohol. And most of my friends from Sundumbili draw strong connections between youth shebeens, alcohol consumption, and sexual encounters.

Right 3: The Right to Live without a Man

Throughout the twentieth century both white and African patriarchs conspired to keep women under the authority of men. They failed: from the birth of the first towns there were always some women who lived independently of male patrons. But in the 1980s a new wave of rural- and sometimes urban-born women moved into informal settlements. Some think that the new word "umjondolo," meaning roughly "shack," evolved from the word "umjendevu," a spinster, and this association suggests that gender relations and meanings were being reorganized as a growing number of women lived without male patrons. Adding to this upheaval in gender norms, legal changes in the 1980s granted women certain property rights, making it easier for them to access housing in urban areas. And in the post-apartheid period, for the first time, a large number of single women gained access to low-cost RDP housing provided by the state.

But—and this is the key paradox—these new rights have been bestowed on women just as many single women are growing more economically dependent on men. This is most seen in Mandeni in the jondolo settlement, where a clear link, probably the most obvious in the area and for this reason worth emphasizing, presents itself between women's economic standing, their access to housing, and their approaches to men. And Isithebe's women live in the shadows of not only Isithebe's disappearing factories but the "industrial women" who in the 1980s gained some economic independence through factory work.

In 2004, I asked a young neighbor of mine in his early twenties to conduct a small door-to-door survey of fifty Isithebe imijondolo, roughly half rented principally by men and half by women. Virtually all of the women renting their own umjondolo turned out to be employed in factories. Most chose to live alone, although they often had boyfriends who slept over some nights. In contrast, the majority of the men who rented an umjondolo said that they lived with dependent girlfriends; from them they got sex, companionship, and help with domestic activities such as cleaning and cooking. The women who lived with these men were typically the newest to the area and had the most difficulty securing formal work. These findings, consistent with research in many settings, confirm that women who have access to employment and housing have more power to navigate intimate relations with men.[19]

The social meanings of housing were further brought to life in a discussion I had in 2006 with three young women, Zethu, Thabile, and Dumi (two sisters and a cousin), who share a small umjondolo about three minutes' walk from mine. The very fact that three women share one tiny umjondolo itself reflects the contradictions of the housing sphere; housing is, in theory, a constitutional right, but access to it is often compromised by economic realities.

Strewn across the top of the jondolo's concrete blocks are rough planks of timber that hold in place a corrugated steel roof. From the timber hangs a light, with plastic tape binding the dangerous strands of an electric cable. Squashed inside their umjondolo is a double bed, a wardrobe, a refrigerator, a large collection of cosmetics, and a two-burner stove. On the floor are large bags of sugar, flour, and cornmeal. Hanging on the wall is a poster of Beyoncé (the lead singer of the band Destiny's Child), a picture of another attractive young lady with the caption "too sexy for my age," and a photograph of one of the women's baby girls (who is being looked after by relatives at the woman's rural home). The whole umjondolo is approximately ten by fifteen feet.

The three relatives work in local clothing factories; each earns about R100 a week, and they split the R70 monthly rent between them. One of their priorities is to send money back every month to their rural-based families; they also visit "home" many times during the year. Born and raised in a rural area approximately two hours north of Isithebe, they have many complaints about the place they migrated to: the imijondolo are too small, pit latrines smell ghastly, queues for water are long, mosquitoes are too plentiful, and salaries are low. When I ask why they share a single umjondolo, they explain the temptations women, especially new arrivals, face if they do not stick together. "Some come, they don't know anyone, they see a man on the road and go with him."

The three women elaborated on their profound cynicism about men. Zethu stated boldly, to the nods of the others, "They are not good . . . they are not truthful." Everyone laughed. "They fight you about every small thing that is wrong. They want food, everything, and they drink too much alcohol. Living alone is better. Boyfriends confuse you. It is better that they visit." The women express a dominant theme among working women in the jondolo settlement: men are needed for companionship, sex, fatherhood, and sometimes financial support, yet they can frequently *hlupha* (disturb) women by, for instance, having other girlfriends, taking their money, trying to control them, and putting them at risk of catching AIDS. Thabile comically described how a suitor came to her one day with a borrowed suit and a Bible to convince her of his good character. Sharing a tiny umjondolo prevented these three women from falling into dependence on men, like many new arrivals to the area.

Right 4: The Right to Children

The new government's introduction of a child support grant in 1998 was surrounded by controversy. Young women, some critics argued, would get pregnant just to gain access to this small monthly stipend. This prejudiced view was quickly rebutted by researchers.[20] But the opposite view—that childbirth is completely separate from the reality of making a living—is equally unjustifiable. More accurate is the statement that children and childbirth are immersed in complex material and emotional worlds, a tension that needs to be explored from the perspective of women themselves. Indeed, many young women see themselves as having certain rights over childbirth and their children in matters from contraception to the naming of a child. Let me give some historical context before elaborating on this point.

The twentieth century witnessed the coming together of a number of powerful forces that reduced fertility levels: agricultural labor declined in importance, Christianity became more influential and promoted the nuclear family, contraception became more widely used, and, after 1994, abortions became available in state hospitals. The decline in fertility rates appears to have begun in the 1960s, and it received a sharp boost in the 1970s when the state introduced an ambitious family planning program aimed at stemming the "black peril."[21] In the 1970s, African women gave birth to an average of six children; by 1998 this figure had halved, and by 2003 it had fallen further.[22]

Although male condoms afford lovers very good protection from sexually transmitted infections, they have not been a favored form of contraception in South Africa. When the apartheid government introduced population control in the 1970s, it encouraged the use of contraceptive injections (especially Depo-Provera) that gave no protection against STIs. Some women thought that such injections were convenient and, in addition, allowed them to conceal birth control use from partners and family members. The country's 2003 Demographic and Health Survey found that among sexually active women aged fifteen to nineteen, 44 percent used injectable contraceptives, compared to 17 percent who used the male condom.[23] It was only later in the 2000s that condom use increased significantly: a study conducted in 2008 found that 62.4 percent of South Africans over fifteen years old had used a condom in their last act of penetrative sex.[24]

Another noteworthy feature of South Africa's fertility decline is the unusually long times between births, compared to other countries. Demographic studies have shown that the median birth interval is now greater than five years; one report notes, "Often, women would appear to use contraception to delay childbearing until some distant and uncertain point in the future."[25] Of course, it is rare, in South Africa and elsewhere, for married couples to space children by five years. But these "uncertain" points and resultant staggered births are consistent with the changing political economy and geography of intimacy outlined earlier. This is marked by predominantly non-marital and sometimes multiple concurrent relationships, as well as significant levels of geographical movement.

While conducting research in rural Hlabisa, KwaZulu-Natal, Thembeka Mngomezulu and I rather accidently gained a window into negotiations around childbirth when discussing the naming of children born to unmarried parents. The Africa Centre, with which we were affiliated, provided us with detailed information about the occupants of each household we visited. We were not surprised to find that the surnames of children often differed from the mother's; however, we expected that the reason for this was because the father had paid ilobolo or inhlawulo (a fine for illicit pregnancy), giving him rights over his child. The reality was murkier.

To explain, I need to give some more historical background. In the early twentieth century, ilobolo ensured that certain rights to a child were transferred to the father's family (signified by the child's adoption of the father's *isibongo*, clan name). Over the course of the century, as premarital pregnancy became more common, just paying inhlawulo typically became enough for a child to take a father's surname. Today, a number of fathers I know vigorously oppose their daughter's child taking its father's surname if the man has not paid inhlawulo. Yet we found in Hlabisa (and I found elsewhere too) that even if inhlawulo was not paid, the daughter generally supported her child being given its father's surname. For instance, the mother might be a Mhlongo, but the child and father would be Mkhizes. Though some women did not want the child to take its father's name, in general young women appeared more likely than their parents to want to name their child after its father.

The giving of a child's surname is invariably closely tied up with maintaining good relations with amadlozi, or the ancestors, whose wrath can affect the child's health. This can justify both naming a child after its father and not doing so. A man who has not paid inhlawulo has not (yet) upheld tradition; yet to refuse to give the child his father's surname is also to neglect tradition.

These intense spiritual discussions, however, overlap with the material consequences of naming a child. In particular, if a child takes its father's surname, the mother is better able to make claims on the father and his family. If the child becomes a Mkhize, the mother has claims on the Mkhizes for various forms of support.[26]

Also inseparable from these dilemmas—ones that etch social change into a person's very name—is women's often strong emotional attachment to the father of a child (*ubaba wengane*). These men are often positioned as "main" (as opposed to secondary) boyfriends, and women have greater hopes of marrying them, or at least staying in the relationship for a long time. The wish to maintain a relationship with the father of a child (especially the first child) is one reason why having children with more than one sexual partner has more negative consequences for women than men. Of course, love is nothing if it is not unpredictable, and circumstances often mean that the father and mother lose contact; yet women's approaches to love and sexual relations—including the use of condoms, which also offer protection against STIs—cannot be separated from their attitudes toward childbirth and children's social construction. And the politics of naming suggest that younger women themselves are influencing changes in practices in ways revealing of wider processes.

To bring these points together—and much more will be said about condom use and main/secondary lovers in chapter 9—although statistics show a dramatic drop over time, fertility is still important to the meaning of womanhood. The scornful word *inyumba* (barren woman) indicates the emphasis that society places on childbirth. But seismic changes are hidden behind the general proposition that fertility has a high status. In the early twentieth century a barren woman could watch the ilobolo cattle given for her being ignominiously returned to her father's homestead. Childbirth stirred emotions and molded femininities, but it did so partly because of the links between families it represented. Today, childbirth takes place within new kinds of intimate relations, ones where marriage is rare and contraception has given women more control over having children—the ability to separate sex from childbirth.

Put in still another way, at the beginning of the twentieth century a predominantly agrarian society was led by male heads of households and ilobolo was closely tied to women's fertility. But by the end of the century women had greater control over their children, albeit in a period characterized by labor market insecurity, new forms of geographical mobility, and a decline of marriage. These forces drive a different set of tensions around children and sex. Men can abandon children and frequently do, and yet contraception has given women the ability to covertly control their fertility. Women make new claims on men's families by giving their surnames to their children but, in doing so, can put themselves in conflict with their own fathers. Children can create enduring links of love and obligation between lovers, though this frequently does not happen. For a young unmarried woman in modern-day South Africa, children are very much part of "making a living."

Right 5: The Right to Multiple Male Lovers

I turn now to a key paradox of "AIDS and rights" discourses: some women are using the language of "rights" to argue that now they—just like men—are entitled to have multiple concurrent partners. Men are unreliable, they say, and so why should women not have many boyfriends? While the It girls are able to embark on this path from a position of economic independence, this is typically not the case for poorer women.

In the early twentieth century, as I noted in chapter 3, migrant labor and Christianity reshaped masculinities and femininities to give men a greater entitlement than women to multiple partners. Today, "isifebe" is still a very insulting term used to deride "loose" women. But some women claim forthrightly that their poor economic circumstances and men's unreliability gives them a greater right than they had in the past to have multiple partners. In a climate where men fail to marry or support women, narratives of modern rights bring into sharp relief the hypocrisy of men's double standard for multiple partners.

Central to women's claims to the right to plural lovers is the tremendous sense of conflict that dominates relations between men and women. I've heard young women say, "I have more than one boyfriend because I was annoyed when I caught him [being unfaithful] for the first time, so I thought, let me find myself another lover." Others explained that "the majority [of women] do it because they say, 'you can't stand on one foot.'" A twenty-two-year-old township woman put it like this: "It is your right because he doesn't give me anything, he didn't pay inhlawulo for our child." In Bongi's sewing room in the jondolo settlement, I heard one self-employed woman joke to a visiting male friend twenty years her senior, "You only have one ugwayi [penis]; how can you have more than one girlfriend?"[27] As these comments show, women today use the language of equality to challenge men's sole entitlement to multiple partners in revealing, sometimes comical, ways.

In a climate of acute gender tensions, few men will not have heard women calling multiple boyfriends their "ministers of finance, transport, and entertainment" (more common in the township) or saying that they have "one for

money, one for food, and one for rent" (more common in the informal settlement). Even if women usually do not call their lovers by these terms to their
faces, the language circulates widely. Here, men are objectified as providers of
gifts that merely meet women's material needs: missing from relationships, it
is implied, is men's more enduring and public commitment to women—one
symbolized by ilobolo. The phrases therefore constitute a kind of sardonic
play by women on men's inability to fully enact provider love by giving ilobolo
and supporting a wife. Such comments also retaliate for the objectifying terms
that men use to describe women, such as *icherry* for a girlfriend.

Condemning young men's unreliability, young women can turn to older,
richer men for support. Despite media representations of sugar daddies as
predatory, I found it revealing that many young women seemed to view these
men as respectable patrons and contrasted them favorably to younger men,
who were typically unemployed.[28] When sugar daddies are spoken about in
Mandeni, they are invariably closely associated with men who work at the
SAPPI paper mill, the firm that launched Sundumbili as a company town.
SAPPI men, as we saw, were the first to secure housing in the township and
gained the status of respectable "founding fathers." Some SAPPI men are
undoubtedly sugar daddies, but the connection between sugar daddies and
SAPPI men also exists because the firm represents everything young men,
most of whom are unemployed, cannot provide to women.

In 2003 I discussed sugar daddies with three women in their early twenties: Busi, Philile, and Sindile. They launched a tirade against men of their age,
who they said were philanderers and unable or unwilling to support women.
But when I began to ask about sugar daddies, the mood in the room took a
more positive turn. "Old men who like [to have relationships with] children,"
the women said almost simultaneously.

"Why do women have sugar daddies?" I asked.

"*Awu*, they give a lot of money," Busi replied.

"Are there many in the area?" I asked.

"Ohh, too much, many at SAPPI," Philile said.

The other two women chimed in with another reason to have a sugar
daddy: "If you kiss him and he is satisfied, he won't grab you like a little boy."
Busi had actually been involved with a sugar daddy for four years; they met
from time to time, and he bought her clothes and even medicine when she was
ill. In addition to her sugar daddy, Busi also had a younger, and poorer, lover.

Another young woman put the advantages of sugar daddies to me in
an even more straightforward way: "Why use a pencil when you can use
a Bic?"

The Good Woman, Re-inventing Tradition

If all periods of history produce conflicts between men and women, democracy in South Africa brewed a specific cocktail of tensions: new narratives of gender equality clashed with chronic unemployment that rendered many young men unreliable. Nevertheless, not all women are openly hostile to young men. Questions of love will receive attention later; for now, I note that some "traditions" retain great, if always reworked, worth.

One day in 2003, I was sitting in Bongi's shack in the informal settlement. Sewing machines purred as the seamstresses made school uniforms and other clothes on special order. Mthunzi, one of the seamstresses, was being lobola'd for the standard amount of eleven cattle, although I inferred from her complaints about men that she was unsure about her boyfriend's commitment to her, as he had only paid the equivalent of a few cattle. I was chatting about the high cost of ilobolo. "What did people think about it?" I asked. Mthunzi replied, "Even R3,000 is enough, because today people don't have money."

Since R15,000–R25,000 is a more common cash equivalent for ilobolo cattle, I pushed the women: "Would you marry someone for R3,000?"

Mthunzi replied, "I don't know. Oh, for so little money, *hhayi, hhayi* ["no, no"]."

I asked, "Who do you know that paid that?"

She replied, "Oh, Bongani [a friend], he paid R3,000 in secret. It was a family thing, it was a shame, *hawu, hawu, hawu.* . . . [I would want] at least R5,000 . . . unless he fills a big house with everything."

Even if these women agree that ilobolo should be reduced (though they are more enthusiastic about this being done for other women than for themselves) they, like most women from Mandeni, vigorously defended ilobolo. Over the course of the twentieth century this payment came to be seen as a sign of love, because of the sacrifices and pain a man endured to marry his girlfriend. Being lobola'd raises a woman's status in ways that simply have no comparison. Indeed, young women still consider finding a good husband to be of paramount importance, even if it means that substantial payments go mainly to their families in the form of ilobolo rather than directly to them.[29]

Certainly, the vast majority of women I knew in Mandeni said that they wished to find a man to pay ilobolo and marry them—although most wanted wedlock to be on more equal terms than it was for their mothers' generation. In 2003, I chatted with three women in their early twenties in the township house of my research assistant, Nonhlanhla. The conversation revolved around the advantages and disadvantages of a 50/50 relationship with a man. All three young women espoused gender equality, but MaBongi rejected the language of 50/50 and preferred to see herself as subordinate to a future husband—providing, that is, that she was allowed to work:

> Ntombifuthi: Me, if I marry, I want to work like him; everything will be 50/50.
>
> MaBongi: Me, if I marry, I want to get a person who works like me, we help each other; but the way we help each other is not 50/50, but 50/25.
>
> Nonhlanhla: Why do you only want 25?
>
> MaBongi: The man [she used the word "ubaba," literally "father," a respectful term for a man] is above you, and it is necessary I am always below.
>
> MH (to Ntombifuthi): Why don't you want that?
>
> Ntombifuthi: It is because if you are under him, he wants you to do whatever he wants. . . . He will end up asking you to leave work, saying, "Stay at home, 'cause you think you are clever."

One reason why MaBongi only wants a 50/25 marital relationship may be that she will be able to make demands on her husband on the grounds that he is the head of the household. A household head is typically expected to provide for and protect a wife and their children. Such ideals, forged by capitalism, are usually interpreted as being associated with past "traditions." But the devotion that is often required of a woman who accepts a man's patronage is very much a part of navigating relationships in the modern world.

Once upon a time in Sundumbili township a good man, Nhlanhla, and a good woman, Nomusa, got engaged. (I knew Nomusa reasonably well, and it is from her that I heard this story.) Nomusa, in her early twenties, lived in her family home in Sundumbili and saw herself as a good woman, the antithesis of an isifebe. Her body manifested her self-respect: neatly clothed and not too sexually suggestive, it reflected her Christian upbringing and reasonably comfortable background but also her attempt to shape it through "bodily labor."[30]

Nomusa's mother was a quiet lady and remained faithful despite her husband's philandering. Nomusa's sisters, one a teacher and one a nurse, were doing well and helped Nomusa financially. The teacher and her husband even had enough income to buy themselves a house in the former white suburb of Mandini. Nomusa's confident but respectful attitude toward men paid off, because she was widely seen to have landed a good man. However, she had some sympathy for other women who had multiple boyfriends; she too might have followed that path if things had worked out differently.

The "goodness" that led the couple to recognize each other's sincerity was embedded in years of "bodily labor" but not in circumstances of the body's own making, and their life paths were unpredictable. It is stories like this one, whose protagonists live "happily ever after," that legitimize narratives of love and show female township residents that not all men are bad and that it is possible to secure a "good man." In order to do so, women are typically required to partially reject the "sexualized femininity" associated with dominant youth culture, adopting instead practices associated with hlonipha (respect). Before returning to the story of Nomusa and Nhlanhla, I want to give a few examples of ways that women can present themselves as being of good character.

Virginity testing is a practice whereby older women inspect a young woman's hymen. Until recently, it had been in decline. My purpose is not to explore its reinvention at the time of the AIDS pandemic, or human rights groups' opposition to it on the grounds that women's and children's rights are being violated by "culture."[31] Instead, I am interested in how it creates a space in which women can perform rituals of bodily purity and call forth notions of hlonipha (respect). In Sundumbili township in 2002, the charismatic MaMfundisi, wife of the priest, organized a virginity testing ceremony at the church where her husband preached; as we have seen, Christian and "traditional" efforts at controlling women's purity are deeply entangled. MaMfundisi is one of Sundumbili's most vigorous opponents of sex-positive AIDS prevention messages (e.g., "sex is okay, just use a condom"). She told me that young people in the township were "sex mad."

It was a warm summer day in 2002. In the front courtyard of the church, the virgins—aged, I estimated, between ten and twenty—were encouraged to *ukusina*, or perform "traditional" Zulu dances. The group chanted, moving rhythmically from one foot to another in a circle, until one girl entered the center, danced, and ended by swinging her leg high over her head—a move that characterizes Zulu dancing.

Aware that traditional dances had a somewhat limited appeal in the township, the church had also hired a DJ who periodically blasted pop music in the courtyard of the church to sustain the youths' interest. The relatively quiet clapping and singing that accompanied the traditional dancing was therefore periodically drowned out when the DJ blasted out the love song of the moment, Mafikizolo's "Ndihamba Nawe" (I Go with You). Only then did the occasion feel like a party, as participants and onlookers erupted into more animated dancing.

As the crowd grew in numbers, one could almost feel different meanings of the body collide at this public event. The virgins danced bare-breasted as a sign of their piety and respect for the tradition of virginity testing. Yet just outside the church's grounds was a line of teenage male onlookers whose body language suggested that they read the flesh in a more sexualized way.

That men's virginity is not valued in the same way as women's speaks to how "the girl's active desire . . . is the intended object of control here."[32] And inspection of a women's hymen is, of course, an imperfect way of investigating her virginity. But virginity testing can help women reposition their bodies as chaste and respectful—wipe clean the slate of bodily image. This was apparent the morning after the ceremony, when I attended a Sunday service organized by the same church. Several hundred people packed into the church to watch fifty or so women be invited up to the stage to receive certificates of virginity. The mood was that of a graduation ceremony; once received, the certificates were proudly clutched to the chests of their smiling recipients.

The virginity certificate publicly signaled the women's chastity, but its validity could also be challenged. Several months later, I interviewed an elderly resident in the township. Her daughter asked to see me in private. She had noticed me at the virginity testing ceremony and, in hushed tones, told me that some of the "virgins" had actually had full sexual relations with men. She seemed to be outraged because the women were beating the system, cheating to get a badge of virginity when in fact they were just as bad as everyone else.

There are other ways to mark the body as chaste and pure at a time when residents are, in the words of MaMfundisi, "sex mad." The annual Zulu reed dance—in which hundreds of virgins parade in front of the Zulu king—attempts to re-associate Zuluness with women's purity. Yet, in a sign of the power and speed of the global image industry, scandal hit the ceremony when photographs of bare-breasted virgins were discovered on Internet pornography sites.[33] Women also present themselves as respectful by worshiping at the popular Shembe church—in the hope, some say rather jokingly, of finding a man who would take them as a second or subsequent wife (polygamy is allowed by this African initiated church). All of these examples show that bodily practices, styles, and knowledges, although partly unconscious, can in certain circumstances be redirected so that a woman can position herself as a "good woman" of pious, and thus marriageable, character.

We return to the love story. Nomusa's good man, Nhlanhla, was tall and in his early thirties. He had a quiet demeanor, and appeared somewhat aloof from other men. Born in a rural area, Nhlanhla did not drink, was a Christian, and worked as a "backyard" car mechanic. On one occasion he sealed the leaks in my car that had amused residents for months (when it rained heavily, my feet and head got drenched, so I had to wear a coat with a hood while driving). He was quiet and unassuming, and his sometimes shy demeanor partially insulated him from masculine practices that could burn disposable income, such as drinking, womanizing, and spending money on flashy consumer items. He sacrificed these trappings of masculinity for the long-term goal of marrying, preserving the resources to pay ilobolo over time.

When they were becoming interested in each other, Nhlanhla and Nomusa each spent months collecting snippets of information about the other from mutual acquaintances. Before they were formally dating or had had penetrative sexual relations, he came with the *abakhongi* (negotiators) to see her father and pay imvulamlomo (the fee paid to begin ilobolo negotiations). The negotiations centered not on the amount of ilobolo to be granted—eleven cattle was the set amount, since she did not have a child and, even more, was a virgin—but on its cash equivalent. Over the course of a long day, the two families discussed the exact value of each cow and arrived at an overall figure of around R38,500, two cattle being valued at R5,000, two at R4,500, two at R4,000, one each at R3,000 and R2,500, and three at R2,000.[34] Nhlanhla paid R13,000 immediately.

After this meeting, Nomusa spent more time with Nhlanhla, and he worked tirelessly to save for the rest of the ilobolo. He paid a second installment of R10,000 after roughly nine months, leaving the cash equivalent of three cows remaining. The two lovers then moved into an umjondolo in the township. The temporary umjondolo, part of a group of eight imijondolo in the backyard of a township house, was not a place they particularly liked living, but it gave them some freedom. Here they had a place for their own furniture and could develop their own relationship. Nomusa told me that she liked not only Nhlanhla's respect for tradition but also his modernity. She was willing to cook and clean for him and happy to abide by his preference that she not wear trousers; in turn, when they parented a child, she was proud to say that he changed its nappies. Occasionally he even cooked, like a good modern man.

Although Nhlanhla was unable to save enough money for a wedding ceremony, and the couple remained engaged for the several years that I knew them, his ilobolo payment elevated his status to that of an *umkhwenyana* (roughly, fiancé). Ultimately he became a man whom other men I knew respected. However, their relationship was disrupted by a dispute over the sacrosanct agreement they had on mutual fidelity. Nomusa had long told her partner that she would dump him or cheat on him if he betrayed her. But a woman had phoned his cell phone, and Nomusa had answered and drawn the conclusion that he was having an affair. She threatened to leave him, although he insisted that the woman who called had gotten his number from another person. To persuade her of his fidelity, he drank a liter of gasoline and collapsed next to his car with a note declaring his love for her. The choice of gasoline was significant: unlike alcohol, it symbolized his work and not his frivolousness. It powered his battered and frequently malfunctioning car, an item that was crucial to his livelihood and his ability to pay ilobolo. Their relationship stabilized.

I tell this story partly to show that non-marital relationships with several lovers are by no means universal. Even women who speak of having many lovers often recall an earlier stage of life when they hoped to marry a good man. They might be only justifying their current actions, but it would be wrong to assume that long-term relationships—which can take a variety of forms— have been simply abandoned. Indeed, as I show later, even multiple-partnered relationships typically include a main lover on whom the hope of marriage is most likely to rest.

<hr>

If Kuli Roberts speaks for no-nonsense up-and-coming women, a defining feature of middle-class women is their ability to define the terms on which they will interact with men—to have pleasurable sex but, in theory, always "safe sex." Yet one gendered figure that stands symbolically at the other end of the social spectrum is uzendazamshiya—a single woman literally left behind. This is a painful reminder not because all women desire to marry, but because it reflects women's inability to control their intimate lives in the way that dominant narratives of rights describe. Indeed, young women expect something better in their economic and intimate worlds than what their mothers experienced under apartheid.

After 1994, the granting of rights to women became a key aim of activists, and undoubtedly this is an important goal. In particular, a better legal system to address sexual violence could reduce HIV infection rates. But the relationship is complex; rights cannot solve all evils, including backward "traditions." Women, as we saw, can even creatively draw on rights language to argue that they too have the right to multiple partners. And by drawing on this language, women not only challenge men, but sew themselves into the very fabric of dominant masculinities—the topic to which I now turn.

EIGHT

Failing Men:
Modern Masculinities amid Unemployment

I wanted to cry like a bereaved woman. But I am a man. A man never cries. He bows his head and listens to the pain deep inside him. The making of a man is the ability to contain tears even when they try to force their way out.

—SIPHIWO MAHALA, *When a Man Cries*

In November 2004, I started my rusty Mazda and drove toward MaDoris's tavern in Sundumbili township. The warm sun had yet to set; it was still early to go out. Residents sauntered along the narrow pavements, lost in conversation; streets serve as an indispensable point of social interaction in overcrowded townships. I collected three young male friends, all in their early twenties, at a crossroads where they washed and vacuumed cars in exchange for a few rand. In the car, Bheka, Vusa, and Msizi responded to my enquiries about their well-being in a familiar way: *"Awukho umsebenzi"* (There is no work). The only news seemed to be that one mutual friend had gone back to stealing cars. After a pause, Bheka turned to me and said "We are *umnqolo*." The sharp alveolar click of the *q* filled the word with intensity and purpose.

An old meaning of the term "umnqolo" is an unmasculine rural man so timid that he won't even herd cattle. Here, Bheka used the word to describe an unmarried man who lives with his family or, to exaggerate the point, his mother. The ignominy of being a woman of marriageable age but still living with one's family has long been expressed in the figure of "uzendazamshiya" (an unmarried woman, a woman left behind). However, "umnqolo" captures the sense that men too are not progressing in life.

The term "umnqolo" hung in the air as we took in the township's physical geography on our way to the tavern. We weaved through the rows of four-room "matchbox" houses that the SAPPI paper mill had granted to its early male employees. In the 1960s, many men accepted these houses reluctantly, afraid that taking one would signify the abandonment of a rural home. Forty years later, the same houses represent a significant asset. In their courtyards, imijondolo are rented out, usually to young men and women, while spaza shops, small retail establishments, are sometimes built against a house's wall. Some houses have been extended with a garage or an extra room. In the most extravagant remodeling projects, concrete blocks and fresh paint have transformed the original matchbox into an eight-room or larger structure.

We pulled up outside KwaMaDoris Tavern in a narrow street of Chappies, a residential part of the township. I had met the infamous MaDoris during previous visits: upon hearing that a white man was present, she usually invited me to join her in the living room within her house, an offer which I politely declined. The tavern, attached like a noisy limpet to the side of her house, had as its main drinking space a room approximately thirty square meters in size. On one side was a deafening jukebox, on another the bar, on the third men's and women's toilets, and tables and chairs occupied the fourth. Accessible from the courtyard was a slightly quieter two-room extension that joined the other side of the bar through a hatch in the wall. The courtyard served as an overflow for these rooms.

KwaMaDoris's was the most popular of a new wave of township taverns that openly embrace young clients: visitors averaged about twenty years old that night. Men's most common drink was Black Label, a lager marketed to the "working man" because of its strength. "Hot stuff" such as brandy and cola provided a more potent alternative. We sat close to the toilets, and every ten minutes or so a couple would enter them together; Bheka told me that they were mostly just kissing. Unable to hear one another because of the deafening music, we collectively devoured some monstrously good meat and "stiff pap" (cooked cornmeal). Outside, neighbors cursed the loud music. One woman whom I danced with asked, "So what?" when I told her that I had a partner elsewhere. Almost all young township residents link casual sex and drinking to taverns and shebeens.

As the night wore on, the young township dwellers who had come of age in the era of political freedom jived to the tavern's rhythms. A favorite tune that night was Mafikizolo's latest love song, "Emlanjeni" (At the River). Since the jukebox had a shortage of CDs, when a track like this one became popular it was played dozens of times in a night.

Several months later, I returned to the tavern. During a lull in the music, I learnt a surprising fact: Bheka told me, with amusement, that Msizi had just started a relationship with a "sugar mummy," and that woman was MaDoris, the shebeen owner, who was in her fifties. He was her trophy. Tapping into post-apartheid youth culture, she had managed to translate the resulting

income into the bricks, mortar, paint, and furniture of her remodeled house—
and also into the power to attract a much younger man.

"The Pick Is Coming": Drinking in Isithebe Jondolo Settlement

Returning from a night out in the township, I often stopped off at the
tavern run by my adopted family in the jondolo settlement. New regulations
had forced the owner to build a wall to separate his alcohol business from the
adjacent shop. Before this, alcohol and other goods had been sold together.
Working occasionally at this shop prior to the partition, I was able to estimate
that nearly half of all purchases involved liquor: only bread, *amaloose* (loose
cigarettes), mosquito coils in the summer, and candles when the electricity
failed rivaled beer in the volume of their sales.

As in the township, men in the jondolo settlement mostly drank together.
Men tended to buy single quarts (750-milliliter bottles) and share them with
friends. In this setting, male camaraderie gave unemployed men the opportunity to make demands on those with an income; I was sometimes encouraged
to buy a beer and pay for the occasional game of pool.

I saw several differences between the taverns and shebeens I visited in
Sundumbili and those I knew well in Isithebe jondolo settlement. I was not
aware, for a start, of any dedicated youth shebeens or taverns close to where I
stayed in Isithebe. Nor was it common to find women in these drinking places.
Sundumbili township had a more prominent youth culture, whereas residents
of the jondolo settlement were generally a little older and maintained strong
ties to the rural areas they still considered home. Notions of "traditional"
hlonipha (respect) circulated more freely and positioned women who visited
taverns as izifebe (loose women). It was one thing for a woman to work in a
factory and live alone in an umjondolo, but another for her to lose control of
herself through alcohol. Her independence rested on a culture of work and
not one of public partying. Many women I knew from the jondolo settlement
did drink, but they did so in private or in all-female groups, sending children
to the shebeen to buy liquor.

Another difference between the two areas is that large amounts of alcohol are brewed in the jondolo settlement. The most notorious such drink
is a potent home-brew spirit called *isiqatha* or, as it is called locally, *isipikili
siyeza* ("the pick is coming," meaning that the drinker's grave will soon be
dug) or *ukhakhayi lwemfene* ("crown of a baboon," because it makes peoples'
hair fall out). This intoxicating brew is made from brown sugar, brown bread,
yeast, malt, and—rumor has it—battery acid. For R2.50 (US$0.30), a man can

buy a liter of this concoction, get drunk for the whole day, and forget all of his problems. The popularity of this cheap, dangerous cocktail shows that for Isithebe men, most of whom had migrated from declining rural areas, alcohol can signify not political freedom but desperation, an escape from the hardships of everyday life. Men had come to the jondolo settlement for one simple purpose—work. Instead, they found only casual employment, if any, and some women earned a steadier wage than they did.

Masculinities

Today, the quickening pulse of alcohol consumption captures not only young men's new freedoms but also their stresses.[1] Alcohol bestows courage and sometimes leads to violence but, in excess, it can render a man helpless. This dialectic of men's power and failures—one that becomes embodied through the physiological changes resulting from alcohol consumption—is an important entry point into modern masculinities, and I emphasize it throughout this chapter.

How to frame male violence amid poverty is a major dilemma for researchers. Racial stereotypes of violent black men are omnipresent worldwide and negate the violence of racism itself. At the same time, it is not possible to simply blame intimate violence on "apartheid," "poverty," or "emasculation."[2] To navigate this difficult terrain, I consider the profound tensions within today's masculinities alongside the rereading of apartheid gender relations I developed earlier. Apartheid's form of racial rule, I argued, did not simply emasculate men, but worked through the patriarchal home and created patterns of respectability amid plural ideas of manhood. These meanings are reconfigured in the current period of chronic unemployment in varied ways, including in attempts by some men to reassert control over women.

A further thread to my argument is that residents encounter this apartheid past in the spatial practices of everyday life: every step through Sundumbili township's geography bears witness to its planners' fantasy of heterosexual couples living in four-room houses. A rural equivalent to this demasculinizing urban terrain is perhaps the depopulated isibaya, the cattle kraal, that once sat prominently at the center of the umuzi (homestead). The few, if any, cattle in most isibaya today, like the many tiny shacks in which unmarried couples live in urban areas, signify the failure of the work-lobola-marriage path and its ritual and emotional ties.[3]

Multiple expressions of manhood developed on South Africa's turbulent terrain. Powerful forces that shaped manhood include the agrarian economy, the rise and fall of the Zulu Kingdom, colonialism, the anti-apartheid movement, and industrialization. I emphasize here the following somewhat selective contemporary themes: masculinities and growing class inequalities, the changing construction of the isoka (a man with many girlfriends), and men's debates about providing love and fathering children. Finally, I turn to two areas of prominent recent discussion—violence against women and same-sex relations—and try to place these practices in the context of always changing masculinities.

Respectable Masculinities amid Growing Inequalities

Colonial officials, missionaries, business leaders, and employers—in short, those with the most power in the region—were overwhelmingly white men. The emasculating effects of racial hierarchies can still be seen today when some white men, women, and even children refer to African men as boys. Certainly, after a decade and a half of democracy, the reins of economic power in South Africa are still largely held by white men. At the same time, a significant group of black men are now prospering in the democratic era. Like the It girls discussed earlier, they highlight the importance of social class as well as race to modern masculinities.

We take a short diversion from Mandeni to capture this development through a magazine called *BL!NK*, launched in 2004; while few of Mandeni's residents read *BL!NK*, and the magazine folded after only three years, similar images circulate elsewhere in the media. The men depicted in *BL!NK* represented a world of conspicuous consumption, male respectability, and independence from white rule—themes that Thabo Mbeki, South Africa's president from 1999 to 2008, actively promoted through speaking of an "African renaissance" and "black economic empowerment."

According to its twenty-eight-year-old first editor, Siphiwe Mpye, *BL!NK* was established to "paint a new face for the black man," who is associated with "abuse and desertion."[4] The first issue features a cover photo of Zam Nkosi, one of the first black T.V. presenters in the new South Africa, and on page twenty-four he is pictured with a confident smile, wearing a casual white shirt and trousers. One hand holds a newspaper and the other raises a straw hat. Nkosi has what *BL!NK* describes as a "classic cosmopolitan New York–style dress code."[5] He talks passionately to the reporter about changing nappies, and the article suggests that his wife is richer than he is, running her own clothing label.

The *BL!NK* man is not as fit and healthy as the men depicted in *Men's Health*, perhaps his nearest equivalent in the international magazines. However, *Men's Health* has an egalitarian tone to its pages, because even the poorest men can develop a "six-pack." In contrast, the South African *BL!NK* man is more elite. He is a success story of the post-apartheid era, and his status is determined primarily by his wealth and his modern outlook, not his bodily strength or good looks.

The *BL!NK* man's desire for "the rebirth of the true self," as the title of the article on Nkosi puts it, bears clear similarities to the aspirations of the independent "It girls." One difference, however, is that *BL!NK* men need have only wealth, not beautiful bodies as the It girls must. Another is that It girls like Nomakula Roberts can celebrate remaining unmarried and yet sexually active. In contrast, the *BL!NK* man enthusiastically embraces his role as the head of the modern nuclear family. Yet only a minority of black South Africans can enjoy high-paying work, the most important social basis for this masculinity.

A Painful Social Differentiation

Mandeni did not foster the rise of a high-earning black business or professional class; consequently there are few prosperous *BL!NK* men in the area. Nevertheless, the gap between the rich and the poor is larger and, most men would claim, more painful among men than women. When men are without stable work, their ability to become real men—to marry and make certain demands on women and junior men—is threatened.

Labor market changes have created new hierarchies among African men in Mandeni. Broadly speaking, at the top are industrial men and a few professionals such as teachers. They are usually older, and some run informal businesses such as taxis or rent out imijondolo. While many live in Sundumbili's four-room houses or the former white town, Mandini, others bought land in the jondolo settlements in the 1980s and 1990s. Then there are men employed in low-paid work but who have some security, perhaps through owning a house. Finally, there is a large group of only casually employed or unemployed men; most of this group rent imijondolo or stay with family members.

Thulani and Phila, whom I was introduced to by a mutual friend, were members of the second and third groups. Both worked at a factory that manufactures plastic bags and earned about R800 a month when I spoke with them in 2006. But their different levels of prosperity reveal particularly well how important a man's date of arrival in Mandeni is to his economic security and status. Thulani arrived first and had bought land and built a small house, while Phila, a more recent arrival, rented a small umjondolo.

When I interviewed Thulani, who was in his early thirties, he sat on his bed in his two-room house and I sat opposite him on a plastic garden chair purchased from a local factory shop. I placed the voice recorder on the iron-

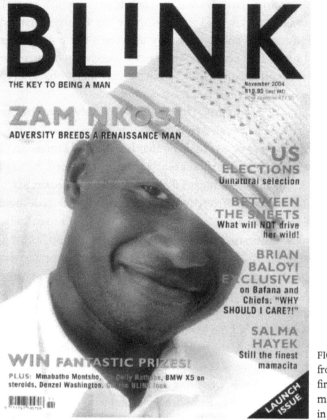

BL!NK

THE KEY TO BEING A MAN

November 2004
R19.95 (incl VAT)
Hard copy price R17.00

ZAM NKOSI
ADVERSITY BREEDS A RENAISSANCE MAN

'US
ELECTIONS
Unnatural selection

BETWEEN
THE SHEETS
What will NOT drive
her wild!

BRIAN
BALOYI
EXCLUSIVE
on Bafana and
Chiefs. "WHY
SHOULD I CARE?!"

SALMA
HAYEK
Still the finest
mamacita

WIN FANTASTIC PRIZES!
PLUS: Mmabatho Montsho, Dolly Rathebe, BMW X5 on
steroids, Denzel Washington, the BL!NK look

LAUNCH
ISSUE

FIGURE 8.1. The front cover of the first issue of *BL!NK* magazine, launched in 2004.

ing board next to a charred electric iron. The house, built on a gentle rise in Isithebe's jondolo settlement, was constructed using concrete blocks and had a corrugated steel roof. It was relatively spacious and well kept, although the green-painted plaster peeled away untidily from the walls.

Raised in a rural area, Thulani had worked on temporary contracts in Mandeni since 1997. He had managed to "buy" some land from a neighbor for R 2,500, and it cost him R12,000 to build the house in which he now lives. Discussing the advantages of his social position compared to that of people living in rented imijondolo, he said that owning a house allows a man to gradually improve his life, and cited his kitchen cupboards, refrigerator, and oven—all bought on credit—as evidence of how he had done so.

Thulani said that he had lived with one woman—*umama wengane* (mother of his child)—since 1997. They met in the area, but his inability to lobola her meant that he had never visited her rural-based family. Hearing this made me recall a time when I gave a male friend and his cohabiting girlfriend, both in their forties, a lift to the woman's rural home. Just before we arrived, a look of panic crossed the man's face and he told me to stop the car. He disembarked and walked to the home slowly and deliberately, arriving a full ten minutes after his partner and I did. This act of deference was necessary because he had not paid ilobolo to his girlfriend's family; even his visit was probably only tolerated because the woman's father had passed away.

Demonstrating similar sentiments, Thulani looked firmly at me before saying with conviction that he intended to pay ilobolo (*"kufanele ushade, kungumthetho,"* it is the law to marry). He told me that he had paid inhlawulo (a fine) for their child. Especially in the rural areas where he was born, he said, marriage wins respect: a man who is married "can't be told what to do."

Thulani is typical of men who arrived in the area on the cusp of its decline; his life was a kind of shrunk-down version of that of the "SAPPI man" who found work in the 1960s at the paper mill and was granted township housing. He earned considerably less than men working at the largest factories, who took home around R4,000 a month, but was better off than the newest arrivals, who were lucky to secure even casual work.

Phila, on the other hand, arrived in 2005, only one year before I spoke with him. Twenty-eight years old, he lived in an umjondolo with a woman he had recently met: as we talked, the woman peeped periodically out of the door, wringing out the clothes she was washing and overhearing fragments of our conversation. Phila said that it was not easy to accept that women were working, but that he still preferred to live with a woman who earned money: "Then we can add a hundred rand and a hundred rand and buy food." He noted that in modern relationships, "You can't go to a woman's house with nothing. They expect something—air time [for a cell phone], or cosmetics, or money." Neither, he said, can a man return to his rural home without bringing food or other gifts for his kin.

Most men, Phila said, like to stay with a woman to ensure that someone will wash, iron, and cook for them. He cracked open a beer and told us, without much prompting, that drinking is one reason why men can violently beat women. Although he acknowledged the high level of domestic violence in the area, he still fondly discussed the prospect of marriage "if she works or not, as long as I love her and she loves me."

Isithebe men's frustration at the poor employment situation usually simmers in the background, or is buried in alcohol, but sometimes it explodes. I had known Andile for four years on and off. His mother and father were *izakhamizi* (locals) and lived close to me in an umuzi in Isithebe which comprised three small mud, stone, and wood buildings. He did not drink, and his conscientious demeanor reflected his commitment to improving his life. As a sign of this, he had managed to become fluent in English despite the poor local schooling, and he told me that a local taxi owner was planning to hire him as a driver in the future.

At twenty-four years of age, Andile moved out of his family home to stay in his own small umjondolo, not far from his parents. His rent, he told me, was paid by an absent male friend who wanted Andile to look after his belongings in the umjondolo. In 2004, he found a temporary job in the same factory at which Thulani and Phila worked. But although his supervisor promised him full-time work, this never materialized and he remained a casual employee on low pay.

After being injured twice in the factory, Andile quit. He then sent his CV to many local factories and even to firms as far away as Johannesburg, without any response. He asked me continually about working overseas, and I found it difficult to explain why residents of former colonizing countries could travel relatively freely around the world while residents of the former colonies had virtually no chance of being allowed to work in the West. One day in 2006 he was really at the end of his tether. He showed me an impersonal letter that the local municipality had sent him: his name and address entered on a standard form saying that it had no vacancies. I wondered how many disappointed residents of Mandeni owned similar letters.

Beginning to walk out of his umjondolo, Andile stopped suddenly in the doorway. Facing toward the sugar plantations to the east of Isithebe, he said, "I am not supposed to be living in umjondolo. I am twenty-five; even the bread you see, it is paid for by my girlfriend, it is not supposed to be like this." His eyes welled up and overflowed; this was one of the few times that I had seen a man (anywhere) cry. Witnessing his desperate state made me feel uncomfortable. "Sometimes I think of suicide, but then I think of what my family will have to face," he told me.

Marriage, Courting, and the Isoka

Earlier, I made the argument that the beginning of the century saw a growing distinction between an isoka (a man with many girlfriends; the plural is *amasoka*) and an isifebe (a loose woman). Although this coincided with women's new ability to move to and survive in urban areas, it reflected men's greater power over courting as a consequence of both wage labor and prudish Christian notions of "sex"—a term by then used more widely in society. Despite polygamy's quite rapid decline in the early twentieth century, men actively drew on its symbolism to justify having multiple intimate relations. This shift was uneven and did not mean that all young men had many partners and all young women did not; moreover, being an isoka was only a kind of phase in the life of a man, since to become a real man he had to marry. But over the last few decades we have witnessed another shift: many amasoka do not marry or work.

In the 1980s, anti-apartheid struggles pushed into view masculinities that celebrated honor and sacrifice but also violence, and nowhere more so than in KwaZulu-Natal, a province wracked by IFP-ANC political violence to which sexual violence was closely linked. Although there were multiple masculinities evident during this period, rising unemployment and men's failure to become abanumzana (heads of household) reconfigured masculinities around court-ing. Democracy freed young men politically, but rising unemployment and falling marriage rates meant that few men were able to invest resources and energy in building a marital home, which has historically been a key anchor of masculinities.

In 2000, at one of Sundumbili's run-down schools, Sipho and two other young men explained the isoka figure to me. (Sipho was the student who gave me information on his classmates' life paths, as mentioned in chapter 6.) We had begun by talking about the school itself, but the conversation drifted onto the subject of courting—the shift was doubtless easier because we were all men. As we discussed the figure of isoka, in a mixture of English and isiZulu, Sipho spotted my cell phone and gave me a dismissive glance:

> With your Alcatel you will not get the *amacherry* [girls] most of the time. If you come with an Alcatel it is like the thing of a child. . . . They want an expensive one, like a T28 or a 6110. If you come with the little Nokia, they are going to hlonipha [respect] you. If you come with the small Siemens, the C2, they hlonipha you, they can see that you're the boss, you have money. . . . That's [where] AIDS comes from. . . . I'm not playing, if you get money, you have an expensive cell phone, you will be tempted, you won't avoid it . . . [because with women] there is competition: if he has six [girl-friends], I want seven, then he wants to have eight.

The concept of "hlonipha," used by Sipho to describe the respect won by owning a pricy cell phone, is, as we have seen, saturated with historical significance. In the early colonial period the inhlonipho a man deserved was primarily determined by the position he had managed to attain: husband, elder, or chief. Of course, these social categories were dynamic. A wealthy man gained status because of his ability to marry several wives, and this high status enhanced his ability to accumulate more ilobolo cattle.

When migrant labor gave young men the ability to make their own ilobolo payments, notions of hlonipha were dramatically reconfigured. But marriage nonetheless remained a central way for men to attain the status of umnumzana, a head of household. Today, by comparison, low marriage rates and grinding unemployment make inhlonipho harder for young men to win; though there are still many ways to win respect, this difficulty helps to explain why some men value conspicuous consumption and having multiple girlfriends.

Earning inhlonipho historically required a man to exert self-discipline, judiciously indulging in potentially hazardous aspects of masculinities like drinking and womanizing. In excess, these habits could lead a man down a path that did not lead to marriage or supporting a home, and the shame involved in this failure is powerfully evoked in the derisive verb "ukubhunguka," to abandon a home. Consequently, in the mid-twentieth century an isoka was a man who attracted multiple women but was aware of limits; he was expected to marry to become a full man, an umnumzana. Respectability required partially trading in his life as an isoka for the status of married man (even if doing so did not prevent men from having extramarital partners). Signifying this, isoka lamanyala (amanyala means "dirt" or "a dirty act") was a term for a man who "wasted" marriageable girls by having many lovers for his own satisfaction.

But the present era has witnessed a shift in the limits of masculinities. The term "isoka lamanyala" still denotes an unacceptable masculinity, but the concept has become partially delinked from marriage—it is no longer so common to hear men being lambasted for having many girlfriends with no intention of marrying them. In the isiZulu media, "amanyala" refers to any disgraceful act by a man: it has recently been used to describe a seventy-one-year-old African man's rape of a five-year-old African child and a twenty-six-year-old white man's rape of a fifty-year-old African woman.[6] In the opinion of many men I knew, an isoka lamanyala was simply a man who went too far, for instance by spreading diseases or sleeping with a girlfriend's best friend. These shifts in meaning capture how isoka-hood is no longer a stage of life, a playboy period that must be superseded by marriage if a man is not to be disgraced. Being a kind of perpetual isoka can be a more central part of men's identity today.

Two young men in their twenties whom I interviewed in Sundumbili township spelled out the difference between an isoka and an isoka lamanyala:

MH: Can you explain what an isoka is?

Khetha: Isoka is someone who greets a girl and then she gets
excited. . . . When he starts to shela [woo] a girl he doesn't
expect her to agree now, but she is excited, and if someone

> comes to shela that same girl . . . she will only think of that isoka.

MH: What is isoka lamanyala?

Thanda: Someone who doesn't choose, he takes a girl even if she has one eye. If he sees a girl on the street he says, "I love you" no matter how dirty she is. He just loves any girl.

Why do men perpetuate the dichotomy between the isoka (a man successful with women) and the isifebe (a loose woman)—a dichotomy that denigrates a woman's sexual conquests but celebrates a man's and, in doing so, literally kills him (and his sexual partners) today? The longstanding, if waning, practice of polygamy in the region is probably men's most common justification. Such cultural claims, in turn, frequently intersect with biological declarations about the naturalness of men's sexual appetite. In turn, biology and culture gain authority through images of philandering men sourced worldwide, from Britain's James Bond to the macho men of Latin America. And, to be sure, images of manhood travel in all directions: Zuluness is a global symbol of a warrior-type manhood, and therefore constitutive of masculinities both inside and outside of South Africa.

As these points suggest, masculinities that celebrate men's sole right to engage in multiple intimate relations are inevitably about much more than simply "sex" (a concept itself, as we have seen, with a fluid meaning). Just as English and American men employ the words "slut" and "whore" to maintain gendered hierarchies, South African men have long drawn on the term "isifebe" to prevent "good" women from gaining an education, taking paid work, and avoiding domestic duties. And although I source the masculinity partly in rising unemployment, social practices are not sealed within neat groups—richer men also draw on the authority of the isoka. Put simply, masculinities are, at one level, always connected to male power, and power is not readily given up.

The status of the isoka faces heavy challenges today from rights-bearing women and also men, especially as a result of AIDS; these contestations are discussed further in the final chapter. Yet, in general, men of all ages tend not to challenge the core tenet of isoka, the naturalness of men's desire for multiple women. Instead, they question its limits and whether or not men should indulge their desire. At times, for instance, a man can publicly support the isoka masculinity but not practice it. About a year after my interview with Sipho, I arranged to meet him in Durban, where he was pursuing tertiary education. I bought him a burger and sat eating mine, although he wanted to keep his as a present for his girlfriend. I placed my cell phone on the table and we joked about how the Nokia 6110, the cell phone so revered when we first spoke, had come to be disparagingly called *ummbila* (a corncob) for its clumsy size.

We chatted about this and that, including relationships, and during the course of the conversation he revealed (to my surprise, given his previous celebration of isoka) that he was still a virgin. He said that he was scared of pregnancy and AIDS. He had one girlfriend in Durban and a more serious one in Sundumbili. A few months later, he introduced me to his Sundumbili girlfriend, whom he said he was keeping an eye on to see if she behaved well and thus was marriageable. Sipho came from a quite well-off family that could afford tertiary education, and his opportunities were therefore relatively good. Although he defended isoka as men's custom—one that clearly gave him power in relationships, including his ability to have two lovers—he had not yet had sexual intercourse with either of these women. He associated the isoka lifestyle with the threat of AIDS and saw it as distracting him from the sacrifices he needed to make in order to get on in life and repay his family's commitment to him.

Providing Love Today

Sipho's seemingly trivial act of saving a burger for his girlfriend enacts men's frequent statement that disposable income and—a signifier of this—consumption are vital if a man is to attract a girlfriend. The system of migrant labor meant that men had to work for many years to save money for ilobolo and then, once married, to build a home. Yet it gave young men new power over girlfriends, because only they could initiate marriage and legitimate childbirth. Today, the core element of men's past contribution to the patriarchal bargain—providing for the household—is ironically turned against men. Women can strike a poor man down by labeling him *isahluleki* (a failure), a word historically used for a migrant man who failed to support his home but used today for any man who fails to support a lover. Men can also overhear, whether from their sisters or friends, the everyday question that women ask themselves: "Should we wait for a 'good man' or milk multiple men for gifts?"

As a consequence of the increasingly winner-takes-all sexual economy —in which wealth can secure many girlfriends and poverty none—men marginalized from the productive economy also face marginalization from the sexual economy. Indeed, poorer men can be extremely resentful of richer men, not simply because disposable income drives conspicuous consumption, but because richer men consume many of the area's women. Even without money, I heard some men say, women can still satisfy their sexual needs; however, in the same position, men struggle to attract women. Or, as I heard quite a few times, a younger man might have to accept sharing a girlfriend with an older, richer man. This close connection between money and sex reveals that class consciousness, long searched for on the shop floor, is constructed today in the sexual and not simply the productive economy.

The emotion-laden connection between money and sex was revealed to me one day in 2000 when I was walking around Isithebe's factories talking with *abafesi* (those looking for work). Outside one furniture factory I found a group of unemployed men playing cards. The men began the discussion by expressing anger at being asked to pay bribes to secure employment. Over time, the discussion shifted to a more emotional topic: how difficult it was for poor men to attract girlfriends. To outbursts of laughter from the crowd, one man said that he had not had a girlfriend for three years. As he spoke, and as if to underline his lack of *ubudoda* (manliness), a woman burst in to tell me, "They are not men if they don't work."

One consequence of today's strong links between money and sex is that men can play intricate games of fraud to conceal their lack of wealth. In late 2000 I accompanied my friend Thami (whom I introduced in chapter 2) to a funeral in rural KwaZulu-Natal. It was a sad affair, but some mourners were dressed attractively, and Thami had his eye on a woman who, I heard, was about six years his junior, fifteen. She wore a low-cut red dress and smiled with a hint of flirtation. Thami used his charm to good effect: soon she was laughing openly at his jokes. Seizing the moment, he asked for her cell phone number. But instead of putting it straight into his phone, as was common practice, he wrote it down on a piece of paper.

She turned and asked in a suspicious voice, "Where is your cell phone?" He looked defensive and replied, "It is being repaired." She continued her interrogation: "Where do you work?" He replied, "For the municipality." My mind spun, trying to reconcile this statement with Thami's informal work as a car guard who earned a few rand every now and then from people whose shopping bags he carried to their cars. Then I recalled that he had a fading bib provided to him by the municipality, making this statement not a total untruth. This scene of a woman testing a man's material worth has been played out millions of times across the world; what makes it different in South Africa is that it takes place at a time when male unemployment is at unprecedented levels.

Given this materiality of everyday relationships, I was surprised to learn that a man's reputation could be harmed if he drew too obvious an association between money and sex. A person who writes his telephone number on a hundred-rand note and gives it to a potential lover, I was told, is the antithesis of an isoka: an isishimane, a man too scared to talk to women. (Jacob Zuma used this term in his trial to justify his claim that he had no need to rape a woman.) An isoka, therefore, was celebrated not because he could simply bribe women, but because he attracted girlfriends through his wit and charm.

In determining acceptable male behavior in respect to gifts, age plays an important role. As suggested earlier, one reason why sugar daddies are not more criticized in the community—and could even be revered as amasoka—is that they are rarely seen as simply bribing younger women for sex. Indeed, to do so would make them appear weak, even feminine. Few would deny that it is these men's money and not simply charm that attracts younger women. Nevertheless, sugar daddies' age allows their gifts to be understood more as a form of help than as a bribe. And, since they are typically already married, sugar daddies are not derided for not marrying their girlfriends, as younger men may be.

For example, a relatively wealthy man I knew, who was in his late fifties, once tried to seduce Nomusa, the "good woman" whose story was told in the previous chapter. Discussing his advances, Nomusa told me that she thought that her father tacitly approved the relationship, because of his constant adulation of his friend around that time. It is certainly difficult to believe that this high-status suitor would have risked his reputation if his advances were not at least somewhat approved by the woman's father—who, in turn, stood to gain from his daughter's having disposable money.

That sugar daddies are not immune to public criticism, however, is apparent in the fall from grace of one of Mandeni's past mayors. Most residents will say that his political career was damaged because of his relationships with several schoolgirls. Certainly, sugar daddies have a double image that reveals deep tensions in manhood itself: on the one hand they can be chastised as exploiters of young women; yet on the other they can be positioned as respectable men who, unlike most young men, provide for the women with whom they have relationships.

Fathering

Everyday disputes surrounding fatherhood reveal tensions within manhood particularly well. "Ubaba" (father) is an isiZulu term that implies respectability and seniority. I used it many times when talking to men, especially those who were my seniors: together with deferential bodily actions, such as moving and talking slowly and deliberately, the word helped me avoid evoking the long history of white men belittling and emasculating African men. When I visited a man's home, in addition, I always made sure that I showed respect by recognizing isihlalo sikababa (father's chair) and sitting in another seat. The care I took indicates the complexities that surrounded my own social location as a researcher. I often felt a need to respect certain patriarchal customs as an anti-racist statement, and yet in doing so I could reinforce practices ultimately rooted in gender hierarchies.

Most young men I knew would agree that fathering a child symbolizes sexual virility and improves a man's social status. Yet if biological *fathering* is relatively easy to achieve, requiring only penetrative sexual intercourse, fulfilling the social role of *fatherhood* is much more challenging. Today, many men are unable to pay inhlawulo, and almost none can afford ilobolo.

If the poorest men invariably do not pay anything to the women they have impregnated or their families, insights can be gained from the dilemma of men who have some resources. These men have to decide whether to pay inhlawulo, support their child, begin ilobolo payments for marriage, or reject the child and spend money in other ways. Each choice has repercussions for masculinity. The highest-status option is to marry their child's mother, but this is also the most costly. Another path, supporting a child but not marrying the mother, boosts a man's image as a good provider, even if it is a constant drain on resources. (Government legislation, although weakly enforced, requires men to support their children at least somewhat.) Abandoning a child allows a man to spend money to boost his masculinity in other ways, but it can lead to feelings of guilt: many young men suggested to me that they would like to support their children, or at least to pay inhlawulo. The problem is their lack of *amandla* (power, or in this context money).

One further possibility is for men to deny paternity altogether. In Sundumbili one day Mdu, a young man in his early twenties, explained to me why this might happen. Like many men in South Africa and elsewhere, he did not see prevention of pregnancy as a man's responsibility. Yet in his testimony the connection between the denial of paternity and economic difficulties became apparent:

> [Denial of paternity] is caused by different things. Maybe you are in love with someone you don't trust, maybe you met her at a bash [street party] or at bad places like that, maybe you become lovers when she already had someone else. When you slept with her maybe she is already pregnant . . . and then when you count the date that she slept with you, if you are clever you will see that it's not yours, especially if you don't trust her. But sometimes the reason [for denial]

is because you are scared of your family. What are they going to say or do about a child? Maybe you are still in school, so you have to leave school to work in order to support the baby. Sometimes you don't deny your baby because you want to, but because of the situation.

Men like Mdu might accept that they are irresponsible in not supporting their children. But these men can also draw on gendered discourses to position unmarried mothers as "loose," in other words as responsible for their pregnancy. Here again it is evident that masculinities are contradictory, punishing men and yet being used by men to discipline women.

As shown earlier, the magazine *BL!NK* countered stereotypes of African men as irresponsible fathers by advancing images of respectable parents. In Mandeni, I saw men acting with sensitivity and love toward their children, cuddling them and bestowing on them great affection. The man of the migrant-labor era provided for his family, but to do so he had to be absent for most of the child's life. But today, especially in townships where movement rates are relatively low, men tend to live close to their children and yet are often unable to financially support them. Dominant descriptions of masculinities as simply irresponsible tend to silence the potential significance of this reversal. Instead, it is perhaps more useful to consider how many young men's identity in relation to their children is defined by the two new factors: their frequent proximity to their children and their inability to support them.

Violence: Straightening Women

Rather than providing a full review of sexual violence, my aim here is to concentrate on one theme, the connection between men's violence and women's questioning of gendered hierarchies.[7] This connection does not explain all aspects of sexual violence, including the much publicized rape of children.[8] But it does help to situate contemporary violence within long histories of men trying to "straighten" women.

I begin by considering women's seemingly mundane act of wearing trousers, articles of clothing associated with men. In a high-profile case in 2007, one woman from the T-section of Umlazi, a sprawling Durban township, defied a local ban on wearing trousers and was forced to walk the streets naked—a punishment that activists challenged through rights-based equality legislation.[9] Typically positioned as a modern-day battle between tradition and rights, this violent attention to women's clothes in fact has a long history. In the late 1970s and early 1980s in Mandeni, as discussed in chapter 4, oqonda or abelungisi men (those who "straighten" or "put right") sought to discipline rebellious women, including those who wore trousers. At this time, "industrial women" were arriving en masse from rural areas and finding work, albeit for very little pay; a few women were even becoming householders of four-room matchbox houses. Hence, oqonda's opposition to women wearing trousers represented wider struggles around women taking over men's roles.

Disputes over trouser wearing today, therefore, demonstrate that we must always keep in analytical tension past gendered contestations and those that appear to be new; I develop this point when considering gang rape below. But the 2007 trouser incident in Umlazi is also consistent with men's more recent claims that the freedom of democracy demands increased disciplining of women.

That modern rights are themselves a focal point for violence, or at least are used to justify violence, is clearly seen in an interview I conducted with three young township men. One of the most controversial legislative acts of the post-apartheid government—and one opposed by most parents I knew in Mandeni—was the prohibition of corporal punishment within schools. Although the practice is still widespread, Khetha and Joe, men of twenty, portray such legislation as productive of gender and generational disorder. They look back favorably to the (imagined) days when disciplined women completed school and entered respectable professions such as teaching or nursing. Now that rights are overturning established paths, they suggest, women need to be disciplined in more direct ways. Controlling one's girlfriend with violence is positioned here as almost a duty, a way to straighten out a morally crooked society.

> MH: When is it bad to hit a girl?
>
> Khetha: To hit a girl it's okay and it helps, because before . . . there was this thing called corporal punishment for those who didn't do schoolwork; they were hit, and those people that got hit, they are now nurses and teachers. After the government said teachers mustn't hit the students, children stopped learning, they are now doing what they want, they are pointing guns at the teachers. As well as your girlfriend; if she is naughty you have to slap her a little.

Men's collective disciplining of women takes perhaps its most violent form in gang rape. In 2001, I heard of a terrible example of this violence in Mandeni. Zinhle, a woman whom I knew in passing, was a good friend of my research assistant. She had grown up in an informal settlement and had not graduated from school; she was rarely able to find work and became dependent on a boyfriend, with whom she lived. When this boyfriend discovered her infidelity, however, he punished not her lover but Zinhle. Together, both men raped her and washed out her vagina with soap. The men saw her as an isifebe—as betraying women's purported duty to be chaste and respectful. She said that this was not an isolated incident:

> They come together, they say let's hit this isifebe. Others, they will sleep with her, all of them. Others, they will get all of the soap—OMO, SURF, Sunlight—and will tell her to wash her vagina.

In trying to understand the historical context of high levels of rape in South Africa, I looked at dozens of rape cases, mostly from the mid-twentieth century; I found it difficult, however, to draw conclusions about how the number of reported rapes changed over time.[10] Yet comparison of past and present rape cases supports the notion that there have been qualitative changes in sexual violence, including a dramatic increase in "jackrolling," or gang rape, such as the incident noted above and the one recalled by journalist Fred Khumalo (and mentioned in chapter 4). One estimate is that a third of reported rapes involve gang rape.[11] This increase is certainly consistent with an unmooring of gender norms at a time when many men failed to find work and marry. Women's move into the labor force and the virtual ending of the "patriarchal bargain" centered on marriage made male-female relations more contested, and gang rape is linked to these contestations in complex ways.

As discussed in chapter 4, the oqonda or abelungisi men who "straightened" trouser-wearing women in the 1970s and early 1980s were middle-aged married men, many working at the SAPPI paper mill. They saw themselves as respectable men who wanted to *lungisa* (put right) moral wrongs in the community. Today, gang rape itself must be seen, in part, as a violent way men seek to straighten women, although today the perpetrators are often youthful and jobless. In both instances, men's collective disciplining of a woman engenders strong homosocial bonds.

Yet as terribly violent as this disciplining is, we cannot fully understand it without recognizing that it is laden with tensions that derive from within masculinities themselves. Men can be ashamed of their sexual violence if it goes too far, for instance by injuring a woman as opposed to "teaching respect."[12] Notions of respectability, deeply linked to men's role as husbands and providers, can also set certain limits on violence.

Male Violence and Same-Sex Rights

One high-profile legal right today in South Africa is the constitutional protection of same-sex intimate relationships. Yet, paradoxically, homophobic violence seems to have increased after apartheid.[13] Seeking to understand opposition to same-sex relations, David Halperin has argued that the strength of homophobic discourses lies partly in their incoherence.[14] Following this point, we can recognize not only overriding sexual hierarchies (heterosexual/homosexual) but the multiple, not necessarily coherent, institutional and discursive practices affecting homophobia: for instance on rights, gender, class, and female-male marriage.

The legal domain is one important realm affecting same-sex relations. While the apartheid state actively oppressed those engaged in same-sex intimacy, in the years leading up to democracy activists successfully linked lesbian and gay rights to anti-apartheid and human rights narratives.[15] (I use the terms "gay" and "lesbian" here not uncritically or because they assume singular identities, but since they were employed at the time.)

This rights-based strategy yielded great success: in 1996 South Africa became the first country in the world to protect sexual orientation in its constitution. And ten years later, the demand for full citizenship rights was realized in the Civil Union Act of 2006 that made it possible for gay and lesbian couples to marry. This landmark granting of formal rights undoubtedly opened up many new spaces and protections for intimate diversity, ones materialized today in gay shebeens, gay beauty pageants, and gay pride marches.[16]

Unlike past same-sex practices, however, these new claims for gay and lesbian rights rest on a clear definition of an oppressed group, those who *identify* through sexual categories. Citizens have to "come out" to claim rights. This foregrounding of same-sex identities and rights, while necessary to challenge institutionalized heteronormativity, is attracting new forms of opposition. As South Africans link sexual rights to citizenship, some men can react violently. There are clearly many dynamics at work here, but, tellingly, some men try to justify this violence by arguing for the naturalness of male-female relations in the face of what appears to be a full frontal attack on heterosexual-identifying men after democracy. The liberal essence of the modern rights framework, for instance, can be opposed on the grounds that same-sex relations are "un-African," a type of claim that has been made in many different settings.[17] Ironically, Christian notions of sexual morality can buttress this position.

The contours of this homophobia are also gendered today in many ways. One extreme example of this is the disproportionate targeting of lesbians in acts of violence. Women who refuse to engage in sexual relations with men are a powerful affront to the values of isoka and a sign of men's reduced power. Between 2006 and 2008, at least ten lesbians (the term used in the media) were killed in hate crimes carried out by men across the country.[18] And same-sex intimacy and homophobia are also classed. As Swarr and Nagar argue, poor lesbians in Soweto have less of a voice in nationwide gay-rights organizations than middle-class (often white) lesbians.[19] In South Africa's postcolonial setting, therefore, rights challenge heterosexual masculinities, but in uneven ways.

A further example of the need to think about the multiple histories of homophobia was brought to my attention in 2009. I was interviewing a group of men about Jacob Zuma a few weeks before he was swept into the presidency. Trying to understand the reasons for his popular support, I was writing a paper that located women's and men's adulation of him in the context of shifting gender relationships and chronic unemployment.[20] Many people I spoke with said that he was popular because he was an isoka and not an isoka lamanyala. In other words, he liked women but was a respectable man who married and supported his girlfriends rather than discarding them. And one group of young men with whom I spoke added that men supported Zuma more than Mbeki because "It's Mbeki that made that law so that that people of the same sex can marry." Indeed, unlike Mbeki, Zuma had controversially asserted that same-sex desire is incompatible with African culture.[21] To these young men, Zuma seemed to represent a reassertion of heteronormativity, as symbolized by the "traditional" family.

After the interview we dug into some Kentucky Fried Chicken and continued chatting. We were talking about the language used to describe same-sex relations. At one point, a young man called Zakhile turned to me and said with a casual laugh, and to my surprise, that he had had a relationship with an older man to obtain monetary gifts. Zakhile did not, however, identify as being "gay," or with any other related term, such as *isitabane*. This latter term, which is usually derogatory, is commonly used to identify men who engage in same-sex relationships, although it can also mean an effeminate man or hermaphrodite.[22] Instead of identifying as isitabane, however, Zakhile said that he had been "loved by isitabane."

I asked how he could have had a relationship with this man, given his previous negative attitude toward same-sex relations. His reply began with the word *isimo*. This word means roughly "situation," and I have heard it used many times to explain actions taken because of a person's relative powerlessness (for instance, a woman's having many boyfriends). He continued that he was not in love with the man, who, in any case, knew that he had a girlfriend. I asked his two friends, "Did you know about this relationship?" His friends replied, "Yes . . . they were not loving, he wanted money." They did not see his actions as unmasculine, because poverty had forced him into this situation (both his parents had died and he had found only casual work repairing the roofs of houses).

I do not, of course, know the kind of pleasure (if any) Zakhile gained from the relationship. He told me that he did it for money and that they had just "baby kissed" on the cheek, although he believed that some other men had had anal sex with izitabane for money. A first conclusion that can be drawn from these statements, however, is that the materiality of everyday sex, a central driver of AIDS, encompasses relationships between men as well as between men and women.

But Zakhile's discussion of connections between class and intimacy raises wider questions around same-sex relations. In the AIDS policy world, it is now common to recognize that men who identify as heterosexual sometimes have sex with other men. The term most commonly used for these men today is "men who have sex with men." However, like many concepts that become institutionalized in policy narratives, it can easily be oversimplified; policy makers can construct "MSM" as a discreet and homogenous group in need of interventions, and the acronym facilitates the process of rendering the concept technical. In contrast, my discussion with these three young men did not support the identity/behavior binary that lies behind this concept; Zakhile might not have identified as being "gay," but neither were his "behaviors" somehow insulated from wider classed, gendered, and sexualized meanings that must be explored.[23]

The fact that all three men excused Zakhile's actions as being driven by poverty certainly suggests that dominant masculinities are heteronormative. But—and this is another important point—the men's opposition to the new rights-based legislation appeared to be primarily due to its legitimization of same-sex marriages. Indeed, Zakhile actually defended his lover's sexual preference, saying that he was born gay.

This conversation cannot be taken as typical. But it certainly suggests that to understand the multiple roots of homophobia and its many inflections today we need to know much more about how the historical construction of same-sex relations and heterosexual marriage are related—and I have mainly discussed the latter in this book. Certainly, as already noted, many men had same-sex relations while working at the mines and saw this as compatible with returning to a rural wife; in Cato Manor informal settlement, in turn, men could marry each other. Such histories challenge statements by leaders like Zuma who deny a history of same-sex intimacy in the region. Yet it is much harder, but equally important, to show how past same-sex practices—ones not defined through today's sexual categories—shape the contours of, and contradictions within, homophobia today. Excellent work is now being been done in this area, but what is clear is that the rush to use categorizations like MSM risks obscuring these important questions in the name of public health.[24]

More than any other slogan, the shout of *amandla ngawethu* (power to the people), accompanied by a raised fist, came to symbolize youth-led struggles against apartheid. Yet now that democracy has been achieved, it is more common to hear young men exclaiming "*Anginawo amandla*" (I don't have power). The phrase can refer to physical frailty, but also to social or material weakness, including—perhaps most pointedly—a man's inability to pay ilobolo or inhlawulo. It captures the dilemma at the heart of this chapter: understanding masculinities and male power at a time when many men, especially the poorest, clearly perceive themselves to be disempowered.

Indeed, viewing male power as simply an expression of patriarchal traditions can downplay the complex changes to masculinities over the course of the twentieth century. My stress on history in understanding these processes is not to suggest that a return to past gendered patterns is possible or desirable. In the 1980s, as we saw, the model of the male-led household faced fundamental challenges as "industrial women" found partial economic independence in factory work, bought land, and fostered a healthy skepticism toward marrying. But deindustrialization partly cut this woman-led model down. Though masculinities are changing across the country today, the middle-class *BL!NK* men are one group vigorously charting a new path in the democratic South Africa. Poorer men, unable to achieve adulthood by marrying and finding housing, often remain unemployed. They may live indefinitely in their family's four-room house, dependent on family members, or move to a tiny umjondolo.

For these reasons, rather than thinking in terms of "rights versus tradition" (or a "crisis in masculinity," another common phrase), we need to recognize how masculinities and femininities are *interrelated* and *constantly changing* when so many aspects of getting by—from housing to domestic responsibilities—are recast and contested in a context of tremendous inequalities and a world with limited work. And, even further, we need to think through how this world, like masculinity itself, is not natural but powerfully produced.

NINE

All You Need Is Love? The Materiality of Everyday Sex and Love

When I began living in Mandeni in 2000 I was struck by an apparent paradox: everybody I knew discussed the close connection between money and sex, and yet they said that few "prostitutes" lived in the area. In my attempt to explore the materiality of everyday sex, I talked to factory managers and unions about job losses and declining wages. I looked at how rents had increased relative to wages and how migration to the area had increased despite job losses. I probed census data and found that only 14 percent of "Africans" living in the municipality were married. I searched for a way to describe the material relationships I saw, and found that scholars called them "transactional sex."

But there was something missing. I became frustrated with the inertia of the concept of "sex" and the way it framed my emerging questions, such as, how had sex become "commodified"? And how had "sexual culture" changed? Over time I began to think that a better set of questions emerged from stepping back and exploring how resource flows, embodied emotions, and social meanings transformed in a shifting political economy. Doing so yielded insight into how the gendered labor market coincided with, and influenced, far-reaching demographic shifts, including rising population mobility and falling marriage rates—but it also took me into the realm of love. Indeed, in everyday conversations, narratives of sex's materiality coexisted with the widespread celebration of love. In turn, love's normative value as "good" made it a powerful symbolic anchor for a cultural politics of intimacy.

Recognizing the particular interweavings of money and love, I argue, can help to explain the most intimate moments between young people, including condom use—a very effective protection against HIV infection. Love in South Africa, as everywhere, has many historical strands, but for analytical clarity I have stressed two forms of love: provider love, rooted in men's payment of ilobolo and support of a wife, and romantic love, which represents, in Lawrence Stone's words, a historical shift toward "affective individualism."[1] Today, key to understanding the materiality of everyday sex is not love's absence from relationships but how money and love have come together in new ways.

Promiscuous Capital and the Materiality of Everyday Sex

Residents' most common explanation for why money and sex are linked in Mandeni is that "factories have closed," rendering women more dependent on men. Intimacy, these testimonies reveal, is firmly encased in today's foot-loose capitalism that creates inequalities wherever it goes—and whenever it leaves. There is, according to Cindi Katz, "a threat at the heart of capitalism's vagrancy," namely that "an increasingly global capitalist production can shuck many of its particular commitments to place, most centrally those associated with social reproduction, which is almost always less mobile than production."[2] Mandeni's very history reveals capital's promiscuity in the era of "globalization." In the 1960s, the SAPPI paper mill helped found Sundumbili township and promoted plans to build tennis courts and a swimming pool for residents. By the early 2000s, however, most employers in the area were Taiwanese garment factories that hired women at very low salaries and threatened to leave if workers joined unions; when workers did unionize and win pay increases, many firms followed through on their threats and relocated to lower-cost sites.

In a climate where some men earn ten times the wages of women, sex has an immediate materiality. I collected dozens of stories that graphically revealed how the closure of factories and constant in-migration fueled a pattern of men providing gifts to girlfriends. And, as I noted earlier, across the country the materiality of sex is widely recorded: labor market inequalities may be particularly pronounced in Mandeni, but unemployment, gender inequalities, and a virtual absence of marriage among the young are widespread in South Africa, as well as in some of its neighbors.

One long-term resident of the informal settlement, Mrs. Ndlela, explained to me in November 2000 the difficulties women face. In doing so, she evoked (with a hint of romanticism) the independent "industrial women" who came to the area in the 1980s in more favorable economic circumstances:

> Before, people didn't rely on anyone, they were having money; now they have to rely on other people. . . . Some see this man today, this man tomorrow, and that man the following day. . . . Some men are working in factories, some outside, like taxi drivers. . . . Today the situation [*isimo*] pushes them to this thing. . . . They are scared [of

AIDS] but sometimes they just say that there is no such thing, they just ignore it.

Yet, however unrelenting capitalist enterprises are in their pursuit of profit, however ruthless they are in exploiting gender inequalities, penetrative sex is not traded like a commodity. Residents are adamant that a man who gives gifts to a woman is a "boyfriend" (denoted by terms like *iqonda*) and his lover a "girlfriend" (*intombi*). Women, I was told, qoma (choose) a lover, whereas a prostitute will *dayisa umzimba* (sell her body). Though the word "isifebe" can mean both a prostitute and a woman who has an excessive number of boy-friends, there are a number of distinct words for a prostitute, such as *umdayisi* (a seller) and *umqwayizi* (a winker). Such women, I was constantly told, were active mainly in large towns like Durban. Sex has not become commodified in the sense that it is traded impersonally for money; instead it is enmeshed in new forms of emotion and reciprocity—exchanges more akin to gift relations, marked by mutual, if uneven, obligations that extend over time.[3]

I opted to use the word "prostitute" rather than "sex worker" above because it better reflects the disparaging comments aimed at women who overtly sell sex. In contrast, gifts given by "boyfriends" to "girlfriends" are more commonly talked about as a form of "help." Lindiwe, a young woman living in the township, explained that men's "help" can take many forms, including clothing and cosmetics.

MH: Why do women have many partners?

Lindiwe: Some, they tell themselves that they are going to get money; women who don't work, they tell themselves that they are going to be helped by men that they love.

MH: What do the men give the women, then?

Lindiwe: Some, they buy them anything, like clothes, or give a woman some money so that she can buy cosmetics.

I spoke with Mrs. Buthelezi in her house in Sundumbili, where she was drink-ing beer with two other women. She is fifty years old and extremely hos-tile toward men, saying that boyfriends had let her down many times. She described the difference between the materiality of everyday sex and prostitu-tion and gave a sense of the power relations that underpin gifts:

MH: Did those people see themselves as prostitutes?

Mrs. B: It's different; let me say here, at the township, the level of unemployment is high. The girl comes from Nongoma [in northern KwaZulu-Natal] looking for work, she can't find

work and she gets a boyfriend who will pay her rent, another
to buy her food, another one who is going to give her money,
and the other will help her for transport. . . . The situation
forces her.

MH: Do women cheat more now than in the past, or did they
always cheat?

Mrs. B: Now they cheat more.

MH: Why?

Mrs. B: Because we want money.

Another township resident, a woman in her fifties, described how some women
have multiple "boyfriends" as a kind of "business." She went on to explain that
women provide men not only with sex but with other "comforts of home":[4]

MH: How is it like a business?

INT: If I'm staying in my umjondolo I know I have five boyfriends;
maybe one is going to come in the morning and sleep with
me because he is working the night shift. When his payday
comes I will demand some money from him: "Do you think
I got food for *mahhala* [free] here in this umjondolo; in this
house you have to pay for the food you are eating here. I need
two hundred rand." One boyfriend again who's doing, like,
the day shift, he is sleeping here the whole night. "How come
you are sleeping here for the whole night, five days, and you
don't want to pay anything here, do you think there's anything
for mahhala?" I also demand something from him. . . . One is
night shift, one is day shift.

The stereotype of naïve rural women leaving home and being forced to sell
their bodies is a strong one, sometimes played on by informants, but many
accounts show that rural-born women are aware of the kind of relationships
that they are likely to have to embark on in Mandeni. Indeed, both people
and information have flowed steadily between Isithebe and rural KwaZulu-
Natal over the last three decades. One young lady in her early twenties from
Hlabisa district, Kheti, told me, "They hear that there are people [in Isithebe]
who stay with their boyfriends and that it is nice to do so. They too want to
stay well. They tell their parents that they want to find work, but they know
that they want a man."

Gift exchanges between men and women are patterned by geography in
other ways. Though, as Mrs. Buthelezi indicated above, Sundumbili township

hosts some rural-born migrants, most residents were born in the township's family houses. In this formally planned urban space, young women tend to have boyfriends less as a means to gain access to accommodation and more for access to consumer goods. The distinction between subsistence and consumption is, of course, a hazy one, but Sundumbili township does have higher average levels of income and a less mobile population than the surrounding informal areas. The most immediate requirements of life are therefore more accessible.

Isithebe jondolo settlement, by contrast, is a place where rural-born migrants are in more urgent need of accommodation and subsistence. Women might stay with a relative in a tiny umjondolo when they first arrive, but rarely do so for long. Moreover, virtually all jondolo settlement residents maintain close contact with rural kin who typically expect remittances, especially when they are looking after a resident's child.

Love in the Time of AIDS

AIDS policy documents are replete with categories such as "transactional sex," "sex work," and "sugar daddies." And, at one level, intimate relationships are certainly marked by their materiality and by great distrust. Is love in South Africa, then, just a façade, a romantic utopia in a country where links between sex and money are common?[5]

Love certainly seems to have sped up in recent years. Text (SMS) messages, with their quick beeps upon arrival, have emerged as the quintessential way of communicating love in South Africa. In 2005 around 120 million text messages were sent during the Christmas and New Year period alone (almost three per person).[6] When they concern intimate matters, as they frequently do, text messages suggest the fleeting nature of love: that love proposals can be quick, replies brash, and unwanted contacts immediately deleted. In a clever marketing move, cell phone service providers offer free "please call me" messages for those who want to communicate but have no airtime; receiving calls is free. Anybody with a cell phone can communicate for nothing—but only with a richer friend; it is tempting to see here an analogy for democracy's uneven reach across the different classes.

Bongi, my friend from the jondolo settlement, often received text messages from male suitors. She has an elegant demeanor, a youthful smile, and an infectious laugh. Often upon meeting a man of status—such as, for instance, when we were once stopped by a traffic cop—she is told *"Ngicela inombolo yakho"* (I am asking for your number). Sometimes a text message follows, one or two lines asking for a meeting or telephone conversation.

The enormous popularity of text messaging today makes older forms of communication seem almost antique—and for this reason highly valued. One day I was sitting on a bench in Bongi's workplace. She is a self-employed seamstress and sews clothes, especially school uniforms. A young man entered quietly and delivered a letter from his friend, her suitor. The letter was handwritten, mostly in isiZulu, on light green writing paper. Its author, whom Bongi knew, was employed by a well-paying factory. His invitation to her to help build an umuzi was a clear reference to marriage; the letter's style—elegant and poetic—contradicted common stereotypes of Zulu men as masculine and violent.

> Since I started to see you I could feel my stomach boil because of the trepidation I had. But I trust that you will feel sorry for me, my mother's child. . . . I have deep emotion in my heart because of you, my lady as white as the sand from the sea. My heart is beating like a fire if I think about you. My hands are soft like a banana ["My heart is beating like a fire *uma ngicabanga* about you. *Izandla zam zisoft* like banana"] . . . I want a woman to build up my family's home.

Bongi eventually dismissed the poetic letter, saying that she didn't find the man attractive, but I asked if she would help my research by collecting other love letters in the jondolo settlement. The shack where she conducted her business was located at a busy taxi stop, and thousands of people passed by it each day. Sitting on the wooden bench inside this small room for hours at a time over many years gave me a revealing window into the social networks in which women were immersed. I often wondered how Bongi herself managed to work with so many people dropping by, so much laughter, so many phone conversations, and such frequent text messaging. I began to realize that making a living for Bongi required constant "emotional labor": managing emotions to make or foster connections between people.[7] I patched together her life story from observations as well as numerous conversations with her and with mutual friends.

Bongi was born in Isithebe in 1970, only one year before Isithebe Industrial Park was established. Since her parents were poor, Bongi's aunt volunteered to raise her in a rural area about an hour's drive north of Isithebe. In her final year of secondary school, she became pregnant. Soon after her daughter Busi's birth, however, she split up with her lover, who moved to Durban and eventually married another woman. Nevertheless, he took responsibility for their child, eventually sending her to a former white Model C school in Durban.

Bongi talks with pride about her daughter. Once she told me that she had *hlola*'d (tested) her virginity, and she was reassured that it was still intact. When

I visited Bongi's rural home in 2000 I met the girl, then aged ten. She appeared quiet and averted her eyes from adults, a sign of deference. But the next time I saw her, some nine years later, she had a quite different demeanor: revealing the way that privileged schooling inscribed itself on the body, she conversed confidently in English with a tell-tale Model C accent that signaled prestige.

When Bongi moved back to Isithebe in the early 1990s, she began a long relationship with a well-known taxi owner. This boyfriend paid for her to live in Durban for a year and study to become a seamstress. They parented two children together, a boy and a girl. Bongi and many mutual friends have noted that she wanted to marry this man and was very distressed when he persisted in having other girlfriends. Although they broke up because of his infidelity, I have often seen her show great respect to him when talking on the phone. She told me many times that she hopes he will eventually send their two children to a former white model C school.

One reason Bongi felt especially strongly about the importance of education was because their son appeared to be following in his father's footsteps—already, at a very young age, showing a liking for guns and cars. Indeed, Bongi's former lover had a fearsome standing as an enforcer of a local "community policing forum"; he was said to have once tied a local thief to his car with a rope and dragged him through the jondolo settlement. I always felt a bit scared when I met him—making an enemy of such a person could swiftly end my fieldwork—but he seemed to approve of a white person living in the area and I got the sense that he saw my safety as part of his responsibility. I felt that, by publicly showing respect to him and his family (he now lived with another woman and their children), I added to his authority rather than challenging it.

For women arriving at Isithebe and knowing perhaps only one or two relatives in the area, Bongi was a superlative guide to the harsh environment. By the 1990s, jobs in the nearby factories were becoming rare and surviving through the informal economy was extremely difficult. As a consequence of the growth of large retailers, many women fought over unprofitable informal trading opportunities, selling items such as fruits, onions, tomatoes, and boiled ummbila (corn) on the streets. The most lucrative informal trading niches in which women gained dominance were illegal; these included trading *dagga* (marijuana) and brewing isiqatha (a notoriously potent spirit described in chapter 6). To navigate this hostile world, relationships of various kinds with men were necessary, and no one was a better source of information about the status and attributes of the area's men than Bongi.

Bongi was widely described as *hlankaniphile* (clever), and her streetwise intelligence was demonstrated by her encyclopedic knowledge of local people, institutions, and rumors. While much of her wisdom came from living for many years in the area, I watched her quickly master the newer domain of local politics. Especially after local municipal elections in 1996, she became acutely aware of the opportunities provided by "development" and built connections with members of the Inkatha Freedom Party, the African National Congress, and the Democratic Alliance, the three main local political parties. We sometimes joked that she was IFP Monday, ANC Tuesday, and DA Wednesday, and at various times I accompanied her to visit high-profile members of all three parties. In 2004 this effort bore fruit when a development project granted her five industrial sewing machines. These were meant to be used to train women to enter the trade, but she also used them to hire subcontractors, expanding her own business.

Bongi's gregarious personality and expert sewing skills ensured her financial independence, but only because of her location in Mandeni. Formal schooling provided credentials such as matriculation certificates and English-language skills that were valuable anywhere. In contrast, Bongi's knowledge was more spatially grounded, and this created problems as well as opportunities. Invariably, when the social networks she confronted in Mandeni extended upward in power and wealth, it was men she asked for various kinds of help.

When Bongi interacted with richer men in the community, she typically adopted a kind of friendly deference. Her own status as an isakhamuzi (local, resident) and a businesswoman allowed her a certain informality. At the same time, she drew on idioms of hlonipha (respect), to which her image as a dignified woman gave credence. Entering webs of patronage was an unpredictable business, and being a woman allowed her to play on men's sense of self-worth through flattery—but it also disadvantaged her at times.

In 2000, the owner of a shop from whom she rented a workspace rather abruptly told her he needed it for another purpose. She went to talk respectfully to a man of high status and wealth who owned another nearby shop and had a spare room; that I gave her a lift to the meeting marked me as a silent party to the negotiations. The man agreed to rent the room to her, and she began to mobilize friends to break open the wall and put in a new door to the outside. However, as the hole grew, the landlord increased the rent significantly and, in disgust, Bongi promptly bought a pile of concrete blocks and paid someone to fill the hole back up. Although she was furious, her actions toward this man were kept in the idioms of hlonipha (respect). Mobilizing other connections, she then moved her business into the small shack I described earlier.

My interest in Bongi's "emotional labor" was especially pertinent because ethnography is itself an emotional exercise; the fostering of friendships is inseparable from the work of collecting "data." Although I had a number

of good male friends in the township and the jondolo settlement, most men
either worked for many hours a day in formal employment or were unemployed. I knew no men in circumstances like Bongi's: with a lot of time to
socialize, a safe and sociable place to hang out, and financial independence.
These circumstances, as well as our similar ages, seemed to narrow the social
gaps between Bongi and me: we sometimes jokingly referred to one another
as *mpintshi* (mate). Bongi never asked me to loan her money, whereas unemployed men occasionally did, or at least asked me to share a beer with them.

As we became closer friends, Bongi did ask me for favors, especially lifts.
At times I became irritated when she would ask me to drive her halfway across
the often muddy informal settlement on an errand. I usually said yes, though;
I was so grateful for the way that she aided my research. In any case, as in the
relationships I studied, it was hard to separate material expectations from feelings of friendship, trust, and guilt that had their own momentum and bodily
gravity. More generally, I believe that residents like Bongi were well aware
that they held a certain power over me because I required their support for
my research project and especially for my safety. She knew that while violence
could uphold social hierarchies, bullets and knives did not discriminate: many
powerful and wealthy men, usually taxi owners or politicians, have been killed
in the area by rivals. With power comes vulnerability, and I was always grateful
when Bongi told anyone who listened that I was a student who was not rich
like other whites. "Look at his *iskorokoro* [beaten-up car]," she would say.

Since Bongi and I spent so much time together, rumors occasionally
surfaced that we were having an affair. At first I was worried about these
and wanted to rebuff them, scared that I would be seen as a rich white man
exploiting a poorer black woman. However, I soon came to realize that they
were repeated with more amusement than venom, and I was sometimes asked
about them in quite a matter-of-fact way rather than judgmentally: "Oh, you
mean that Bongi [or any other women I knew] is not your girlfriend? But I
always see you together."

Any resentment of my apparent ability to enter into relationships with
women was more likely to come from men, who were painfully aware that
money was a gatekeeper for their intimate encounters. On one occasion, driving Bongi home through the muddy shack settlement, I saw an unemployed
man I knew clutching a beer bottle and heard him mutter, *"Sawubona mkhwe-
nyana"* ("Hello, fiancé") as we drove past. *Umkhwenyana* is a respectful term
for a man who is lobola-ing a woman; its ironic use here drew attention to the
connection between my wealth and my ability to attract girlfriends in ways that
could raise my status. The stark differences between my life and the lives of the

poorest male residents were highly visible to them because I represented, not only white privilege, but also male privilege they should have enjoyed.

Love Letters and Changing Connections

The archetypal love letter from South Africa's era of male migrancy can be found in Isaac Schapera's 1940 ethnography *Married Life in an African Tribe*. The touching note was penned by a migrant man in Johannesburg and addressed to his rural-based girlfriend. Describing the pain of separation, he writes, "I still think of how we loved each other; I think of how you behaved to me my wife."[8] But while similar romantic notes are found in Isithebe today, their context is quite different. They reflect women's own movement out of rural areas, the rise of unemployment, and the rarity of marriage.

One letter Bongi collected for me was written by a man to Themba, a woman in her late twenties. Themba had arrived in the area with hardly any money or contacts, and Bongi had helped her as a kind of patron, giving her a place to stay in her family home in Isithebe. Bongi's family were longstanding residents and therefore had access to a small plot of land on which were built three mud, wood, and stone structures, two for her mother and brother and one for her; Themba stayed in Bongi's house.

Outwardly at least, Bongi and Themba's relationship appeared to be somewhere between that of an elder and younger sister and that of a husband and wife. When I dropped Bongi at her home, Themba would sometimes emerge to greet her with Bongi's two children, as if she were a loyal wife waiting for her husband. Once I asked Bongi whether Themba and she were lovers; Bongi laughed in apparent shock, saying candidly that she desired a man's penis and not a woman's body. Themba was a kind of social wife in an arrangement that reflected growing economic gaps between women in the area as well as between men and women. She diligently undertook domestic duties while Bongi supported the household financially, as a man had done previously.

Themba's poverty typified the dismal economic circumstances of newer migrants to the area in the recent period of industrial decline. Nevertheless, her intimate encounters with men represented more than the narrow exchange of money for sex. One day a man in his fifties shela'd (proposed love to) Themba in a letter written in isiZulu. He began by informing her about the death of his children's mother. He then tried to allay any fears that because of his age he might be sexually impotent, an embarrassing topic that a letter could most easily address. His mention of sexual performance suggests that even relationships that crossed very large age differences can be built in part on sexual satisfaction or procreation and not simply on gifts from men to women:

> I am happy if you are still alive. I am not well, and you know my problem: that the mother of my children left me. I tried to tell you everything but you ignore me. I do not intend to play with you but I love you with all of my heart. . . . Don't worry, as my penis is still working, I am not that old. Your food, you'll find it still full, it is yours only, I don't give it to anyone.

Themba was very ill when she received this letter. A few months later, as her health worsened, she went to stay with her brother in Inanda, an informal settlement close to Durban; returning to stay with one's relatives is usually a sign that someone is close to death. On my way to Durban one day, I visited her in the mud and stick umjondolo that hugged the crooked hills of Inanda's informal settlement. Her thin body lay limply on the bed, and on the bedside table sat a bottle of powerful *umuthi* (medicine) from a famous *inyanga* (traditional healer) in Umlazi township. As I said goodbye, her brother, mistaking me for a medical doctor, showed me the painful-looking shingles blisters on his own back (shingles is an opportunistic infection often associated with the early stages of AIDS).

Themba eventually recovered and returned to Mandeni, putting on weight and beginning to look healthier. Such slumps in health followed by a quick improvement were not uncommon. One day, however, Bongi told me that Themba had fallen ill briefly and had been tested for HIV and found to be infected. When I heard this news I tried to introduce her to the Treatment Action Campaign, the organization at the center of treatment activism in the area. It was 2004 and antiretroviral drugs were about to become available. Themba, however, argued that her health was getting better and refused to take medication.

A year later, while I was in the United States, I phoned Bongi one day and she told me that Themba had passed away. She had become pregnant by the suitor who sent her the letter, who also gave her significant financial support. However, she had not wanted to risk giving birth to an HIV positive child (although clinics by then provided drugs that reduced the chance of mother-to-child transmission, it could not be eliminated). In an attempt to abort the baby, she had drunk a large amount of *Jik* (bleach), which had caused her death. Themba's story represented a tragic case of someone who came to the area and formed social and sexual connections from a position of weakness. She also fell ill before the government had fully implemented its program to provide antiretroviral drugs to HIV positive people.

During 2004, Bongi collected three more letters, this time from Mr. Mathe, thirty-six, a neighbor and friend of hers who had a quite high-paying factory job. (In rural areas, where gender and generational boundaries are more policed, it would be less common for a man and woman of similar ages to discuss love affairs.) Mr. Mathe sent the first letter to a woman in her thirties whom Bongi knew. The second was intended for another woman, and the third was received by Mr. Mathe from a third woman. Taken together, these three letters (all sent within a short period) indicate that multiple forms of relationships can exist, all with different requirements, expectations, and emotional characteristics.

In the first letter, Mr. Mathe proposed love to a woman living in the jondolo settlement: "Please be specific from now on, please accept me and you know that I love you, your heart knows that I worship you, my lady." He wrote the second to end a relationship with a woman in very direct terms, saying that she was isifebe, a slut. "I am tired of you, can we please break up because you are a slut that gets around using her vagina on the floor. Indians, Coloureds and Blacks it's you being a slut, you slut. There is already a girl that I am involved with so stay away with your slutness. I don't need an answer." He showed this letter to Bongi, and she persuaded him not to send it. The third was from a woman with whom he had a child, informing him that she wanted to end the relationship because she was marrying another man.

> I write this letter and I have tried many times to reach you but didn't succeed, I tried calling you on the phone and there was no response. The bad news as you know that I go to the Nazareth church and I have told you before that I want to get married. I have found someone to marry me, in other words I don't want you anymore. No one is allowed to do anything to me, the other family is coming the next Monday [to begin marriage proceedings].

The reference to the Nazareth (or Shembe) Church is significant because the church allows polygamous marriages.

Love and Money

In Mandeni the famous Beatles lyric "Money can't buy me love" is far from true. In fact, it is a global falsehood, because marriage and dating are always mediated by class, status, and many other factors. One day in 2003, I had a conversation with three young women, Dumazile, Qondeni, and Hlengiwe, who were in their early twenties and lived in Sundumbili township. This discussion, held at my research assistant's house, captures the way that gifts can sometimes foster feelings of love, but at other times signify lovelessness. At one point, Dumazile appears to approach men through a crude instrumentalism, categorizing them by what they give her, and showing the power of money in determining love.

> MH: Do women sometimes have more than one boyfriend so that they can get lots of things?
>
> Dumazile: There are some that say this one will buy me clothes, this one will buy me cosmetics, and this one will give me money.
>
> MH: But it never works like that though, does it? They say that, but really men give them money, don't they?
>
> Dumazile: Yes, this one gives her money and she will go and buy the things by herself. Some women do these things because they have no money. She loves the one who is already her boyfriend, but the problem is that he does not do anything for her. Then another man will shela her and she discovers that this one has money, so she will love him too.

What does Dumazile mean by saying that when a man has money, a woman will love him? Despite the importance of gifts to relationships, I believe that she uses the verb "ukuthanda" to indicate an emotional bond. The nature of intimate connections varies from relationship to relationship, but sex is not simply exchanged instrumentally: the two lovers are "boyfriend" and "girlfriend," not "prostitute" and "client."

To understand the coming together of money, sex, and emotion today requires returning to the concept of provider love I outlined earlier. Historically, provider love developed because a man paid ilobolo for and then married and supported a woman. But marriage is rare today, and great mistrust ensnares many relationships. Consequently, a diminished form of provider love can be seen in gifts from a man to a woman, such as cosmetics or money. To put these recent changes in a different way, men have moved from being "providers within marriage" to less reliable and less esteemed "providers outside of marriage."

Certainly, ilobolo and marriage still cast long symbolic shadows over relationships. If sex were simply commodified, women and men would have equally uncommitted relations with different partners. But in fact, people in multiple concurrent relationships typically differentiate between a main lover and secondary lovers. This ranking structures these sexual networks both emotionally and materially. A woman's main lover, described by various terms—*istraight* or *iqonda* (straight), "number one," or umkhwenyana (fiancé, if he has begun to pay ilobolo)—is the one with whom the relationship is most serious and might one day lead to marriage. In the rare cases when ilobolo payments have been initiated, the status of a woman's main lover is raised substantially. Such payments are the most decisive symbol of commitment and, most residents would say, obligate a woman to be faithful to that man.

Secondary lovers—that is, lovers who are not "istraight"—can, at times, be casual partners with whom relationships are brief. Yet although surveys of sexual behavior commonly distinguish between "main lovers" and "casual lovers"—the latter term resonating with a number of English concepts such as "fling" and "one-night stand"—secondary lovers are rarely the same thing as casual lovers; relationships with them can persist for some time. To understand why, we must conceptualize relationships as reciprocal—as "gift relations," in anthropological language. A relationship's secondary status is typically determined not by how long it is expected to last, but by the lesser obligations and expectations it creates and by its more secret nature; for instance, a secondary lover can be called an *ishende* (secret lover) or umakhwapheni (under the armpit). The primary determinant of a relationship's status is not its duration, but the nature of its bond.

Such differentiation, as we have seen, was apparent earlier in the century, too, when rural-based women distinguished between their ibhodwe (pot, or main lover) and isidikiselo (top of a pot, or secondary lover). These secondary relationships were often entered into during a husband's absence. Yet they were not casual, but could persist for many years. Indeed the word "isidikiselo" is still in circulation and typically provokes laughter as well as disputes over its meaning. If women can use it to justify having multiple partners, men are more likely to argue that doing so was exceptional in the past, and not due to desire for consumer goods.

Today, a good example of a secondary lover is a sugar daddy, and most young people would agree that there is little expectation that such relationships will lead to marriage. Sugar daddy relationships, then, are secondary because they are not likely to lead to marriage—and yet they are not simply "casual" in a temporal sense, because they can last for months and even years. Notably, sugar daddies today appear to be positioned quite differently from the umathandezincane (man who likes young women) of an earlier period, who might have married his younger girlfriend.

As we have seen, the structural distrust between many young people today, rooted in the painful dismantling of a patriarchal bargain, provides some justification for young women's having a sugar daddy. Similarly, men's "failures" allow women to link different men to specific expenses (e.g., "one each for money, food, and rent" or "ministers of finance, transport, and entertainment"). The lack of a husband's support allows a woman to characterize her day-to-day dependence on men in ironic terms. Yet rather than being directly told that they are a provider of food or money, men are more likely to be made aware that they are a primary or secondary boyfriend, as Dumazile noted earlier. A linear ranking of boyfriends or an itemization of what each provides is less important than whether each is the main, generally public, lover or one of the secondary ones, more likely to be secret. Qondeni elaborates:

> MH: But do the boys know what the girls say about them, namely, this one is for food, this one is for clothes; do the boys know that?
>
> Qondeni: When he comes to me he will ask if I am involved. Then I will either tell him that I am single, or that there is someone I am involved with and that he will be the second one. Then to the third one I won't say that he is the third; I will say that he is number two.

As these examples make abundantly clear, monetary or other gifts often ensure a man's status as a lover. Yet material expressions of love are not always the most important. For a start, a man's financial situation can change; a young, poor boyfriend can find work and then repay his girlfriend's loyalty during tough times. Moreover, romantic love's claim that "love conquers all" creates its own emotional inertia. Hlengiwe expressed the romantic view when I asked her what would happen if a number-one boyfriend lost his job: "If you really love the number-one boyfriend truly, there is nothing that can change, because you love the others for their money only."

If women typically have a single main lover but sometimes other lovers, how do men approach multiple-partnered relationships? Young men I knew also discussed the intense love they felt for some women, especially their main lover. Like women, men may use the words "istraight" and "iqonda." But dominant masculinities exert less pressure on men to remain sexually faithful and therefore to have a single public lover. While a man gains status by lobola-ing a main lover, he—unlike most women—can also raise his status by having multiple sexual partners. Hence, men are more likely than women to brag about the number of partners that they have. As Simone de Beauvoir pointed out many years ago, "The word *love* has by no means the same sense for both sexes."[9]

Negotiating Love

In 2002 love came to South Africa with a bang in the form of the T.V. show *All You Need Is Love,* which depicted the delivery of messages of love and recorded the recipients' responses. "Lost love, long distance love, unrequited love, looking for love, fragile love, forgotten love, star crossed lovers . . . you name it, *All You Need Is Love* will find it and try to fix it," proclaimed its website.[10] The show quickly attracted two million viewers, and soon after its launch friends of mine in Mandeni began to enthusiastically dissect its every episode. The question on everyone's mind was whether love can prevail. Would a touching message of love surmount the problems faced by the couple featured on the show? At times the answer was no, and the camera awkwardly dissected the reaction of a rejected suitor. But more often than not the audience was able to cheer—and the loudest applause was reserved for a public proposal of marriage.

Resting on the seeming universality of love, the popular T.V. show celebrated not only heterosexual sex but same-sex love (although only between men, in the episodes that I saw). Its success captures a certain optimism about love that emerged in the jet stream of democracy; indeed, the "better life for all" promised by the ANC in 1994 extended to all spheres, from the economic to the interpersonal. Especially in the early years of democracy, love became something of a metaphor for uneven new freedoms: just like the rapid social mobility enjoyed by a few South Africans, love is unpredictable but potentially life-changing. Yet, in turn, the program's cancelation several years later perhaps reveals the fickleness of love and, by association, social mobility after apartheid.

The high regard for love, evident in programs like *All You Need Is Love,* means that one way Mandeni's residents mark inappropriate behavior is by presenting it as loveless, or as corrupted by the wrong kind of love. Both men and women declare adamantly at times that "love no longer exists" (*alusekho uthando*). The claim echoes longstanding contestations of love in the country. Accounts going back to the 1930s reveal a sense that a new and passionate force of love was appearing that could, for instance, lead to premarital pregnancy.[11] A truer love, from this perspective, rested on a man lobola-ing and then supporting a woman. In similar ways today—although in the new context of unemployment and the scarcity of marriage—women can complain that men are only interested in love that results in immediate sex. And men can equally often claim that women will only love boyfriends with money.

A good example of today's nostalgia for a purer, more moral love is the popularity of Mafikizolo's 2003 hit "Emlanjeni" (At the River). The song depicts a woman waiting for her absent boyfriend, who, we might presume, works as a migrant laborer and is saving money for ilobolo. The lyrics begin, *"Yandlula iminyaka ngingakuboni, yandlula iminyaka ngingakuboni, isoka lam"* (Years have passed and I haven't seen you, my boyfriend).[12]

Mafikizolo's tune, a rewriting of an older song, evokes nostalgia for "meeting at the river," where rural men and women used to court, and suggests the integrity of past relationships, when a man would patiently save to pay ilobolo and marry his girlfriend and a woman would not trade sex for gifts. In the slow swaying of people dancing to this song, which I have witnessed at many shebeens and other venues, this melodic and emotional tune reifies a past genuine love: both provider love and romantic love. Yet what is important to listeners is not so much the specificity of past forms of love as the song's regret at the absence of love today—and its hint that love may nonetheless suddenly appear.

In such an uncertain world, how do you know that you are in love? The verb "ukuthanda" (to like or to love) is widely and ambiguously used in everyday conversations. Bodily sensations are difficult to read, and relationships unfold in unpredictable ways. Love can come from the heart, but can also be promoted by money. So too can love potions stimulate love, as they did in the past. A Sundumbili woman in her twenties whom I knew well swore that her father had been bewitched by his lover, who, she said, was milking him for money. How else could he not see what a manipulative woman she was? Just as biomedical and spiritual explanations of health coexist, so too can romantic love jostle and yet overlap with accounts of love as stemming from umuthi (traditional medicine).

The most genuine expression of a man's love for a woman, I have argued, is his payment of ilobolo. But this payment is rare today. Ilobolo is very costly, and women's families typically require a large initial payment. As noted earlier, residents do debate the high cost of ilobolo, and families sometimes accept smaller amounts. I have also come across churches sanctioning reduced payments. But reducing ilobolo inevitably invites suspicion that the man is not really in love with the woman. On one occasion I heard residents gossip, somewhat maliciously, that a female teacher had given her unemployed lover the money with which to pay ilobolo for her.

Feelings of love can nevertheless be manifested in everyday acts of reciprocity, affection, and desire, which help to cement intimate relationships. My female research assistant collected text messages from friends in reasonably long-term relationships, and these messages capture how love is expressed in sometimes mundane, sometimes sensual acts of intimacy and support. They also bear traces of negotiation, as couples chart out a path that is simultaneously material and emotional.

> *Sthandwa sami anginayo imali yokugibela* this week *emsebenzini* pls help I love you (my lover I don't have money for transport to get to work this week pls help I love you) [woman, 24, to man, 24, 11-month relationship].

> I'm all alone in bed hoping you will join me, naked I'm dying to have sex with u. Reply pls. [woman, 26, to man, 27, 1½-year relationship]

> *Sthandwa ngilambile ngicela uzopheka ukhiye kwanextdoor* see you after work I love u. (my love I am hungry please can you cook the key is next door see you after work I love u.) [man, 30, to woman, 26, 2-year relationship]

> Baby *ngithi angikwazise ukuthi ngiyakuthanda, ngicela uziphathe kahle.* (Baby I want you to know that I love you, please behave yourself.) [woman, 23, to man, 24, 6-month relationship]

Love and Care

The final message above suggests a fundamental tension within relationships: "I want you to know that I love you," the woman says, suggesting unconditional caring, and then she ends with "behave yourself," which implies his potential for wrongdoing, especially sexual. How much does love, here and in other relationships, involve caretaking? An enormous amount of caretaking takes place in the midst of an AIDS pandemic, often in private and through kinship networks. South Africa, in short, is a very caring society. But boyfriend-girlfriend relationships are often not characterized by care "no matter what." This is graphically shown in the case of a man who fell ill and died of AIDS in Sundumbili township.

I had known Dave, a mechanic, in passing for five years. My friends always gossiped about his *isoka* activities; he owned a car and was rumored to have a host of girlfriends. But in 2006, when I entered his house to visit his father, I saw him lying in pain on a makeshift bed on the lounge floor. His two sisters, who lived there as well, chatted to me and did not even mention the person dying in their midst. Dave yelled for me to help him, but one sister ushered me away. They were irritated because he had not provided any support for the family when he was earning money, preferring to travel around as a philandering isoka; now they were expected to look after him.

Once surrounded by female admirers, Dave was now dying in a state of ignominy, his shame worsened by his constant dirtying of his clothes through diarrhea. "Where are all his girlfriends now?" one sister asked. "Not one has called. It is us, the family, who are left to take care of him." It was as if his choice to concentrate on sexual escapades rather than long-term relationships had become realized in his humiliating illness.

One day his constant screams for help led him to be admitted to the hospital, but Dave was too much for the nurses and was quickly discharged. He refused to take ARVs despite their availability. I have no idea how he experienced his illness, but it is not uncommon for understandings of the cause of AIDS to jostle between the biomedical (a virus) and the social (witchcraft), and in the latter case the disease is typically seen as deliberately caused by malice, often jealousy.[13] His frequently soiled body, looked after by unenthusiastic relatives, did not give him grounds to believe that relationships of any kind could be easily mended; he was too ill, physically and socially. In agony, he was taken again to the hospital and eventually died a painful death.

Dave's experience reveals that none of his relationships with his girlfriends created an obligation of care on their part. Once he became ill they abandoned him; his family had to provide care. (It is possible, of course, that some of Dave's former girlfriends were also ill or had died.) But his kin were not enthusiastic about doing so, because he had never helped them, though they didn't deny their obligation. Thus, while gifts and sex are very much an accepted part of non-marital relationships, care tends to be organized in the first instance by kin, and also by friends, perhaps constituted in groups such as churches.[14] This has important implications, as we see below.

To Condom or Not to Condom

Condoms are extensively advocated in global AIDS campaigns and are given away free by Sundumbili's clinic and other institutions in Mandeni. The "ABC" campaigns preach three ways of preventing AIDS: abstain from sex, be faithful, or use a condom—the latter especially with casual lovers. Condoms were increasingly used by young people in the 2000s, and there are many reasons for this, as well as for their non-use. Indeed, diverse meanings attach themselves to condoms, including whether their "fat" (lubricant) itself infects people with HIV. Here, I only explore connections between love, money, and condom use.

One common reason given for the non-use of condoms in South Africa —as elsewhere—is that dominant masculinities promote risk-taking and pleasure at all costs. This is readily displayed in the phrases men use to celebrate "flesh-to-flesh sex," such as "you can't eat a sweetie with its wrapper on." Foregrounding the power relations that underpin these comments, gender activists have fought a long and important battle to make female condoms more available.

Yet men's opposition to the use of male condoms, while certainly important, does not fully explain why women themselves sometimes advocate not using them. Most men I spoke with were adamant that women as well as men opposed condom use at times. Moreover, while gendered poverty certainly affects a woman's ability to "negotiate" condom use, women often explained that they did not use condoms because they were "in love."

Since fertility is still highly valued, one reason why some women may be reluctant to use condoms is that they prefer to chance "falling pregnant or falling positive."[15] Parenting a child creates material and emotional links between the parents, and when marriage rates are so low, these permanent links can signify love. But this cannot entirely explain why condoms are not more widely used. As we have seen, from the 1970s contraceptive use accelerated in South Africa, although the most common form, until very recently, was Depo-Provera injections. Clearly, then, condoms have not been the most typical means by which women avoided childbirth. So we return to the question, why are many young women and men not using condoms?

To go further in addressing this question, we must conceive of relationships as characterized not by a narrow commodification of sex but by reciprocal bonds based on exchanges and affection. That poverty and "unprotected sex" play out through the medium of love was made clear to me one day by Thandi, twenty-one. An attractive lady with a gap in her front teeth from a fight with a former boyfriend, Thandi related at my research assistant's house the harsh social conditions that she, like many young South African women, face—she had recently lost a parent and had a child to support. Yet unlike other young women, who depended on local boyfriends, Thandi maintained that she preferred to "sell her body" (*dayisa umzimba*) as a prostitute or sex worker in Durban. Boyfriends, she said, wouldn't wear condoms, but she could insist that clients oblige. For much of our discussion, she appeared quite positive about selling sex in Durban; however, at one moment tears came to her eyes, betraying her vulnerability, especially when her earnings from sex were low. Thandi said that payments were not fixed, but ranged between R30 and R100 (US$3.75–12.5) for sexual intercourse.

This somewhat counterintuitive fact—that the most instrumental sex-money exchanges are most likely to lead to condom use—has been noted elsewhere.[16] For "boyfriends" and "girlfriends," in contrast, condomless sex can signal and be felt as love. It can differentiate main from secondary lovers, open up a relationship to the prospect of permanence, provide greater intimacy and pleasure, and increase the man's obligation to support his girlfriend. Sex without condoms is not, therefore, a simple expression of "male power" in the sense that men don't want to use condoms and women do, but is motivated more subtly, through embodied sets of obligations and flows of material resources. This has important implications. Condom campaigns typically target "casual" relationships, and by this they mean short-term, "loveless" encounters. The reality, however, is that partners are usually distinguished by the obligations that each relationship creates, rather than by its duration. If varied but definite feelings of love permeate most relationships and yet condoms are constructed as signaling casualness (and thus a lack of love), is it any surprise that lovers don't use them?

. . . and Then There Is Care

Still, these explanations leave unanswered questions concerning risk and care—ones with resonances in many geographies. Why does a lover, especially a "main" lover, take the risk of infecting his or her partner, and perhaps a child, with HIV?

We can turn for possible answers to some recent accounts of what love is or is said to be becoming. For British sociologist Anthony Giddens, modern relationships are becoming characterized by a kind of "rolling contract," according to which individuals can enter and leave them more freely.[17] This he sees as driving a more egalitarian form of "confluent love": less hindered by the male-dominated institutions of marriage and the constant threat of pregnancy, relationships can yield always-contingent pleasures.

Giddens's model rests on a particular vision of an autonomous body able to defend itself from undesirable expectations and obligations. And his modern subjects bear many similarities to the rights-bearing individuals that AIDS campaigns sometimes try and promote in a bid to empower women in poorer countries. Here, too, women's right to choose can be championed through advocating a kind of "confluent love." Yet Giddens's vision of intimate equality in the West rests, crucially, on women's growing access to work and contraception. In contrast, many relationships in South Africa embody stark inequalities in power and resources, although there are exceptions (perhaps best symbolized by the "It girls").

Let's look at this point again in a slightly different way. Some AIDS interventions champion, in Giddens's term, a kind of "pure relationship"—in which relationships can be ended at will—as capable of fighting the disease. The reality, however, is that in settings of great poverty, love can rarely be severed from a world of dependences: when money and sex are closely connected, love is often more embedded within relationships, not less.

A second—and in my view more useful—approach to love rebels against the shallow and consumer-driven notions of romantic love that particularly emanate from Western capitalism. Feminist writer Mary Evans argues that "the proposal is not that we abandon love in the sense of care and commitment, but we abandon it in its romanticized and commercialized form."[18] For Evans, "care" is not intrinsic to most modern ideas of love and yet should be its guiding tenet. As we noted, in South Africa most non-marital intimate relations today are not premised on care, although they are always emotional and often involve a sense of care. Intimate relations between men and women are structured by great conflict: key to this is the sense of betrayal caused by the unmooring of gendered assumptions based on the "patriarchal bargain" of men working and supporting women.

With these points in mind, we can extend the already stated critique of much AIDS policy. When campaigns do talk about love, they tend to present it as a way to promote individualistic notions of choice. The youth AIDS NGO loveLife, which I discuss in the next chapter, uses romantic love to celebrate individuals' ability to move in and out of relationships at will and to choose a partner regardless of race, religion, and sex. The very fact that loveLife discusses love sets it apart from many AIDS campaigns. But the love it presents is more viable for the sassy middle-class people who frequently appear in its advertisements.

In contrast, many young people in places like Mandeni enter relationships structured by reciprocity and yet great inequality. The fact that they often involve gifts does not mean that they are not also loving: these relationships entangle love with gifts and sometimes, as we have seen, with violence. It is tempting to see highly material relationships as simply loveless; I did at first. But we must take more seriously the way people often understand their lives as simultaneously material and emotional despite, or perhaps precisely because of, the existence of profound inequalities.

Furthermore, the idea of love as care—protecting others as well as one-self—is rarely promoted by AIDS campaigns or popular culture. The latter is particularly influenced by images of romantic love on T.V. and in magazines. With so many people falling ill in society, an enormous amount of care is carried out; but this is typically organized within kin relationships rather than boyfriend-girlfriend ones.

———————

Bringing love into tension with its apparent opposite—material exchanges linked to sex—reveals how love structures relationships, is a site of struggle, and therefore must be taken more seriously. Material and emotional practices are always intertwined; sex and love are always material—worldwide, at all times. What is unique to South Africa today is the shockingly high levels of inequality and unemployment; this results in everyday intimate relations being highly material, very much a part of "making a living," or social reproduction. By presenting "main" relationships as safe, loving, and long-term, AIDS campaigns frequently ignore the fact that relationships, including those where people have more than one sexual partner, are typically marked by very fluid obligations, some material and some emotional. It is within ever-shifting relationships partly based on love, and especially in those between "main" lovers, that condoms are often least likely to be used.

To the extent that care is promoted in South Africa, the state has typically reiterated its association with kin, for instance by promoting "home-based care" as a way to reduce government spending. This is a problematic approach when the country has widening gaps between the rich and the poor; at worst, it essentially amounts to telling the poor to look after themselves.[19] Yet other models of care draw deeply on South African history. Bishop Desmond Tutu, anti-apartheid activist and former chair of the Truth and Reconciliation Commission, is a passionate advocate of connecting care to love—and attaches both of them firmly to questions of social justice and social struggle. Tutu has been a consistent spokesman on a range of moral issues, from the existence of poverty amid riches to homophobia. He draws on the tremendous moral authority of the anti-apartheid struggle, focusing conceptions of "freedom" less on consumption and more on equity, care, love, and justice. In Tutu's words, "Evil, injustice, oppression, all of those awful things, they are not going to have the last word. Goodness, laughter, joy, caring, compassion, the things that you do and you help others do, those are going to prevail."[20]

South Africa's unique history of social struggle is embodied in figures like Tutu, and provides important, often forgotten, lessons. Images of love tend to flow from Hollywood to Soweto, from New York to Durban, getting reworked along the way, but nevertheless portraying love as firmly embedded in individualism and consumption. But Tutu argues that care and love must be attached to a more equitable political economy. Moreover, the notion of personhood to which he subscribes draws from *ubuntu,* an ethical philosophy holding that individuals are not autonomous beings but are formed through relationships with others. Of course, ideas of personhood in the West and Africa are never static, and the search for an authentic African (or Euro-American) personhood is fraught with difficulties.[21] But Tutu's South African use of love decenters love's attachment to individualism and choice. And perhaps his notion of a love that combines political economy, care, and social justice could be exported from South Africa and help to recast key concepts of intimacy circulating in the AIDS world.

PART 3

Interventions

TEN

The Politics of Gender, Intimacy, and AIDS

"It is important that we all should recognize the fact that it was very deliberate that we chose this community of Mandeni," Jacob Zuma told a Mandeni crowd in July 2001. "We do so to highlight our serious concern about the scale and ferocity that HIV/AIDS is engulfing our rural communities and youth in those communities."[1] Zuma, then the country's deputy president, was speaking at the opening of Mandeni's loveLife youth center, set up to stem the high HIV rates in the area. I stood next to the large function tent, admiring the pomp and ceremony. The center was a beaming, bright purple, postmodern building that couldn't have contrasted more with the monotonous, apartheid-era, four-room houses in the adjacent Sundumbili township. That was precisely the aim: to create an island of positive sexuality and motivation in an area known to be badly affected by AIDS.

Established in 1999, loveLife quickly became the largest AIDS intervention program for youth in South Africa, and Mandeni's youth center was one of sixteen it established. Running through loveLife's institutional veins was a bold philosophy: it wanted to advance "a new lifestyle brand for young South Africans, promoting healthy living and positive sexuality."[2] In this spirit, love-Life argued that bland ABC programs (advocating abstinence, being faithful, and using condoms) had failed to appeal to its target group of twelve- to seventeen-year-olds.

Certainly, young women in particular were becoming infected with HIV at a shockingly high rate: a 2003 study found that HIV prevalence rose from 4 percent among fifteen- and sixteen-year-old women to 31 percent among twenty-one-year-olds.[3] If this most at-risk group is to be convinced to practice safe sex, loveLife argued, campaigns had to be relevant and fun. To this end, its strategy built on what it regarded as "the fundamental aspirational optimism among South African youth."[4] By tapping into this optimism, it could help youth overcome negative peer pressure and deadly silences around sex. Parents, for their part, would talk openly to their children about sex—or, as the organization put it, "love them enough to talk about sex."

In addition to the network of youth centers, loveLife sponsored hundreds of billboard advertisements (more than two thousand in 2002), ran a busy telephone hotline, and ran numerous T.V., radio, and newspaper advertisements. The organization was generously funded (mostly by foreign donors), especially at first. Consequently, visitors to Mandeni's youth center were greeted by an array of expensive equipment: a fully operational radio station, a clinic, a sports and recreation department, and a computer center.

From the outset, LoveLife attracted criticism. Skeptics quickly derided it for glamorizing sex and producing overly cryptic advertisements that few young people understood.[5] I do not intend to provide a full review of the institution. My argument thus far is that AIDS emerged rapidly in the area because of the fissures caused by rising social inequalities and unemployment. I focus on loveLife, therefore, because it typifies a response to AIDS that links rights and intimacy in ways that appeal most to socially mobile young people. I develop this theme by considering loveLife alongside the Treatment Action Campaign (TAC), the other main AIDS organization in Mandeni in the 2000s. In sharp contrast, the TAC's approach linked health and socio-economic rights to advocate for citizens' access to health services and AIDS drugs; a majority of its activists, in turn, were poor African women.

These are certainly two very different types of organizations, with different aims and constituents. Indeed, the context they operate in speaks to broader power relations shaping social movements and NGOs in a globally unequal world. The loveLife program was initiated to reduce HIV prevalence among young people; it was funded by both the government and foreign donors, and it would therefore have been difficult for it to promote redistributive programs. The TAC, in contrast, advocated greater health equality but it did so, in part, through campaigning for biomedical treatment for sick people, an approach that appealed to some public health institutions. What follows, then, is not simply a comparative exercise.

Sex and the Self: loveLife Youth Center

My familiarity with loveLife stems from media reports and volunteering at the Mandeni youth center several afternoons a week for large parts of 2003. Most of the center's activities were run by around ten "groundbreaker" volunteers (who were paid about US$150 a month) and a larger group of unpaid "peer educator" volunteers. Especially in its early days, loveLife's well-funded programs reinforced an institutional culture of opportunity and optimism.

One morning in January 2003, a buzz of excitement consumed volunteers at the center. Leaving the shade of the building and entering the unrelenting summer heat, we made our way to Mandeni's bare grey train station. Here, our eyes widened at the sight of a bright purple "Love Train," a four-carriage mobile AIDS unit that was visiting Mandeni as part of a national tour. I entered an air-conditioned carriage with some volunteers to find a well-equipped radio studio, and we sat down in comfortable designer chairs. The surroundings were salubrious and strangely familiar: it was as though a piece of Johannesburg's trendy media world had been transported to our doorstep.

Recruited from around the country, the volunteers on the train mixed freely with the youth center's staff; together they showed off their talents by taking turns to DJ the country's latest tunes on an impressive sound system. About two hundred young people crowded around, and the volunteers offered activities ranging from playing basketball to learning about "positive sexuality," a way for individuals to exert their right to make choices on sexual matters. Meanwhile, one volunteer "did a motivation," giving a kind of evangelical sermon that exalted the virtues of positive living, self-esteem, and resistance to peer pressure.

The stylish and expensive Love Train symbolized the NGO's uneven influence in Mandeni. Although its community outreach program visited many schools in the area, the hub of loveLife's activities remained the youth center itself. And during the period of my involvement, most of its volunteers lived in the township, the residential area closest to the center. Only one stipend-earning volunteer I knew lived in the poorer Isithebe jondolo settlement, and none came from rural areas far outside central Mandeni—despite the fact that Zuma had supported the youth center because it was located in a rural setting. Nor were visitors to the youth center fully representative of the area's population: like the volunteers, the majority lived in or near the township and only a few came from the jondolo (informal) settlements and rural areas.

Access to the youth center was mediated by social class and geography in several ways. The center's need for infrastructure, including roads and electricity, attracted it to the township. Many township residents walked to the youth center, whereas young people from the poorer jondolo settlements and rural areas could rarely afford the transport costs to get there. The formal and informal qualifications favored by the institution constituted a further filter. LoveLife preferred its stipend-earning "groundbreakers" to have completed high school, and also required volunteers to be competent in the English language. Although volunteers at the center spoke to one another mostly in isiZulu, virtually all of the written material was in English.[6] English was also used when outside visitors, especially the all-important funders, came to the center.

In this respect, loveLife worked through rather than against the contours of emerging class differentials: in Mandeni better-off African parents sent their children to former white and Indian schools precisely because these institutions imparted good English-language skills. Class distinctions also reproduced themselves because parents in relatively high-status jobs, such as teachers, were more likely to encourage some use of English in the home. Moreover, loveLife's embrace of English accorded with the language's rising status among South Africa's new elite, including media celebrities and business people who had graduated from former white Model C schools.

As mentioned, informal lines of exclusion were most firmly drawn against residents of jondolo settlements and rural areas, generally the poorest areas in Mandeni. But loveLife's celebration of optimism and social mobility did not prevent young people from modest and sometimes very poor backgrounds from becoming involved with the organization. Volunteers did not have to have graduated from former white Model C schools, but had to aspire to the confident, articulate, and English-driven cultural styles symbolized by these institutions. If some Model C accents could be heard at the center, most volunteers had studied at township schools; while these institutions had a reputation for offering a lower standard of education than the Model C schools, they were generally more highly regarded than schools in the jondolo settlements and rural areas.

Youth could also absorb the organization's culture and partially remake themselves along the way. Visitors typically served a kind of apprenticeship as unpaid volunteers before they were eligible to apply to become stipend-earning "groundbreakers." An array of in-house training programs across the country taught participants about not only AIDS prevention but the institutional culture of loveLife. Other informal mechanisms existed for youth to embrace loveLife's optimistic culture. One popular book on motivational skills I saw volunteers reading was called *Phila! 150 Success Insights to Excite, Empower, and Energize You* (*phila* means "life" and "health" in isiZulu and isiXhosa).

According to loveLife, volunteers exhibit positive traits that are supposedly natural: they are confident and have a "clear direction of future aspirations."[7] But as the French sociologist Pierre Bourdieu notes, cultural dispositions are inherently power-laden. He famously showed how the aesthetics of culture, such as elite art, helped to maintain distinctions that effected the dominance of the French middle class.[8] In an analogous way, loveLife's trendy and confident cultural style forms part of an emerging middle-class culture premised on English-language communication. Some black South Africans now join this middle class, but social inequality means that most are excluded, and can be relatively estranged from the AIDS messages tied to these cultural forms.

The youth center's emphasis on English meant that it was seen by residents of the jondolo settlement (not entirely accurately) as a place where the socially mobile amaModelC (students of former white schools) hung out. The amaModelC embody in their confident English accents the importance of privileged education to social mobility. But loveLife's allocation of groundbreaker jobs to those with English skills was not the only reason it was seen as biased toward them. Nor did it lead most jondolo residents to oppose loveLife; virtually everyone I knew was happy that the center was located in Mandeni.

The wider point I want to make is that loveLife's elitism speaks to much deeper social fissures in a society where so many young people have been "left behind." This, in turn, raises crucial questions about the effectiveness of AIDS interventions that hinge on young peoples' optimism about social mobility. While loveLife tried to influence young people in the community to practice safe sex by showcasing positive images of the future, clearly optimism was unevenly distributed among Mandeni's residents. And it is ironic that the poorest residents, who live in rural areas and informal settlements (the latter of which have the highest HIV rates), face the strongest barriers to participating in the activities of the area's most high-profile AIDS prevention organization.

The tensions between an ideology of optimism and the reality of chronic unemployment—ones at the heart of the country as a whole—were visible daily in the youth center. According to loveLife, groundbreakers were volunteers and community leaders first, and recipients of small stipends second. In fact, volunteers' stipend was not peripheral but central to their interaction with loveLife. From the groundbreakers' perspective, their one-year nonrenewable contracts gave them status and allowed them to save some money, perhaps live alone, and, as a male volunteer told me, even to attract girlfriends. All of the stipend-earning volunteers I knew were passionate about the devastating effects of AIDS in their community, but they were also aware that the organization provided them with a small wage, some training, and perhaps even the hope of future work.

On several occasions I witnessed loveLife's managers or donors calling on the center, and they were always keen to talk to young people. But I felt that volunteers relayed, in somewhat clichéd tones, stories of motivation and individuals' right to ignore peer pressure, narratives that appeared often in loveLife's own brochures. Outside the youth center, young male volunteers told me several times that they ignored loveLife's core messages and didn't always use condoms. "We say those things but we don't do them," one young man in his early twenties told me. Moreover, when I talked to friends after they had stopped earning a stipend from loveLife, their optimism seemed to have faded. While one had secured a full-time job as a direct consequence of his involvement with loveLife, most remained unemployed, at least for a while; the highs of temporary employment meant that they fell further, and, tellingly, none was enthusiastic about returning to loveLife as an unpaid volunteer. One young man bemoaned having to give up living in an umjondolo and move back with his mother, which he said made him an umnqolo (a sissy).

Former volunteers that I kept in touch with did remain positive about the training they had received from the institution and, over time, they seemed more likely than other young people to attain work. I do not, of course, know exactly how volunteers' interaction with loveLife affected their intimate lives; perhaps it did provide them with a greater impetus to practice safe sex. Given that optimism and English skills are de facto criteria for involvement with loveLife, its message might resonate most with its own volunteers.

But, nationwide, HIV prevalence among the young remained stubbornly high, although some recent data suggest a drop in the infection rate.[9] It is, of course, difficult to determine the effect of one program on young people's behavior.[10] It is also certain that changes in intimate relations preceded loveLife's establishment and operation. Since 2000, young people have told me that they are increasingly using condoms; moreover, as I outline later in this chapter, AIDS creates profound challenges to masculinities that celebrate multiple partners.

Nevertheless, one thing is certain: while AIDS interventions are increasingly differentiating the population by gender, age, and more recently sexual activity (male-female and same-sex; this dimension had long been ignored), there are considerable blind spots around class. These blind spots persist even though the increase in class divisions is one of the most significant social trends after apartheid. What's more, the disregard of class (and, closely related, of geography) exists amid poorer South Africans' growing criticism of amaModelC, the group to whom loveLife's institutional culture most speaks. If South Africans elected the poorly educated Jacob Zuma in part to signify their disillusionment with a new multi-racial elite, isn't it time that AIDS prevention messages began to better address class inequalities? Certainly, a reported 3 percent rise in HIV prevalence in urban informal settlements from 2005 to 2008 suggests that HIV may be becoming more polarized by social class.[11]

Health Activism and the TAC

> But what has happened is that our politics generally has become empty
> of any moral content. . . . And at the same time there is a whole industry
> of people who survive on consultancy fees and a whole range of things to

keep the epidemic going. . . . So my position is based on an understand-
ing that . . . I want the right to life and that I want to live in a political
community in which that right is extended to every person. If such a
political community does not exist and the only reason that you die or you
are allowed to die is because you are poor when you are sick, then I do
not want to be part of such, on a conscious basis and on a moral basis I
couldn't be part of such a community.

—ZACKIE ACHMAT, former TAC chairperson, explaining his
decision not to take ARV drugs (in It's My Life, Icarus Films)

In 1998, a year before loveLife's launch, health activists established the
Treatment Action Campaign and elected Zackie Achmat as its chairperson.
The TAC was a vocal and innovative grassroots movement politicized by the
huge numbers of AIDS deaths despite the existence of drugs that could have
prevented them. When the TAC was launched, the government was already
engulfed in a storm over its support for two AIDS initiatives, an expensive and
unwieldy play about AIDS entitled *Sarafina II* and a supposed AIDS cure called
Virodene, developed in South Africa, that turned out to be an industrial solvent.
Even more controversially, in a series of speeches beginning in 1999 Mbeki
questioned the causal link between HIV and AIDS and the effectiveness of antiretroviral treatment. He drew authority from a small number of dissident scientists from the West, most notably Berkeley biologist Peter Deusberg, whom
Mbeki controversially invited to sit on an HIV/AIDS advisory panel in 2000.

Divisions around HIV exploded in the late 1990s over the issue of treatment. For over a decade HIV medication had been of limited effectiveness. But
all that changed in 1996 with the development of "triple therapy," an expensive concoction of drugs that effectively made HIV a manageable disease. It
is likely that Mbeki's skepticism about mainstream AIDS science is related to
the extremely high cost of these drugs: ironically, 1996 was also the year that
the ANC adopted the broadly neo-liberal plan GEAR (discussed in chapter 6).
The fact that the main reason for the high cost of this life-saving drug therapy
was patent laws also fueled controversy.

Patent laws, strengthened as part of the 1994 World Trade Organization
agreement, meant that unbranded "generic" products could only be sold
when patents on the drugs expired, after twenty years. This allowed pharmaceutical companies to sell AIDS drugs at exorbitant prices, supposedly to
recuperate their investment in the drugs' development. In the 1990s the resultant cost of AIDS treatment was around US$15,000 per person per year, an
amount that virtually no South Africans could afford. Most activists accepted

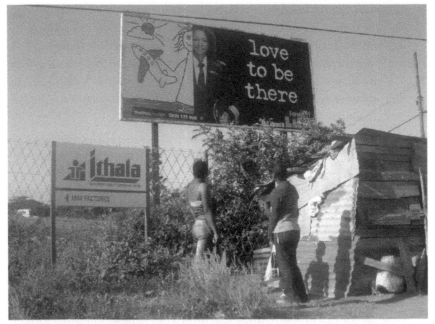

FIGURE 10.1. A loveLife billboard in Sundumbili township, 2004. On the left side is a child's drawing of herself flying a plane; on the right she is an adult, living out that dream. Photograph by Mark Hunter.

that pharmaceuticals should recoup their research expenses in rich countries, but questioned charging such high prices in poor countries. Such reckless protection of "intellectual property rights" came to symbolize massive global disparities in health. Millions of people faced certain death while pharmaceutical companies defended their profits with patent laws—and all in the name of free trade.

In 2001, the TAC formed a temporary alliance with the South African government. With a simple moral message about how drug-company profiteering was causing countless deaths, the TAC shot to international prominence. The immediate issue that brought the TAC and government together was the need to fight in court forty pharmaceutical companies that were trying to use patent laws to scupper South Africa's Medicines Act. This legislation, drafted in 1997 soon after the ANC came to power, aimed to reduce the price of medicines in the country by encouraging the use of generic drugs in South Africa and the "parallel importing" of drugs sold in other countries at lower prices.

The government did not have antiretrovirals in mind when it drafted this bill; it was simply hoping to reduce the country's massive expenditures on drugs. But the TAC quickly saw an opportunity to make ARVs more available to HIV positive South Africans.[12] On March 5, 2001, the opening day of the decisive court case, demonstrations were held worldwide in response to a call by the TAC; I was involved in a protest at a Bayer pharmaceutical plant in the San Francisco area. After the TAC's show of strength, and facing a public relations nightmare, the pharmaceuticals withdrew their case. The victory was momentous: it exposed as ruthless the drug companies' use of patents to keep prices high and thus deny life-saving drugs to millions of poor people. As a result of this and other campaigns, the price of ARVs in South Africa and other poorer countries tumbled.

The alliance between the TAC and the South African government was always fragile, and it collapsed dramatically. Despite having secured a means to lower drug prices, the government outraged the TAC by quickly announcing that it would not provide antiretrovirals through the public sector. Mbeki's controversial stance on AIDS appeared to be the main obstacle to providing the drugs. Why, activists asked, was Mbeki questioning whether HIV caused AIDS when thousands of people were dying from AIDS-related illnesses?

To confront both the government and the pharmaceutical companies, TAC branches sprang up across South Africa in the early 2000s, especially in urban areas, and Mandeni had the biggest branch north of the Thukela River.[13] In 2003, as AIDS deaths mounted, activists embarked on a strategy of "civil disobedience" to push for ARVs to be made available in the public sector. Supporters staged sit-ins and marches, and at police stations across the country activists laid charges of culpable homicide against the minister of health and the minister of trade and industry.

In this period of intense activism, President Thabo Mbeki was increasingly ridiculed for his "AIDS denialism." Yet anthropologist Didier Fassin argues for a deeper understanding of Mbeki's stance, one that recognizes the "inscribing of historical time onto flesh."[14] Fassin notes that Mbeki's skepticism about mainstream science was, in part, a reaction to racist discourses of lascivious Africans and the AIDS industry's often vitriolic tone. As Fassin demonstrates, depictions of Mbeki as a "backward" and "unscientific" African contributed to the stark political polarization in the country around AIDS.

But while Fassin details well the complexity of Mbeki's "denialism," he tends to collapse the views of a myriad of Mbeki's opponents into a blind defense of "science."[15] He ignores, for instance, how TAC activists, some of Mbeki's strongest critics, also embodied the pain of apartheid and—much more directly than the political elite—the contours of post-apartheid inequalities. To TAC activists, many of whom were women and most of whom were

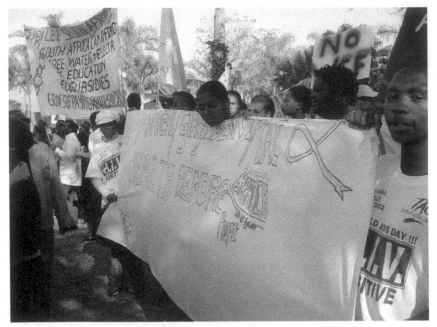

FIGURE 10.2. TAC members from Mandeni demonstrate with activists representing other social justice movements in Durban, June 2003. The banner says, "Mandeni/ Gingingdlovu Branch. Health before Profit." Photograph by Mark Hunter.

HIV positive, the state's violent suppression of political opposition seemed little changed from what it had been before democracy; their bodies remembered the continuities between the apartheid and post-apartheid periods. For example, during a demonstration in Durban in March 2003, the police lost no time in beating protesters and firing a water cannon at them, leaving five people in the hospital (I took a pregnant women to the hospital whose child's life was put at risk by these actions). The TAC quickly mobilized another demonstration to protest this violence; six buses were needed to carry four hundred people from Mandeni to Durban for it.

Indeed, the emergence of the TAC points to important gender and class realignments that demand attention. In the afternoons in Mandeni I sometimes moved between loveLife's well-equipped center and the TAC's small office, rented from the SAPPI paper mill. The TAC's leader in Mandeni, Richard Shandu, was a former employee of SAPPI and always greeted me with a big hug. His stocky body could have allowed him to pass as a boxer, but he had an air of gentleness. In the 1980s, as a SAPPI worker, he would have walked the same land on which TAC activists now met. Then, he would have been shoulder to shoulder with a generation of industrial men who unionized rapidly: their collective aim was to fight apartheid and secure a family wage. In the 1980s many women joined unions, but the assumption persisted that women's salaries supported one person only: the extreme mobility of the garment industry and the discipline of trade reforms from the 1990s naturalized these gendered understandings.

Two decades later, the TAC's rapid growth spoke to the arrival of a deadly new disease in a democratic period when all citizens had rights. But the TAC's mobilization also embodied a no less radical shift in the gendered lives of Mandeni's residents. Men like Richard Shandu tend to hold disproportionately senior positions in the TAC, but the organization became gendered very differently from local trade unions. The TAC's core members were not male wage earners whose political identities were formed through images of a male breadwinner and a heterosexual family: they were predominantly poor, unmarried women.[16] Nationally, the TAC had strong historical links to the gay rights movement; in fact, Zackie Achmat, its leader, had headed the National Coalition for Gay and Lesbian Equality (NCGLE), an organization that had broken away from the politically conservative and white-dominated Gay Association of South Africa (GASA).[17]

The TAC's very office seemed to reflect the declining status of the male industrial worker and the emergence of a new kind of politics of the poor. It was located next to the paper mill's decrepit compound, and the sulphurous fumes and a leaking sewage drain gave it a ghastly smell. Livening up the place, colorful isiZulu-written posters adorned the walls, giving detailed information about AIDS medication. Newspaper articles on the TAC's marches were also displayed prominently. These images and pamphlets advocated a collective struggle for the right to life and demanded that pharmaceuticals and the state take this struggle seriously.

The TAC therefore interpreted rights in terms not of social mobility but of health for all. Taking AIDS matters to the constitutional court in 2001, the TAC successfully forced the government to provide cheap ARV treatment that reduced the chances of HIV being passed on from mother to child. And this call for a health-based citizenship and rights did not stop at drugs. Nationally, the TAC endorsed the growing campaign for the Basic Income Grant, a small payment to all South Africans intended to relieve poverty. The TAC also organized a people's health summit to campaign for a more equitable health system. By representing poorer residents of Mandeni, generally women, the TAC in Mandeni therefore constituted a gender and class politics quite different both from the union and anti-apartheid politics that dominated the 1980s and 1990s, and from the politics of loveLife—an organization, of course, with quite different aims.

The link between social background and AIDS politics struck me further when I attended an AIDS support group of which most members were female teachers, a relatively well-off segment of society. It is widely recognized that women around the world are more willing than men to admit to ill health and seek assistance.[18] Though there are complex reasons for this, it is certainly the case in South Africa, where HIV support groups are dominated by women. Yet none of the female teachers in the group I visited appeared to be living with HIV. Non-disclosure of HIV status is not in itself unusual: a common support group maxim is that people are *affected* by AIDS, not necessarily *infected*. However, one teacher went beyond this and openly stated that she was not infected with HIV; although my presence might have prompted her statement, I have never heard it made so explicitly in other similar settings. It may well be that some of these teachers were already taking ARVs, but they certainly did not want to be seen (at least by me) as HIV positive.

In contrast, many TAC members, generally poorer women, lived openly with HIV. My sense was that the discrepancy between their openness and others' secretiveness was not due just to the TAC's encouragement of disclosure (although it also respected people's right to privacy). If teachers were archetypal pillars of the community, the lower social status of many TAC members meant that in some respects their bodies had less status to lose. Weakening every day, they were dying of AIDS and had no hope of paying for private treatment. Their openness echoes the postcolonial politics envisioned by Franz Fanon in *Wretched of the Earth*, where the revolutionary group is not the pampered union members but those with nothing to lose, the peasants and lumpenproletariat, including shack dwellers.[19]

Indeed, at demonstrations and marches, the TAC spoke for those left behind after apartheid and unable to advance socially, or to access life-saving drugs through private health schemes. Songs, dances, and stories reworked past political struggles. One popular TAC song, for instance, was "Senzeni Na?" (What Did We Do?), a famous song of the anti-apartheid struggle that now directed its message toward the new government and its stance on AIDS. Zackie Achmat, the TAC's charismatic leader, literally embodied the TAC's connection with the anti-apartheid struggle and its dream of freedom. A former anti-apartheid activist jailed by the apartheid state, he refused to take ARVs until the ANC government provided them to the population. Achmat's moral message struck a deep chord, including with Nelson Mandela, who labeled the sick TAC leader a hero and visited him to persuade him to begin treatment.

In late 2003 the government's skepticism about ARVs was finally overturned. In the face of extraordinary pressure from the TAC and critics worldwide, not to mention a looming election, the government announced that it would initiate a nationwide antiretroviral program—Achmat himself began to take ARVs around this time. A new vocabulary emerged around AIDS: the words *ikhambi* (with a meaning somewhere between "treatment" and "cure"), *amaphilisi* (ARV pills), and *amaantiretrovirals* or *amaARVs* were frequently heard on isiZulu radio programs and in popular culture.

In Mandeni, the TAC began to play a key role in directing HIV positive people to health services to get CD4 counts (a measure of the immune system's strength) in preparation for starting on ARVs. From this moment on, AIDS and bodily death were no longer inextricably tied together. ARVs seemed to take weakened bodies backward in time: adding weight, curing skin infections, and reducing incontinence. Many people saw rapid improvements in their health and transitioned from "near death" to "new life," an improvement that bolstered the enthusiasm of TAC's activists.[20] I left South Africa in January 2005 knowing many people on ARVs in Mandeni who were doing well.

When I returned to Mandeni in 2006 to stay in Isithebe for a month, seven hundred people were getting ARVs from the Sundumbili clinic, and long queues were evident. Back at Isithebe, sitting in Bongi's sewing room as I had done for many hours over many years previously, I witnessed a significant change in the topics of conversation. Boyfriends, work prospects, and housing were still on the agenda, but new and important discussion points were ARVs' side effects and the doctors and nurses who administered them. Tellingly, I did not witness the same openness about ARVs in informal male groups I joined. Women's longstanding need to form alliances led them to discuss life-saving drugs. "How can people laugh at others who are HIV positive?" Bongi asked rhetorically. "Who is not positive in Mandeni?" Of course, not everyone who was HIV positive took ARVs.[21] But in January 2009 the minister of health said that more than 700,000 South Africans were on ARV treatment; the number acquiring ARVs from the Sundumbili clinic had risen to 4,000.[22]

At one level, the TAC's success in winning access to ARVs was a remarkable victory by poor people against profiteering pharmaceutical corporations and an intransigent government. However, the case of Brazil suggests the need for caution amid celebration. As far back as 1996, Brazil launched a widely lauded ARV program, partly in response to activists' pressure. But, according to anthropologist João Biehl, this program led to "an incremental change in the concept of public health, now understood less as prevention and clinical care and more as access to medicines."[23] Social issues like economic security and housing, he argued, were pushed aside by civil society's highly visible demands for medicines. Similarly, some fear that, following the TAC's spectacular success in ensuring the provision of ARVs, the group has become a "conservative NGO-type organization."[24] In Mandeni its influence certainly declined in the late 2000s, in part because of reduced funding. With a membership base consisting of the poorest South Africans, the TAC had always been heavily dependent on international donors.

Has the TAC become a victim of its own success, now that ARVs are available in the public sector, or can it continue with its efforts to promote health equality? This question speaks to more subtle global inequalities than those so starkly revealed by different access to AIDS medication. In general, funders prefer to finance biomedical health interventions, such as provision of ARVs, rather than campaigns for health equality; as radicalism and drugs became delinked, the latter attracted the most funds. Many people involved with what is now called "global health" commend the TAC for helping to increase global access to drugs. Yet the TAC's radical messages of health equality have been largely forgotten by the public health industry and its funders.

Despite these points, the TAC's activism clearly did and still does represent a politics that goes beyond simply advocating drugs. In efforts that included leading a global coalition against pharmaceutical profiteering in 2001 and organizing a people's health summit, the TAC connected health to global and national inequalities. And it drew on the language of citizenship and rights to speak particularly strongly to unemployed female South Africans, a group that suffers from the country's highest HIV infection rates and had been "left behind" by the consumption and social mobility of a rising middle class and an economic system that cares little for poor peoples' livelihoods. Although its resources have shrunk, the TAC is still one of the few organizations that campaigns on these issues.

The Politics of Gender and Intimacy

To date, AIDS research has largely connected political economy, gender, and intimacy at a very general level. Consequently, many AIDS intervention programs have tended to inadequately address how societal inequalities affect sexual practices. Yet, rather than seeing political economy as giving context to intimacy or sexuality, political economy and intimacy are best thought of as *dialectical*—that is, in an ever-changing relationship to each another and to other socio-spatial processes. Sex—and other aspects of intimacy, including affection, love, pleasure, and fertility—is always linked in ongoing and multifarious ways to "making a living." These are general lessons, but I have shown that recent dramatic shifts in South African households, marriage, and employment need to be given particular attention. These fueled what I call a changing political economy and geography of intimacy.

The South African AIDS pandemic, I have argued, is rooted not only in apartheid or in an abstract "gender inequality" but in the reconstitution of intimacy as a key juncture between production and reproduction in a period of unemployment and capital-led globalization. Unemployment and inequalities increased starkly in the 1980s and worsened after the end of apartheid; many women have been thrust into a new dependence on men. In the name of white rule, the early apartheid period saw high employment and an active, gendered role for the state; in contrast, the late apartheid and post-apartheid eras have been marked by casual employment or unemployment for many and a techno-cratic (neo-)liberal development project. Of course, it is inevitably problematic to simplify the book's long story in such simple terms; yet while the intricate details of everyday life are necessary to understand intimacy, abbreviations are always needed if the politics of AIDS is not to be lost in this complexity.

Gender and Intimacy's Still-Shifting Grounds

One of this book's key arguments is that colonialism and apartheid did not simply destroy the family and sexuality in a linear way, making the scale of the AIDS pandemic inevitable. The wage-earning umnumzana (male head of household) was a cornerstone of South Africa's racialized capitalism; in both rural and urban areas his wage and his wife's domestic labor instigated a joint but contested project of "building a home." Over time "industrial women" took jobs and challenged this model. But rising unemployment from the late 1970s created new forms of gendered dependence—with, crucially, some men remaining relatively well off.

In turn, as mass unemployment threatened a "patriarchal bargain," gendered conflicts became intensified in new ways. I traced earlier how the figure of the isoka (a man with many lovers) partly emerged with colonialism and migrant labor and took on a new boldness in the era of chronic unemployment; I end my discussion of gender by taking this figure into the realm of AIDS to further show its inherent plasticity. As this shifting figure shows, the coexistence of male power and weakness cannot be understood through either political economy or gender/intimacy alone; an approach is required that incorporates both. And gender's dynamism means that simplistic notions of "harmful gender norms" or decontextualized understandings of "rights" or "tradition" will not take forward our understanding of the gendering of AIDS.

Showing gender's constant restlessness, over the last fifteen years a variety of developments—the AIDS crisis, the creation of a modern constitution
espousing equality, and the appearance of many negative media images—have
forced masculinities to shift in new ways. Writing about Alexandra township,
Liz Walker has shown how men's questioning of dominant masculinities can
be institutionalized in the male-run group Men for Change.[25] In Gugulethu
township, Steven Robins has charted the rise of a support group of HIV positive men taking antiretrovirals. Its members, shocked by AIDS, sought to redis-
cover a more responsible manhood.[26] And in February 2010, a national outcry
forced Jacob Zuma to apologize for fathering a child outside of marriage with
the daughter of a prominent soccer administrator. Union and ANC members,
previous supporters of Zuma's right to engage in polygamy, appeared to force
his hand. In an era of AIDS, Zuma had moved from being seen as a respectable
isoka to isoka lamanyala, a "dirty" isoka who took his masculinity too far.

The time is about 3 PM, the year is 2003, and I am visiting a shebeen in
Sundumbili that has been run by Mrs. Phiri since the 1960s. She serves only
sorghum beer, brewed on an open fire in large steel containers. My discussion
with her mostly middle-aged clients ends when one of the men takes the stage.
Dressed in faded blue overalls and flanked by a thin woman with a tattered sun
hat, he plays the accordion and the whole shebeen begins to sing and dance.
The song is about *ingculaza* (HIV/AIDS), and in isiZulu the "c" is a kind of
"tut" sound, giving the word a haunting ring in songs.[27] The lyrics are "People
are dying, people are dying, God help us, AIDS is finishing people, there are
many graves, there are many orphans, I'm scared of AIDS." I was struck by the
significance of such a song in a space so associated with casual relations. The
music's genre, Maskanda, contributed to the intensity of the moment: born
out of the pain of labor migrancy, it reflects everyday struggles in its powerful
isiZulu lyrics. Today, popular Maskanda singers Shiyani Ngcobo and Shwi also
have songs that warn of the dangers of AIDS, although notably it is women,
not men, who are usually blamed for cheating on their lovers.[28]

Yet these shifts in masculinities generally fall under the radar of intervention campaigns. The English-speaking press is dominated by negative
representations of African men, such as as perpetrators of violent crime. By
contrast, in the isiZulu media men rarely conform to such simple stereotypes.
The newspaper *Isolezwe* carries a popular daily cartoon by Qap's Mngadi. I
saw many people purchase *Isolezwe* at my adoptive family's store in Isithebe
and turn immediately to Mngadi's cartoon. One theme that he persistently
repeats is how men are coming to terms with narratives of gender equality
after democracy. Bhoza, a popular cartoon figure, for instance, is always being

pushed around by his wife, who enjoys her new "rights." Cartoons of Bhoza's life are both a sardonic depiction of women's apparent new powers and a statement about men's sense of disempowerment. Mngadi explained to me that his cartoons grew out of his own observations living in a Durban township where unemployment is rife.[29]

Also revealing of men's insecurities is a letter to *Isolezwe* entitled "Hhayi, Asibesabi, Siyabathanda" (No, We're Not Scared of Them, We Like Them).[30] In this letter (and in many others like it), a man argues that South African men must not be scared to propose love to successful women just because they are driving nice cars and have money. Men, the writer said, must not beat and abuse women, but instead learn to deal with their new powers. Standing at the door of the car in the accompanying photo is a well-dressed woman, suggesting the way that women themselves contest contemporary masculinities.

Perhaps more powerful than these images is the specter of a wasting body and eventual death that haunts masculinities today. Within the first few months of living in Mandeni in 2000, I attended two funerals with my friend Bongi. Lucky, her brother, once a muscular and famous amateur footballer, was among the first HIV positive people whose death I witnessed. When I met him he was already a thin, forlorn man with heavily swollen feet and freckles standing out sharply on his yellow-toned skin. Discharged from a local hospital, he refused to return, complaining that staff had left him to rot in his own feces. Together with Bongi, I carried him to my car and took him to the local hospice. In this place of death, I was struck by how he sought to differentiate himself from other patients. One of the last statements he made before dying was how ill the person in the opposite bed looked. It was as if, to cling longer to his own life, he needed to see that there was somewhere further to sink.

A short while later, Bongi's cousin committed suicide, shooting himself in the head. He was in his early thirties, and his wife had died earlier in the year. I gave Bongi and two other people a lift to the funeral, which was held north of Mandeni (one of these people was Thami, whose attempt to woo a young mourner at this funeral is described in chapter 8). In the early evening, we sat in the dead person's home, a house with all the signs of prosperity: concrete walls, a neat and fenced igceke (courtyard), a gate for a car, and four large rooms. Sitting in the lounge, I listened to guests call out, sadly and rhythmically, his many possessions: "fridge, sofa, T.V., video . . ." It was uncanny to hear him remembered in this way; at first, I felt that this funeral was terribly materialistic. However, the naming of goods served to emphasize that the deceased man had built a large home—his material possessions signified this success. Nothing did so more than the pile of fifty-kilogram cement bags which lay awkwardly in the corner of the lounge as visitors spoke. Here was a true man who had thrown everything away in an act of suicide widely thought to be motivated by an AIDS-related illness.

These deaths were two of the many that occurred with sad regularity in the 1990s, before ARVs became widely available. And day by day, funeral by funeral, AIDS bears down on the isoka masculinity. The symptoms, recognized by even very young children in the township, cannot be more emasculating—and de-masculinizing. Some of the most virile, popular, and independent bodies are steadily transformed into diseased and dependent skeletons, shunned by friends and neighbors. Connell's term "body-reflexive practices" captures how the body sits within—not outside of—the social world.[31] Indeed, it is at the many funerals, as mourners walk in a slow circle around the coffin, taking shocked glances at the deceased's diminished body, that the contradictions of isoka are most tragically played out.

Endnotes: Geographies of Health Inequality

The partial history of Mandeni that I have written shows that the drivers of the epidemic are deeply rooted in the fault lines of the society, and it is these fault lines that need to be tackled. AIDS stands as a symptom of ills rooted in colonialism and apartheid that have not transformed after apartheid.

Why did the post-apartheid government not address the social roots of AIDS? Thabo Mbeki, South Africa's president from 1999 to 2008, a critical period for AIDS, argued that he questioned the presumption that HIV causes AIDS to emphasize that poverty causes AIDS. This view is most resolutely defended by Suresh Roberts, Mbeki's supportive biographer.[32] Mbeki, Roberts suggests, is a misunderstood visionary who wanted to challenge Euro-centric approaches to the pandemic that stressed biomedical interventions (especially antiretroviral therapy) and the emphasis on sex as the sole means of HIV transmission. Yet while Mbeki certainly argued that colonialism and poverty caused AIDS, he did not theorize either poverty or race beyond the fact that they were colonial legacies. Notably, in his criticism of the AIDS industry, Roberts preferred to draw heavily on Franz Fanon's insights into the psychology of colonialism (made famous in *Black Skin, White Masks*) rather than on his critique of the parasitic postcolonial national bourgeoisie (described in *The Wretched of the Earth*).

One reason why Mbeki did not pursue the connections between poverty and AIDS is that to do so he would have had to confront not only how poverty affects intimacy, but the nature of South Africa's unequal transition.

The tragedy of Mbeki's stance, therefore, was not only his "denial" of AIDS science but also his failure to pursue and address the links between poverty and AIDS. These links are by no means straightforward, since richer South Africans can and often do become infected with HIV. Consequently, statistical models favored by public health authorities do not always show a clear link between poverty and AIDS—although high HIV prevalence rates in informal settlements are strongly suggestive of this connection. But statistics can give only an aggregate picture, and they say little about historical processes. If a man earning R4,000 a month in an Isithebe firm passes on HIV to a female migrant earning nothing, statistically the rich and poor are equally affected—but does this mean that poverty does not drive transmission? While the effects of poverty, unemployment, and inequality are sometimes difficult to capture in statistical models, I hope that this historical ethnography has convinced readers of their importance in driving AIDS in South Africa.

Certainly, had Mbeki sought to connect disease with poverty he would have found important lessons in South Africa's scholarship that might have helped him respond to the large AIDS industry he clearly resented. As I noted earlier, the Karks famously showed sixty years ago that the South African syphilis epidemic during the first half of the century was sourced in racial segregationist policies that divided African families and fostered men's circulation between rural and urban areas.[33] In the 1980s, a new generation of anti-apartheid writers detailed the health consequences of South Africa's uneven geographies and of the state's attempts to reform apartheid. Neil Andersson, Shula Marks, Ben Wisner, and Randall Packard all documented the devastating health inequalities in South Africa, especially between white South Africa and the rural homelands.[34] Wisner, for instance, wrote that democracy would not necessarily bring equality: "Ultimately the whole of South Africa's spatial organization—the relationship between towns and villages, the distribution and flow of people, patterns of access to tax revenues and scarce resources—will have to be reworked if majority rule is to give rise to social justice."[35]

These geographical divisions were not significantly reduced after the end of apartheid. And it is perhaps the growth of shacks that best captures the state's technocratic approach to "development" and thus its failure to address the changing political economy and geography of intimacy. Informal settlements are generally overcrowded, with poor water supplies and awful sanitation infrastructure—perfect conditions for any disease. And shacks have multiplied not simply because of a "backlog" or "legacy of apartheid" but as a consequence of the dynamic processes of capitalism, race, gender, and intimacy. For every two-room RDP house that is built, another shack is constructed, as households become smaller and more mobile. Their inhabitants often maintain close links to rural areas and are very rarely married. Imijondolo appear to harbor the highest HIV rates in the country: more than any other structures, they signal a postcolonial geography of AIDS.

Addressing these inequalities, Abahlali baseMjondolo, the shack dweller movement founded in central Durban in 2005, has called attention to the terrible neglect of water, sanitation, and housing in the city's informal settlements.[36] Activists challenge not just the lack of housing but a technocratic housing policy. Although an impressive number of low-cost RDP houses were built after apartheid, these are two-room structures with a minimum size of only thirty square meters, whereas under apartheid "matchbox" houses had four rooms and a minimum size of fifty-one square meters. Because of the high cost of land in towns, the two-room, government-funded RDP houses are often located on the outskirts, where there are few work opportunities.

When I interviewed Sbu Zikode, Abahlali's leader, he told me that "umjondolo" is an "ugly" word and that activists use it to remind people in power of occupants' poverty. And he sees political struggles as extending beyond simply building shacks of better materials than their current flimsy paper, cardboard, wood, and plastic. Even houses in rich areas could be called imijondolo, he said, if they lack basic services: "When you go to Umhlanga or Morningside [rich suburbs of Durban], if you cannot provide water, if you cannot have a sewage system, if there is no electricity, automatically Umhlanga Rocks will become imijondolo, there are no basic services. . . . Even if you get those low-cost [RDP] houses, they will become imijondolo if no one is working in the family, if you cannot pay for your services."[37] Here, Abahlali's leader evokes an alternative to technical, numbers-driven fixes: housing for a dignified life, with access to clean water and other basic services as well as proximity to places of work.

Yet, in sharp contrast to this vision, in 2007 KwaZulu-Natal Province passed a slum elimination act in an attempt to clear urban areas of shacks by 2010—the year, as many pointed out, that the World Cup soccer tournament was to be held in South Africa. In reaction to this move, Abahlali argued successfully in the constitutional court in 2009 that the act should be struck down because it denied citizens their constitutional right to housing. This built on an earlier landmark constitutional court case that prevented the state from razing shacks without providing suitable alternative accommodation.[38]

The state's contested return to the language of "slums" is a reminder not only of the huge social distance between policy makers and the poor but of the way that South Africa's urban segregation often relies on geographical imagery of disease. The government might argue that "slum elimination" will improve the population's health. Yet this would be a deeply ironic argument. As noted, AIDS institutions like loveLife typically cater to better-off urban dwellers; moreover, government AIDS programs, such as Voluntary Counseling and Testing (VCT), usually are not located in communities they see as temporary or illegal. A policy of forcibly clearing shacks also fails to recognize the dynamic processes that lead to shack growth and the fact that ridding towns of these structures and moving their inhabitants to the urban periphery will not address disease's social roots. Indeed, even if shack settlements are risk factors for HIV infection, slum removals are one of the worst possible interventions. People moved to the urban periphery will face higher transport costs to look for work and may even return to insecure and temporary shacks in the city.

What may befall Mandeni in the future is uncertain. Launched into the industrial era in the 1950s by the paternalistic SAPPI paper mill, the area grew massively from the 1970s after state-led "industrial decentralization." But in the current era of "globalization" and democracy, Dubai developers put forward for consideration a R55 billion (US$7 billion) project to build a sports and leisure facility in the southern part of Mandeni. Residents facing removal from former KwaZulu land are opposing the development, and its future is unclear.[39] But, if it happens, what kinds of jobs will it create? To what extent will employers invest in the welfare of workers and not just a quick profit? Will Mandeni become an island of tourist wealth in a sea of poverty?

One of the abiding lessons of health policy in poorer countries, in both the colonial and the postcolonial eras, is that technical fixes to health, whether DDT for malaria or vaccinations for smallpox or ARVs for AIDS, tend to leave the social and economic determinants of health, and the social-spatial relations that underpin them, untroubled.[40] As I bring the book to a close, I remember my last visit to the area, in 2009, and how it was quite different from my first, twelve years earlier. ARVs have greatly reduced the number of AIDS deaths in Mandeni. But while biomedical interventions have transformed key aspects of AIDS, the social roots of this disease remain stubbornly in place.

GLOSSARY

One of this book's central themes is that language is not a static reflection of society but a contested, power-laden domain. There is no single, agreed-upon English translation of isiZulu words, and I demonstrate in the book how concepts like *isoka* (playboy) have shifted over time and remain controversial. IsiZulu is especially fluid in its spoken form. For instance, speakers frequently add English inflections to isiZulu words, such as when women discuss *qoma*-ing men (choosing men as boyfriends). Similarly, sometimes Zulu inflections are added to English words, such as *icherry* (cherry, or girl).

I have not provided here a comprehensive list of isiZulu words used in this book. Instead, what follows is a guide to some of the most important words, especially in relation to matters of intimacy. IsiZulu dictionaries list words alphabetically according to their stem (for instance, under *dlozi* rather than *idlozi* or *amadlozi*). This is because a word's prefix affects its meaning. However, to aid those unfamiliar with the language, I have listed words with their prefixes, as they appear in the text. To retain consistency I have done the same when referencing dictionaries that I quote from (thus when I cite a dictionary's definition of "ukuqoma," the infinitive form of the verb, this will actually be found in the dictionary under "qoma"). I have made one main exception to this rule, in my use of the stem "hlonipha" (respect). I have done this because the concept is particularly relevant to this book, a point that cannot be always relayed through using the noun form, "inhlonipho," or the infinitive form of the verb, "ukuhlonipha." I have used modern orthography; some isiZulu words will have been spelled differently in earlier periods covered by the book.

I have tried to strike a balance in the text between using isiZulu terms and (virtually always imperfect) English translations. IsiZulu words are italicized only at their first use.

amadlozi	human spirits or souls, ancestors
amagoduka	those who return home, migrant men who support their rural families
amakhaya	rural areas, rural homes
amakholwa	Christians, literally "believers"
amalungelo	rights
amaModelC	students of former Model C "white" schools

amaqhikiza	girls of marriageable age, supervisors of younger girls' purity
ibheshi	a street party or "bash"
ibhodwe	a pot, a main lover
icherry	a girl
ilobolo	bridewealth
indlu, pl. *izindlu*	a house
ingculaza or *ingculazi*	HIV/AIDS
inhlawulo or *ihlawulo*	a fine paid to an unmarried woman's family for deflowering or impregnating her
inhlonipho	respect or deference (the general concept is sometimes referred to by the stem, *hlonipha*)
intombi	a girlfriend, a girl
iqonda	a main (straight) boyfriend or girlfriend
isahluleki	a failing person, a failure
ishende, pl. *amashende*	a secret lover
isibaya sikababa wakhe	father's cattle kraal, or woman's genitalia
isidikiselo	the top of a pot, a secondary lover
isifebe, pl. *izifebe*	an immoral or sexually loose woman, a prostitute
isishimane	a sissy, a man who cannot attract women
isoka	a man with many girlfriends, a boyfriend
isoka lamanyala (*amanyala*	an *isoka* who takes his womanizing too far means "dirt" or "disgrace")
istraight	main boyfriend or girlfriend
izindlwana	small huts or houses, an early word for shacks
khuthele	be hardworking, be diligent
phucukile	be civilized
ubaba	father

ucansi	a grass sleeping mat, penetrative sex (often denoted through the phrase *ukuya ocansini*, literally "to go to the grass mat")
ukubhunguka	to abandon home
ukufesa	to queue in search of work
ukuhlalisana	to cohabit
ukuhlobonga	(to engage in) penis-thigh intimacy, typically translated as "(to have) thigh sex" or "(to have) intercrural intercourse"
ukuhlonipha	to show respect, to act with deference
ukukhonza	to pay respects to, to show allegiance to
ukukipita	to cohabit, literally "to keep it"
ukulunga	to be right, to be morally righteous
ukumunca	to engage in oral sex, literally "to suck"
ukungena	levirate marriage, to engage in levirate marriage, literally "to enter"
ukuqoma	to choose, especially to choose a lover (for a woman)
ukuromensa	to romance, to engage in foreplay
ukushela	to propose love, to woo (for a man)
ukusoma	(to engage in) penis-thigh intimacy, typically translated as "(to have) thigh sex" or "(to have) intercrural intercourse"
ukuthanda	to love, to like
umakhwapheni	a secret lover, literally "under the armpit"
umathandezincane	a man who likes young women (but who, unlike a modern-day sugar daddy, might marry one)
umdayisi	a seller, a prostitute
umjendevu	an old spinster
umjondolo, pl. *imijondolo*	a shack or small rented place of temporary residence
umkhukhu, pl. *imikhukhu*	a shack

umkhwenyana	a fiancé, a man who has started to pay *ilobolo*
umlungu	a white person
umnqolo	an unmasculine man or boy
umnumzana, pl. *abanumzana*	a male head of household, later a gentleman or "mister"
umqwayizi	a winker, a prostitute
ushukela	sugar, sex
uzendazamshiya	an unmarried woman

NOTES

1. Gender and AIDS in an Unequal World

1. Robinson, Tabane, and Haffajee, "23 Days That Shook Our World."

2. On the trial and Zuma's resonances with dominant masculinities, see Ratele, "Ruling Masculinity and Sexuality"; for a critique of traditional/modern binaries often used to understand the trial, see Robins, "Sexual Politics and the Zuma Rape Trial." Jacob Zuma was South Africa's deputy president from 1999 to 2005 and president from 2009; he was sacked in 2005 by then-president Thabo Mbeki after Zuma's financial advisor Schabir Shaik was convicted of fraud and corruption. Formal charges of corruption against Zuma have so far failed in the courts. Zuma's supporters claimed that the rape and corruption charges were an attempt by Mbeki's allies to prevent Zuma from winning the ANC presidential elections at the national conference in 2007.

3. Robinson, Tabane and Haffajee, "23 Days That Shook Our World."

4. Controversy, however, surrounds statistics on both rape and HIV prevalence. According to police figures, there were 55,000 cases of rape reported between April 2005 and April 2006. For these figures and a helpful discussion see Vetten, "Violence against Women in South Africa." On HIV infections, until July 2007 India was estimated to have the highest number of HIV positive people of any country in the world; in that month officials revised India's estimate from 5.7 million to 2.5 million. This left South Africa as the country with the estimated highest number of HIV positive people, around 5.5 million in 2006. See Cohen, "HIV/AIDS: India Slashes Estimate of HIV-Infected People."

5. Even before Zuma's resounding victory in the 2009 election, other evidence suggested that he enjoyed considerable appeal among South African women. For instance, the "Friends of Zuma" website set up to support Zuma became filled with literally thousands of positive comments, many of them from African women (http://www.friend sofjz.co.za, accessed January 10, 2007). Demonstrating Zuma's support in urban as well as rural areas, roughly as many women as men indicated their approval of the leader in a 2007 survey conducted in Soweto township. The survey was reported in Terreblanche, "Poor Love Zuma, Study Finds."

6. For instance, Isolezwe, "Ngangingenankinga Ngelobolo: JZ" (I Didn't Have Any Problem with Ilobolo: JZ).

7. The song is performed by Kwaito star Arthur and banned by the national broadcaster.

8. Annual HIV prevalence figures are calculated from anonymous tests on pregnant women's blood taken during their antenatal visits. In 2008 such tests found an average countrywide HIV prevalence of 29%. More detailed trends are calculated from wider surveys of the country's population, the largest of which in South Africa is a household study conducted three times thus far by the Human Science Research Council. In 2002 this found that 12.8% of South African women and 9.5% of men over age two were HIV positive; the 2005 study found that 13.3% of women over two were infected and 8.2% of men; the 2008 study found a rate of 10.9% for the population over two (initial data was not disaggregated by sex). Unlike antenatal surveys, these household studies include men, the elderly, and the young. See Republic of South Africa, Department of

Health, *2008 National Antenatal Sentinel HIV and Syphilis Prevalence Survey, South Africa;* HSRC, *Nelson Mandela/HSRC Study of HIV/AIDS: South African National HIV Prevalence, Behavioural Risks and Mass Media, Household Survey 2002;* HSRC, *South African National HIV Prevalence, HIV Incidence, Behavior and Communication Survey 2005;* HSRC, *South African National HIV Prevalence, HIV Incidence, Behaviour and Communication Survey 2008: A Turning Tide among Teenagers?* For an insightful review of AIDS data in South Africa see Marais, *Buckling: The Impact of AIDS in South Africa,* 25–43.

9. The term "structural violence" was coined by Johan Galtung in the 1960s. See Farmer et al., "An Anthropology of Structural Violence"; Farmer, *Infections and Inequalities: The Modern Plagues;* Schoepf, Schoepf, and Millen. "Theoretical Therapies, Remote Remedies: SAPs and the Political Ecology of Poverty and Health in Africa."

10. Comment in Farmer et al., "An Anthropology of Structural Violence," 318.

11. As geographer David Harvey argued, the body must be considered as a "relational 'thing'" that requires for its understanding a framework combining social and spatial relations and the production of the self as historically and geographically contingent. Harvey, *Spaces of Hope,* 97–116. More generally, feminist writers have pioneered studies of the body within geography. For a summary of some of this literature see McDowell, *Gender, Identity and Place: Understanding Feminist Geographies.*

12. When discussing approaches to or the history of HIV/AIDS I use the term "AIDS"—for instance, AIDS' social roots, AIDS policy makers, or AIDS campaigns. AIDS is the acronym for acquired immune deficiency syndrome. Antiretroviral medication means that HIV (the human immunodeficiency virus) no longer automatically leads to AIDS, and I use "HIV" to speak of the virus, for instance, HIV prevalence.

13. Republic of South Africa, Department of Health, *2008 National Antenatal Sentinel HIV and Syphilis Prevalence Survey, South Africa,* 6.

14. HSRC, *Nelson Mandela/HSRC Study of AIDS 2002;* HSRC, *South African National HIV Survey 2005;* Pettifor, Rees, Steffenson, et al., *HIV and Sexual Behaviour among Young South Africans: A National Survey of 15–24-Year-Olds.* The 2002 HSRC study found a prevalence of 21.3% in urban informal areas as compared to 12.1% in urban formal areas, 8.7% in tribal areas, and 7.9% on farms (over age two). The 2005 HSRC study found a prevalence of 17.6% in urban informal areas, 11.6% in rural informal areas, 9.9% in rural formal areas, and 9.1% in urban formal areas (over age two). The 2008 HSRC study found a prevalence of 20.6% in urban informal areas, 11.1% in rural informal areas, 11.1% in rural formal areas, and 9% in urban formal areas (over age two). I am grateful to Professor Thomas Rehle for providing me with the unpublished 2008 figures. Pettifor, Rees, Steffenson, et al. found a prevalence of 17.4% in urban informal areas, 13.5% in rural formal areas, 9.8% in urban formal areas, and 8.7% in rural informal areas in a 2004 study undertaken for the Reproductive Health Research Unit. It should be noted that spatial data is fraught with difficulties. For instance, informal shacks are often located next to, and sometimes within, formal urban areas. The HSRC and RHRU studies use spatial classifications developed by Statistics South Africa for the census.

15. Katz, "Vagabond Capitalism and the Necessity of Social Reproduction," 711.

16. Only 6.6 million people today are in "core" work, around 3.1 million are in outsourced work, 2.2 million are in informal work, and 8.4 million are unemployed. See Von Holdt and Webster, "Work Restructuring and the Crisis of Reproduction," 28. I use different sources on the labor force at times within this book; although estimates vary slightly, all are in agreement about the high level of unemployment.

17. I follow Von Holdt and Webster in distinguishing between "earning a living" (having regular paid employment) and "making a living" (creating one's own income-

generating or subsistence activities). Von Holdt and Webster, "Work Restructuring and the Crisis of Reproduction," 4.

18. The phrase "the comforts of home" is taken from Luise White's landmark work on "prostitution" and social reproduction in colonial Nairobi, *The Comforts of Home: Prostitution in Colonial Nairobi*. For a review of the large literature on the marital home and social reproduction, see Laslett and Brenner, "Gender and Social Reproduction: Historical Perspectives." On sex work more generally see, for instance, Kempadoo and Doezema, *Global Sex Workers: Rights, Resistance, and Redefinition*. Standing provides an excellent anthropological review of how narrow notions of "prostitution" can be inappropriately applied to Africa. Standing, "AIDS: Conceptual and Methodological Issues in Researching Sexual Behaviour in Sub-Saharan Africa." Other references on "prostitution" are given in chapter 3.

19. Bakker and Silvey, *Beyond States and Markets: The Challenges of Social Reproduction*; Bezanson, *Gender, the State, and Social Reproduction: Household Insecurity in Neo-liberal Times*; Bezuidenhout and Fakier, "Maria's Burden: Contract Cleaning and the Crisis of Social Reproduction in Post-apartheid South Africa"; Katz, "Vagabond Capitalism"; Mitchell, Marston, and Katz, "Introduction: Life's Work: An Introduction, Review and Critique."

20. Republic of South Africa, Department of Labour, *Women in the South African Labour Market, 1995–2005*, 18.

21. Kandiyoti, "Bargaining with Patriarchy."

22. See, for instance, Nattrass, "Poverty, Sex, and HIV."

23. The literature on "transactional sex" in South Africa includes Dunkle et al., "Transactional Sex among Women in Soweto, South Africa: Prevalence, Risk Factors and Association with HIV Infection"; Hunter, "The Materiality of Everyday Sex: Thinking beyond Prostitution"; Kaufman and Stavrou, "'Bus Fare Please': The Economics of Sex and Gifts among Young People in Urban South Africa"; LeClerc-Madlala, "Transactional Sex and the Pursuit of Modernity"; Selikow, Zulu, and Cedras, "The Ingagara, the Regte and the Cherry: HIV/AIDS and Youth Culture in Contemporary Urban Townships"; Zembe et al. "Transactional Sex amongst Young Women at High Risk of HIV in the Western Cape." On transactional sex in Madagascar see Cole, "Fresh Contact in Tamatave, Madagascar: Sex, Money, and Intergenerational Transformation"; for Mali, see Castle and Konate, "The Context and Consequences of Economic Transactions Associated with Sexual Relations among Malian Adolescents"; for Malawi, see Swidler and Watkins, "Ties of Dependence: AIDS and Transactional Sex in Rural Malawi." Since sex-money exchanges are saturated with questions of morality, in-depth qualitative research has been much better than quantitative research in picking up the extent of exchanges that link money and sex—although see Zembe et al., "Transactional Sex," a study of more than 250 young women in Cape Town, which found that 76% of respondents (chosen for having multiple partners) said that they would not engage in a sexual relationship with a man if they knew they would not get any money or material goods.

24. UNAIDS, *AIDS Epidemic Update, December 2009*, 6, 21, 22.

25. On young women's susceptibility to HIV see Pettifor, Hudgens, et al., "Highly Efficient HIV Transmission to Young Women in South Africa."

26. See particularly Susser, *AIDS, Sex, and Culture: Global Politics and Survival in Southern Africa*, chapter 2.

27. Brown, "Suffering Rights as Paradoxes." For further critical discussions of rights see Cornwall and Molyneux, *The Politics of Rights: Dilemmas for Feminist Praxis*; Mamdani, *Beyond Rights Talk and Culture Talk: Comparative Essays on the Politics of Rights and Culture*; Petchesky, *Global Prescriptions: Gendering Health and Human Rights*.

28. Hassim, *Women's Organizations and Democracy in South Africa: Contesting Authority*.

29. Manicom, "Constituting 'Women' as Citizens: Ambiguities in the Making of Gendered Political Subjects in Post-apartheid South Africa," 32, 34 (emphasis in original).

30. Jean Comaroff and John Comaroff, "Criminal Justice, Cultural Justice: The Limits of Liberalism and the Pragmatics of Difference in the New South Africa," 189.

31. Doke et al., *English-Zulu, Zulu-English Dictionary*, s.v. *ukulunga*. (See my comment in the glossary on dictionary citations.)

32. On the colonial government's upholding of certain rights within "traditional" institutions see John Comaroff, "The Discourse of Rights in Colonial South Africa: Subjectivity, Sovereignty, Modernity."

33. Burawoy and Verdery, introduction to *Uncertain Transition: Ethnographies of Change in the Postsocialist World*, 2. Ethnography, however, has been a relatively neglected methodology among scholars drawing on Foucault's concept of "governmentality" to emphasize the discourses through which subjects are governed in liberal societies. To date, writings on "governmentality" have perhaps been most influentially elaborated in the work of Nikolas Rose; see for instance Miller and Rose, *Governing the Present: Administering Economic, Social, and Personal Life*. For a detailed study of rights in Malawi that does utilize ethnography see Englund, *Prisoners of Freedom: Human Rights and the African Poor*. For a fascinating ethnography of "development" in Indonesia that brings together Gramsci and Foucault see Li, *The Will to Improve: Governmentality, Development, and the Practice of Politics*. For an ethnographic account that focuses on rights' contestability in Bolivia see Postero, *Now We Are Citizens: Indigenous Politics in Postmulticultural Bolivia*.

34. See particularly Petchesky, *Global Prescriptions*; Cornwall and Molyneux, *The Politics of Rights*.

35. On constructions and representations of "African AIDS," see Treichler, "AIDS, Africa, and Cultural Theory."

36. Mohanty, "Under Western Eyes: Feminist Scholarship and Colonial Discourse." Influential criticisms of the relevance of Western feminism to Africa include Amadiume, *Male Daughters, Female Husbands: Gender and Sex in an African Society*; Oyewumi, *The Invention of Women: Making an African Sense of Western Gender Discourses*. For an example of collaborative research in India that yielded a fascinating critique of "gender and development," see Sangtin Writers and Richa Nagar, *Playing with Fire: Feminist Thought and Activism through Seven Lives in India*.

37. Mama, "Demythologising Gender in Development: Feminist Studies in African Contexts," 121.

38. Brown, "Suffering Rights as Paradoxes," 239.

39. UNAIDS, *2008 Report on the Global AIDS Epidemic*, 67–76.

40. Scott, *Gender and the Politics of History*, 4.

41. For instance, Connell, *Gender and Power: Society, the Person and Sexual Politics*; Connell, *Masculinities*; Connell, *The Men and the Boys*; Connell and Messerschmidt, "Hegemonic Masculinity: Rethinking the Concept." As writers on "female masculinity" have shown, these masculinities are not simply fixed to male bodies. Halberstam, *Female Masculinity*.

42. Beauvoir, *The Second Sex*, chapter 23.

43. On the need to better integrate studies of masculinities and femininities see Connell and Messerschmidt, "Hegemonic Masculinity."

44. David Valentine puts this well: "Age, race, class, and so on don't merely inflect or intersect with those experiences we call gender and sexuality but rather *shift the very*

boundaries of what 'gender' and 'sexuality' can mean in particular contexts." Valentine, *Imagining Transgender: An Ethnography of a Category*, 100 (emphasis in original).

45. Foucault, *The History of Sexuality*, vol. 1, *An Introduction*, 154.

46. The best historical work on sexuality is, of course, premised on decentering "sex" and showing its entanglement in changing discourses and subjectivities. Although the introductory volume of Foucault's *History of Sexuality* is the most widely quoted book in this series, his two subsequent volumes (*The Use of Pleasure* and *The Care of the Self*) give more attention to the themes of this book, including marriage, love, and masculinities. Other landmark work on sexuality, for instance by sociologist Jeffrey Weeks, is premised on exploring diverse constructions of sex; Weeks also usefully outlines how Foucault himself built on existing studies of the social construction of sexuality. See Weeks, *Sex, Politics and Society: The Regulation of Sexuality since 1800*. Despite this (and more) rich work on sexuality, I still feel that the term "intimacy" can best capture questions around fertility, love, masculinities, and femininities, at least for the topic I study. For an excellent and relevant account of how notions of "sex" and linear narratives of "development" come together in problematic ways see Adams and Pigg, *Sex in Development: Science, Sexuality, and Morality in Global Perspective*. Neville Hoad's *African Intimacies: Race, Homosexuality, and Globalization* sets out particularly well the arguments in favor of using "intimacy."

47. See particularly Hyslop, "White Working Class Women and the Invention of Apartheid: 'Purified' Afrikaner Nationalist Agitation for Legislation against 'Mixed' Marriages, 1934–9."

48. On AIDS and "heterosexual Africa," see especially Epprecht, *Heterosexual Africa: The History of an Idea from the Age of Exploration to the Age of AIDS*.

49. Much has been written on the household in African studies, but see particularly Guyer, "Household and Community in African Studies"; Guyer and Peters, "Conceptualizing the Household: Issues of Theory and Policy in Africa."

50. On Africans as "promiscuous" see McClintock, *Imperial Leather: Race, Gender, and Sexuality in the Colonial Conquest*. On the construction of "Africa" see Mudimbe, *The Invention of Africa: Gnosis, Philosophy, and the Order of Knowledge*; Mbembe, *On the Postcolony*; Ferguson, *Global Shadows: Africa in the Neoliberal World Order*.

51. The 2008 HSRC household study found infection rates of 14% for Africans, 1.7% for coloureds, 0.3% for Indians, and 0.3% for whites. HSRC, *South African National HIV Survey 2008*, 79.

52. Republic of South Africa, Statistics South Africa, *Census 2001: Primary Tables South Africa Census '96 and 2001 compared*, 61, 31.

53. These figures use the broad definition of unemployment, which includes people deterred from actively seeking employment. Republic of South Africa, Department of Labor, *Women in the South African Labour Market 1995–2005*, 4–5.

54. UNHABITAT, *State of the World's Cities 2008/2009: Harmonious Cities*, 72.

55. Studies of love framed particularly in the context of AIDS include Hirsch and Wardlow, *Modern Loves: The Anthropology of Romantic Courtship and Companionate Marriage*; Padilla et al., *Love and Globalization: Transformations of Intimacy in the Contemporary World*; Parikh, "The Political Economy of Marriage and HIV: The ABC Approach, 'Safe' Infidelity, and Managing Moral Risk in Uganda"; Smith, "Love and the Risk of HIV: Courtship, Marriage, and Infidelity in Southeastern Nigeria." In addition, see Cornwall, "Spending Power: Love, Money, and the Reconfiguration of Gender Relations in Ado-Odo, Southwestern Nigeria," and Rebhun, *The Heart Is Unknown Country: Love in the Changing Economy of Northeast Brazil*, for important attempts to go

beyond the love/money dichotomy in Nigeria and Brazil. See Lipset, "Modernity without Romance?" for a fascinating account of how modernity did not lead to romance in Papua New Guinea. On transnational links and love see especially Hirsch, *A Courtship after Marriage: Sexuality and Love in Mexican Transnational Families.* In the West, the false dichotomy between love and money has also faced increased questioning in recent years. See for instance Swidler, *Talk of Love: How Culture Matters;* Zelizer, *The Purchase of Intimacy.* On geography's "emotional turn" see Davidson, Bondi, and Smith, *Emotional Geographies.* This is just a summary of recent literature on love and emotion; more references are given throughout the book.

56. In addition to work mentioned above, one recent attempt to challenge love's absence in writings on Africa is Cole and Thomas, *Love in Africa.*

57. Colenso, *Zulu-English Dictionary,* s.v. *uthando.* This definition of *uthando* was given in the second edition of the dictionary (1878), but not the first (1861). Between those dates, the Natal government legislated that women had to explicitly confirm at their wedding that the marriage was one of choice (see chapter 3). It should be noted that on matters of marriage, as on most others, the colonial voice was by no means unitary: Bishop Colenso himself rebelled against many elements of mainstream settler thinking, particularly the view that Africans should not be allowed to convert to Christianity unless they withdrew from polygamous marriages. On the extraordinary life of Colenso see Guy, *The Heretic: A Study of the Life of John William Colenso, 1814–1883;* on colonial conflicts over marriage and *ilobolo* see Welsh, *The Roots of Segregation: Native Policy in Colonial Natal, 1845–1910.*

58. Radcliffe-Brown, introduction to *African Systems of Kinship and Marriage,* 46. Of course, social anthropology did not hold by any means a united view on love. The classic structural-functionalist account of "the Zulu," Eileen Krige's *Social System of the Zulus,* noted elaborate courting rituals. Among the best sources on love and social change in the early colonial period are Wilson, *Reaction to Conquest: Effects of Contact with Europeans on the Pondo of South Africa* and Schapera, *Married Life in an African Tribe.* For a discussion of how Schapera and Wilson engaged with matters of love see Thomas, "Love, Sex, and the Modern Girl in 1930s Southern Africa."

59. For instance, Little and Price, "Some Trends in Modern Marriage among West Africans"; Vandewiele and Philbrick, "Attitudes of Senegalese Students toward Love"; and Stones and Philbrick, "Attitudes toward Love among Xhosa University Students in South Africa."

60. Stone, *The Family, Sex and Marriage in England, 1500–1800.* Other historians draw somewhat different timelines but still posit a general shift toward individualistic notions of love. See Shorter, *The Making of the Modern Family;* Macfarlane, *Marriage and Love in England: Modes of Reproduction, 1300–1840.* From a slightly different angle, one question anthropologists have considered is whether there exists a universal form of *romantic passion,* a kind of intense passion with an erotic dimension—the answer, in general, is yes. See Jankowiak, *Romantic Passion: A Universal Experience?*

61. Illouz, *Consuming the Romantic Utopia.*

62. Giddens, *The Transformation of Intimacy: Sexuality, Love, and Eroticism in Modern Societies.*

63. Gillis, "From Ritual to Romance: Toward an Alternative History of Love," especially p. 88. Gillis draws on the work of Francesca Cancian to make these points.

64. See Packard and Epstein, "Epidemiologists, Social Scientists, and the Structure of Medical Research on AIDS in Africa." More recently, Stillwaggon argued for the sig-

nificance of nutrition, parasites, and other co-factors to the spread of AIDS in Africa. Stillwaggon, *AIDS and the Ecology of Poverty*.

65. Centers for Disease Control and Prevention, U.S. Department of Health and Human Services, "The Role of STD Prevention and Treatment in HIV Prevention."

66. These and other inequalities are well documented in publications by the Health Systems Trust. See, for instance, Health Systems Trust, *South African Health Review, 2003/4*. The ANC has supported, in principle, the establishment of a national health insurance program for many years. Such a program is intended to close the health gap between the relatively small number of privately insured people and the rest of the population. In the late 2000s the proposal gained traction although, at the time of writing, a plan has not yet been implemented.

67. Zikode, "The Third Force," 1.

2. Mandeni

1. Mitchell, "Death City," 8. The story pertained mainly to Sundumbili township, although it made references to other parts of Mandeni.

2. Republic of South Africa, Department of Health, *2008 National Antenatal Sentinel HIV and Syphilis Prevalence Survey, South Africa*, 10.

3. Republic of South Africa, Statistics South Africa, *Stages in the Lifestyle of South Africans*, 1.

4. In 1996, following the ANC's victory in the local government elections, the name of the municipality was changed from Mandini to Mandeni. In 2000 municipal boundaries were extended to incorporate previously rural homeland areas. When the Inkatha Freedom Party won the local elections in 2000, the Zulu Nationalist party renamed the municipality eNdondakusuka, after a hill on the eastern side of the municipality that was the site of the famous battle in 1856 in which Cetshwayo defeated Mbulazi to gain dominion over the Zulu Kingdom. The ANC regained control of the council in 2004 and in September 2006 changed the name back to Mandeni. I use "Mandeni" throughout to refer to the present-day municipality, and "Mandini" to refer to the former white town in present-day Mandeni.

5. Residents of the former Zululand "went to the [sugar] farms as employers of the last resort." Jeeves, "Migrant Workers and Epidemic Malaria on the South African Sugar Estates, 1906–1948," 117.

6. This and other statistics relating to Mandeni municipality are calculated using online interactive tools applied to the 2001 census data. See Statistics South Africa, "Interactive and Electronic Products," *Census 2001*, http://www.statssa.gov.za/census01/html/C2001Interactive.asp (accessed February 10, 2008). Hereafter, I will simply reference these statistics as "Census 2001 Mandeni data" and refer to the website.

7. As apartheid segregation heightened in the 1970s, the state removed African people living on the Mangete land and relocated them to nearby homeland territory. Since 1993 some former residents of the "coloured" Dunn land have mounted land invasions to reclaim parts of this land; these incursions were instigated, it is usually said, by the chief who oversees the land to which former residents of Mangete were moved.

8. I employed one full-time research assistant, whom I call Nonhlanhla, a woman who was in her early twenties when I first worked with her in 2000. Seven people from different parts of Mandeni helped us find people with whom to talk. When we had more formal discussions with groups or interviews of single people, Nonhlanhla actively

participated, asking questions, and she is quoted in some of the dialogues that follow. Nonhlanhla also undertook a small number of interviews, usually when she had a close friendship with an informant.

9. I find Hofmeyr's and Moore and Vaughan's work to be invaluable guides to how to combine social history and sensitivity to the discourses through which informants, ethnographers, and the archives speak. I. Hofmeyr, *"We spend our years as a tale that is told": Oral Historical Narratives in a South African Chiefdom;* Moore and Vaughan, *Cutting Down Trees: Gender, Nutrition, and Agricultural Change in the Northern Province of Zambia, 1890–1990.* For an insightful discussion of oral histories in African Studies see White, Miescher, and Cohen, *African Words, African Voices: Critical Practices in Oral History.*

10. On space as "produced," see Lefebvre, *The Production of Space;* on interconnections between places, see Massey, *Space, Place and Gender.*

11. Feminist geographers' critiques of local/global binaries include Massey, *Space, Place and Gender;* Nagar et al., "Locating Globalization: Feminist (Re)Readings of the Subjects and Spaces of Globalization"; Gibson-Graham, *The End of Capitalism (As We Knew It): A Feminist Critique of Political Economy;* Rosner and Pratt, *The Global and the Intimate.* In a somewhat related move, critical anthropologists have sought to shift away from seeing culture and place as isomorphic and to envision the faraway place as "remotely global." See Gupta and Ferguson, *Culture, Power, Place: Explorations in Critical Anthropology;* Piot, *Remotely Global: Village Modernity in West Africa.*

12. For general accounts of shifting identity among isiZulu speakers see Morrell, *Political Economy and Identities in KwaZulu-Natal: Historical and Social Perspectives;* Carton, Laband, and Sithole, *Zulu Identities: Being Zulu, Past and Present.* Instead of the rather rigid terms "Zulu people" and "Zulus," I mainly use the term "isiZulu speakers." Of course, not all isiZulu speakers identify as of Zulu ethnicity, and one can identify as Zulu without speaking isiZulu. Moreover, isiZulu itself is a constructed language emerging from constant interactions and social change. Yet this is exactly the point: the term "isiZulu speakers" suggests the kind of fluidity in ethnic belonging (a belonging constituted through practice) that I believe is important to emphasize.

13. For an overview of the study and its context see Lawson, *Side Effects: The Story of AIDS in South Africa.*

14. Actuarial Society of Southern Africa, *Summary Statistics, ASSA2003.*

15. For an overview of AIDS in Asia see UNAIDS, *AIDS Epidemic Update, December 2009,* 37–47. The same report noted that 5.7 million South Africans are HIV positive (27).

16. On an "African system of sexuality," see the influential article written by Caldwell, Caldwell, and Quiggin, "The Social Context of AIDS in Sub-Saharan Africa." For criticisms see Heald, "The Power of Sex: Some Reflections on the Caldwells' 'African Sexuality' Thesis"; Ahlberg, "Is There a Distinct African Sexuality? A Critical Response to Caldwell."

17. Kark, "The Social Pathology of Syphilis in Africans." In 2003 the journals *Society in Transition* and the *International Journal of Epidemiology* both reprinted Kark's landmark piece without emphasizing changes in the social setting. One of the first accounts to draw attention to the potential connection between male migrancy and AIDS was Jochelson, Mthibeli, and Leger, "Human Immunodeficiency Virus and Migrant Labour in South Africa"; see also Horwitz, "Migration and HIV/AIDS: A Historical Perspective."

18. Critics of *Yesterday* charged that the film plays into stereotypes by presenting rural women as "resilient" but ultimately immobile and sexually passive. See Mbali and Hunter, "Yesterday's Stereotypes Are a Thing of the Past."

19. This is adapted from Hunter, "The Changing Political Economy of Sex in South Africa: The Significance of Unemployment and Inequalities to the Scale of the AIDS Pandemic."

20. See Morris and Kretzschmar, "Concurrent Partnerships and the Spread of AIDS"; Halperin and Epstein, "Concurrent Sexual Partnerships Help to Explain Africa's High HIV Prevalence: Implications for Prevention." Epstein outlines this model in detail in Epstein, *The Invisible Cure: Africa, the West, and the Fight against AIDS.* The importance of differing social contexts of sexual networks has been made clear by Robert Thornton in his comparison of Uganda and South Africa. Thornton, *Unimagined Community: Sex, Networks, and AIDS in Uganda and South Africa.* I consider multiple concurrent partners from the perspective of masculinities within this book and in Hunter, "Cultural Politics and Masculinities: Multiple-Partners in Historical Perspective in KwaZulu-Natal."

21. The case that programs aimed at reducing concurrent partnership patterns worked in Uganda is elucidated particularly powerfully by Epstein, *The Invisible Cure.* This argument has to be taken seriously; yet the data showing changes in sexual behavior and, even more, the link between such changes and a single government intervention program are far from clear.

22. HSRC, *South African National HIV Survey 2008,* 40–41, 31.

23. I have no real evidence that Mandeni was the "AIDS capital" of KwaZulu-Natal when this statement was made in 1997: HIV prevalence has long been high across the province. In 2006 the government started disaggregating HIV antenatal statistics by health districts; this analysis found that iLembe (the district in which Mandeni falls) had the fourth (2006), second (2007), and eighth (2008) highest HIV prevalence of the eleven districts in KwaZulu-Natal Province. Republic of South Africa, Department of Health, *2008 National Antenatal Sentinel HIV and Syphilis Prevalence Survey, South Africa,* 15. Swaziland, Botswana, Lesotho, and Zimbabwe have higher reported HIV prevalence than South Africa, although fewer HIV positive people. See UNAIDS, *AIDS Epidemic Update, December 2009,* 19, 27. For an excellent account of AIDS across the continent, see Iliffe, *The African AIDS Epidemic: A History.*

24. On the protection provided by male circumcision see Auvert et al., "Randomized, Controlled Intervention Trial of Male Circumcision for Reduction of HIV Infection Risk: The ANRS 1265 Trial."

25. See particularly Iliffe, *The African AIDS Epidemic.*

26. UNAIDS, *AIDS Epidemic Update, December 2009,* 19.

27. Unemployment rates have risen elsewhere in Africa, partly as a result of "structural adjustment" programs sponsored by the World Bank and the IMF. Implemented from the 1980s, these programs cut government expenditures and encouraged trade liberalization. On the connections between SAPs and AIDS elsewhere in Africa, see Schoepf, Schoepf, and Millen, "Theoretical Therapies, Remote Remedies: SAPs and the Political Ecology of Poverty and Health in Africa." On the disempowerment of unemployed youth in Zambia see Hansen, "Getting Stuck in the Compound: Some Odds against Social Adulthood in Lusaka."

28. Bongaarts, "Late Marriage and the HIV Epidemic in Sub-Saharan Africa." For reasons that I hope will become clear in this book, the concept of "late marriage" often used by demographers does not adequately capture the consequences of a situation in which young people are rarely marrying even as they grow older. On reduced marriage rates and HIV in Namibia see Pauli and Schnegg, "'Blood tests with the eyes': Negotiating Conjugal Relations during the HIV/AIDS Crisis in Rural Namibia."

29. Parikh and Smith show how in Uganda and Nigeria condomless sex can signify love within marriages. Parikh, "The Political Economy of Marriage and HIV"; Smith, "Love and the Risk of HIV."

30. See UNAIDS, *AIDS Epidemic Update, December 2009*, 23, 24.

31. All of the names of individuals in this book, unless otherwise stated, are pseudonyms. In a few cases, to make it harder to identify informants, I have changed small details about their lives. In two cases where I give quite a lot of information about informants' lives, I asked their permission to do so.

32. During my research, the rand/U.S. dollar exchange rate fluctuated enormously, from almost 12 to less than 6. The rate as of August 2009 is just under 8 rand for one dollar. For the sake of brevity I provide dollar equivalents only the first time rand prices are mentioned in each chapter; throughout the book I use an exchange rate of 8:1.

3. Providing Love

1. See for instance Hobsbawm and Ranger, *The Invention of Tradition;* Chanock, *Law, Custom and Social Order: The Colonial Experience in Malawi and Zambia;* Geschiere, *The Modernity of Witchcraft: Politics and the Occult in Postcolonial Africa.* For a useful discussion of debates on customary law and the use of court cases as historical sources, see Mann and Roberts, *Law in Colonial Africa.* For a critical review of the "invention of tradition" literature that demonstrates how stories of Shaka's legendary power were forged in intricate interactions between the colonizer and colonized, see Hamilton, *Terrific Majesty: The Powers of Shaka Zulu and the Limits of Historical Invention.*

2. Colenso, *Zulu-English Dictionary,* 1861 ed., s.v. *ukuhlobonga.*

3. These points are taken from Vaughan's discussion of Foucault in Vaughan, *Curing Their Ills: Colonial Power and African Illness,* 8–12. For a criticism see Stoler, *Race and the Education of Desire: Foucault's "History of Sexuality" and the Colonial Order of Things,* 33. Without getting into the details of this dispute, my point is to simply flag the huge differences between "Western" discussions of the history of sexuality and the project in a setting like South Africa.

4. Pigg and Adams, "Introduction: The Moral Object of Sex," 19.

5. Vance, "Anthropology Rediscovers Sexuality: A Theoretical Comment." See also Adams and Pigg, *Sex in Development.* Richard Parker usefully highlights how AIDS prevention efforts have partially shifted from relying on individualistic psychological models that promote "education" to more intersubjective notions of "sexual meaning" or "sexual culture." Parker, "Sexuality, Culture, and Power in HIV/AIDS Research." For an example of the rich work within this field, see Parker, Barbosa, and Aggleton, *Framing the Sexual Subject: The Politics of Gender, Sexuality, and Power.* When institutionalized in AIDS programs, however, models of "sexual culture" can lose their dynamism and can reify somewhat static models of bounded cultures.

6. See especially Cooper and Stoler, *Tensions of Empire: Colonial Cultures in a Bourgeois World.* A few notes on the simplified story I tell: though Natal and Zululand have quite different histories—the latter being conquered later than the former—I do not explore this further; nor do I explore different Christian denominations, including African initiated churches, although these also affected "sex" in important ways; finally, I do not give specific attention to the way that scientific discourses shape sexuality, for instance through medical categories.

7. I conducted eighty interviews with twenty elderly informants in a rural part of Mandeni; some residents I spoke with in Sundumbili township also discussed their rural

upbringings. Court cases and other official records mainly related to Eshowe, the district in which most of central Mandeni is situated. Many of the Eshowe civil court cases I looked at in the National Archives of South Africa (Durban Archives) were not catalogued and I accessed them directly from the strongroom.

8. See, for instance, Bryant, *A Zulu-English Dictionary with Notes on Pronunciation,* s.vv. *ukushela, ukuqoma.*

9. The best known example of young lovers' rebellion against kin is the case of the *inGcugce* age-set of girls who in the 1870s flouted King Cetshwayo's order to marry an older regiment of men and ran away with their sweethearts. Many of the young rebels were captured and brutally killed. Jeff Guy reviewed court cases relating to the inGcugce girls. Guy, "Love and Violence, Sex and Fertility, in the Zulu Kingdom." Cetshwayo himself testified in the late nineteenth century that forced marriages were not common; Cetshwayo's evidence, given to the 1883 Cape Government Commission on Native Laws and Customs, is published in Webb and Wright, *A Zulu King Speaks: Statements Made by Cetshwayo kaMpande on the History and Customs of His People.*

10. Women's absence, according to Kark's figures, peaked at only 20%. Kark, "The Influence of Urban-Rural Migration on Bantu Health and Disease," 25.

11. Guy, "Analysing Pre-capitalist Societies in Southern Africa"; see also Guy, *The Destruction of the Zulu Kingdom: The Civil War in Zululand, 1879–1884;* Wright, "Control of Women's Labour in the Zulu Kingdom."

12. On the return of cattle because a woman was "without issue," see *Vanganye v. Makanyezi* (National Archives of South Africa, Durban, 1/ESH 2/1/1/2/1, 1907). Giving a sense of the intricate connections formed by ilobolo, court cases in the early twentieth century describe *ukwethula,* to loan cattle, a practice that could entangle ilobolo in complex patterns of debt that stretched over many decades, especially between kin. On ukwethula, see for example *Mxokozeli kaBobe v. Msincomkwenyana* (National Archives of South Africa, Durban, 1/ESH 2/1/1/2/1, 15/1905). In the mid-1950s Vilakazi noted that ukwethula could also mean "to pay tribute." Vilakazi, *Zulu Transformations: A Study of the Dynamics of Social Change,* 19–20.

13. Jeffreys, "Lobolo Is Child-Price."

14. For a particularly nuanced analysis of wedding gifts in Niger that recognizes women's influence over them, see B. Cooper, "Women's Worth and Wedding Gift Exchange in Maradi, Niger, 1907–89." For detailed evidence from Zambia of how migration and money did not break down but reconstituted social relations around marriage, see Moore and Vaughan, *Cutting Down Trees,* chapter 6.

15. According to Bryant's 1905 dictionary, "A married woman *hlonipa's* the names of her father-in-law and all his brothers, the *ama-kosana* or elder among her brothers-in-law, her mother-in-law and all other wives of her father-in-law. Any word containing the radical of such a name would be avoided by her in speech and another word substituted for it. Thus, if these persons were called *u-Muti* (Mr. Tree), not only will this actual word for 'a tree' be disused and the word *um-Cakantshi* substituted, but every other word containing within it the particle *ti,* will be equally avoided." Bryant, *A Zulu-English Dictionary with Notes on Pronunciation,* s.v. *ukuhlonipha.*

16. Bryant, *The Zulu People as They Were before the White Man Came,* 219.

17. The James Stuart Archive gives a sense of the historical and geographical variability of courting and marriage. James Stuart was a colonial official who collected more than a hundred oral histories from informants, mostly men and African, at the turn of the nineteenth century. His archive was translated and published in five volumes by Colin Webb and John Wright. Using this and other sources, Hanretta argues that gender relations were

far from static in the centralized Zulu state established by Shaka in 1816 (which foundered with the defeat of Cetshwayo in 1879). Hanretta, "Women, Marginality and the Zulu State: Women's Institutions and Power in the Early Nineteenth Century."

18. Welsh, *The Roots of Segregation,* 95. Welsh charts the decline of second or subsequent marriages from 44% of all marriages in 1870 to 30% in 1909.

19. Smith, *Labour Resources of Natal,* 35.

20. The vast majority of civil court disputes over the course of the twentieth century revolve around claims on ilobolo cattle, and some even rest on whether couples are, in fact, married. For an example of a dispute over whether a couple was married, see *Yibhepu v. Makwapa Xulu & Ratana Lutuli* (Durban Archives, 1/ESH 2/1/2/1, 80/1937). The commissioner said, "They did not actually go through the ceremonies of marriage but that does not invalidate their marriage as there are numerous instances today where men and women live together and it is presumed they are married." Ilobolo payments were sometimes not fully completed and were frequently disputed, as court cases demonstrate. At times, the bride's family could implicitly or explicitly approve the non-completion of ilobolo: a well-known Zulu saying is *"Intombi ayiqedwa"* (The girl's ilobolo isn't finished). One outstanding cow could leave the groom's family with an almost indefinite ongoing obligation. For a discussion of how anthropological writings on marriage tended to ignore the institution's ambiguity, see John Comaroff, *The Meaning of Marriage Payments.*

21. *Mtiyeni Vilakazi v. Matini Vilakazi* (d/a M. Gumede) is a typical case. Mr. Vilakazi sought dissolution of a customary union, saying that his wife bore two children when he was working in Durban. She claimed that he hadn't been sending her money (National Archives of South Africa, Durban, uncatalogued Eshowe civil cases, 50/54). With the exception of a small number of women "emancipated" from customary law (having applied to a court and typically proven their financial independence and education), women could not directly take a case to court; Joena Zulu therefore was "assisted" by her brother in applying for dissolution of a customary union on the grounds of her husband's desertion. *Joena Zulu v. Tom Zulu* (National Archives of South Africa, Durban, uncatalogued Eshowe civil cases, 38/55).

22. Carton, *Blood from Your Children: The Colonial Origins of Generational Conflict in South Africa.*

23. See especially Murray, *Families Divided: The Impact of Migrant Labour in Lesotho.*

24. Mayer, "The Origin and Decline of Two Rural Resistance Ideologies," 52. See chapter 5 for a fuller discussion of declining marriage rates; obviously there was no mechanical connection between increasing unemployment and changes to the household. Indeed, although unemployment rose in the late 1970s, the full effects of this on the household might not have been felt until later, depending on the region; Mayer's research and qualitative studies referred to in chapter 5 would seem to support this point.

25. Kark, "The Influence of Urban-Rural Migration," 34.

26. Schapera, *Married Life in an African Tribe,* chapter 2.

27. Parle and Scorgie, "Bewitching Zulu Women: Umhayizo, Gender, and Witchcraft in Natal"; Köhler, *Marriage Customs in Southern Natal,* 23–24.

28. In the U.S., urbanization, industrialization, new spaces of consumption, and men's superior position in the labor market engendered new connections between money and courting. Among the working class, at the turn of the twentieth century there emerged the practice of men "treating" women to gifts in exchange for sexual favors; this came to greatly mold later forms of "dating." See Clement, *Love for Sale: Courting, Treating, and Prostitution in New York City, 1900–1945.* On somewhat similar

changes in courting among the middle class (although less overt sexual bargaining) see Bailey, *From Front Porch to Back Seat: Courtship in Twentieth-Century America.*

29. Bryant, *The Zulu People as They Were before the White Man Came,* 566.

30. Republic of South Africa, Statistics South Africa, *Census 2001: Primary Tables Compared,* calculated from table 5.1, 24.

31. Census figures from 1951 are taken from the Eshowe District Record Book (Eshowe Magistrates Court, uncatalogued, 30-4-72), 145.

32. Eshowe District Record Book (Eshowe Magistrates Court, uncatalogued, 30-4-72), 53–55.

33. Simons, *African Women: Their Legal Status in South Africa,* 69.

34. On love letters as a private realm, see Breckenridge, "Love Letters and Amanuenses: Beginning the Cultural History of the Working Class Private Sphere in Southern Africa, 1900–1933"; on schooling and love letters see Thomas, *Politics of the Womb: Women, Reproduction, and the State in Kenya,* chapter 4.

35. Vilakazi, *Zulu Transformations,* 30.

36. Marx, *Economical and Philosophical Manuscripts of 1844,* 122 (emphasis in original).

37. On prostitution and sex-money links in South Africa, see Bonner, "'Desirable or Undesirable Basotho Women?' Liquor, Prostitution and the Migration of Basotho Women to the Rand, 1920–1945"; Jochelson, *The Colour of Disease: Syphilis and Racism in South Africa, 1880–1950;* Van Onselen, *Studies in the Social and Economic History of the Witwatersrand, 1886–1914,* vol. 1. In other parts of Africa, see Barnes, "*We women worked so hard*": *Gender, Urbanization and Social Reproduction in Colonial Harare, Zimbabwe, 1930–1956;* Bledsoe, *Women and Marriage in Kpelle Society;* Bujra, "Women 'Entrepreneurs' of Early Nairobi"; MacGaffey, "Evading Male Control: Women in the Second Economy in Zaire"; Parpart, "Sexuality and Power on the Zambian Copperbelt"; Powdermaker, *Copper Town: Changing Africa; The Human Situation on the Rhodesian Copperbelt;* Schuster, *New Women of Lusaka;* Wa Karanja, "'Outside Wives' and 'Inside Wives' in Nigeria: A Study of Changing Perceptions in Marriage"; L. White, *The Comforts of Home.*

38. See Schapera, *Migrant Labour and Tribal Life: A Study of Conditions in the Bechuanaland Protectorate;* C. Walker, "Gender and the Development of the Migrant Labour System, c. 1850–1930: An Overview." Geographical differences in the decline of rural production, the penetration of schooling and Christianity, and the proximity of potential migrants to well-established traveling routes meant that migration differed greatly by region. Moreover, although young unmarried women were often seen as being among the least likely to migrate, as early as the 1920s Christian-educated women from Phokeng moved to work in Johannesburg to accumulate consumer items before entering matrimony. See Bozzoli, *Women of Phokeng: Consciousness, Life Strategy, and Migrancy in South Africa, 1900–1983.*

39. Wilson, *Reaction to Conquest,* 208.

40. Bryant suggests that there was a heavy penalty among isiZulu speakers for adultery. Bryant, *The Zulu People,* 578. Oral testimonies I collected also support this view. Further, Thembeka Mngomezulu, a nurse in her early fifties who grew up close to Pondoland and then married into a Zululand umuzi, sharply contrasts the freedom of the amadikazi of Pondoland, whom she remembers, to the widows in KwaZulu-Natal who are expected to be chaste (personal communication, December 2003; Thembeka and I worked together on the Hlabisa part of my study outlined in chapter 5). One possible reason for this is that in Natal, but not in other provinces, adultery was a criminal offense, although the law was not always enforced. Simons, *African Women,* 208.

41. Vilakazi, *Zulu Transformations*, 49.

42. Extramarital relations could, as Spiegel notes in the case of Lesotho, be justified by calling on the tradition of polygamy. Spiegel, "Polygamy as Myth: Towards Understanding Extramarital Relations in Lesotho."

43. Simons, *African Women*, 128–131.

44. The authors of dictionaries also drew heavily on previous dictionaries, making distinctions difficult. On language and the creation of ethnic boundaries in colonial Africa see Vail, *The Creation of Tribalism in Southern Africa*.

45. Colenso, *Zulu-English Dictionary*, 1861 ed., s.vv. *ukusoka, isoka*.

46. I found evidence for this in several court cases. In the 1887 murder case *Rex v. Gumakwake* (National Archives of South Africa, Durban, RSC II/1/42, 85/87), one witness, Ncwebu, noted that it was common for women to move quickly between different lovers. "It is usual for a girl to throw up a lover, and to take another lover, when a girl has 'chosen' a man, he and she have external sexual intercourse with each other for a short time and then they throw each other up, and take others: this external sexual intercourse is 'ukuhlobonga' [another word for ukusoma] and it takes place at night—some men go themselves to call the girl, some send for her." See also Ndukwana's testimony in the James Stuart archive (quoted later in this chapter) and Henry Fynn's diary, written in the first half of the nineteenth century, which describes how men who visited a kraal were allowed to *ukuhlobonga* with available girls. "The plan is repeated as often as strangers make their appearance, so that one girl may have 100 sweethearts, as also a man the same." Fynn, *The Diary of Henry Francis Fynn*, 295.

47. On the difficulty of conceptually separating fertility from other aspects of intimacy, see particularly Thomas, *Politics of the Womb*.

48. Webb and Wright, *The James Stuart Archive of Recorded Evidence Relating to the History of the Zulu and Neighbouring Peoples*, 4:299, 300.

49. Doke and Vilakazi, *Zulu-English Dictionary*, s.v. *isoka*.

50. Vilakazi, *Zulu Transformations*, 47.

51. The isoka figure appeared, for instance, in *izibongo*, oral praise poems that described and celebrated the characteristics of successful men. See Koopman, "The Praises of Young Zulu Men"; Turner, "Representations of Masculinity in the Contemporary Oral Praise Poetry of Zulu Men"; Gunner and Gwala, *Musho: Zulu Popular Praises*.

52. On restrictions on women having more than one ukusoma partner see Krige, "Girls' Puberty Songs and Their Relation to Fertility, Health, Morality and Religion among the Zulu," 174; Köhler, *Marriage Customs in Southern Natal*, 32.

53. See *Majozi v. Khuzwayo* (National Archives of South Africa, Durban, uncatalogued Eshowe civil case, 65/63) for a rural setting and *Buthelezi v. Ntuli* (National Archives of South Africa, Durban, uncatalogued Eshowe civil case, 66/66) for an urban setting.

54. Figures from Simons, *African Women*, 278.

55. Vilakazi, *Zulu Transformations*, 49.

56. On the history of African initiated churches see Sundkler, *Bantu Prophets in South Africa*.

57. On the prevalence of syphilis see Kark, "The Social Pathology of Syphilis in Africans."

58. Moodie, *Going for Gold: Men, Mines, and Migration*, chapter 4.

59. Epprecht, *Hungochani: The History of a Dissident Sexuality in Southern Africa*. Zackie Achmat made a pioneering earlier critique of social histories that reduced the sig-

nificance of pleasure in same-sex relationships. See Achmat, "'Apostles of Civilized Vice': 'Immoral Practices' and 'Unnatural Vice' in South African Prisons and Compounds, 1890–1920." Prior to Dunbar Moodie's work, these relations were described in Charles Van Onselen's groundbreaking social histories of the region (which were also subsequently criticized for not considering pleasure). See Van Onselen, *Studies in the Social and Economic History of the Witwatersrand, 1886–1914*, 2:187. Same-sex relations among women have been even more understudied than male-male relations, but see Wieringa, "Women Marriages and Other Same-Sex Practices: Historical Reflections on African Women's Same-Sex Relations."

60. A criticism that Hoad aims at the volume by Murray and Roscoe. See Hoad, *African Intimacies;* Murray and Roscoe, *Boy-Wives and Female-Husbands: Studies in African Homosexualities.* For insightful discussions of writing "homosexual" histories see Halperin, *How to Do the History of Homosexuality;* Houlbrook, *Queer London: Peril and Pleasures in the Sexual Metropolis, 1918–1957.*

61. Marks, "Patriotism, Patriarchy and Purity: Natal and the Politics of Zulu Ethnic Consciousness," 225.

62. Africans outnumbered settlers by ten to one, according to the first Natal census in 1891. Smith, *Labour Resources of Natal,* 9. From 1893 Britain granted Natal's white settlers responsible government. For a recent account of the importance of "indirect rule" to contemporary politics see Mamdani, *Citizen and Subject: Contemporary Africa and the Legacy of Late Colonialism.*

63. Guy, "An Accommodation of the Patriarchs: Theophilus Shepstone and the Foundations of the System of Native Administration in Natal."

64. For vigorous critiques of the effects the Natal Code had on women, see Simons, *African Women.*

65. See Welsh, *The Roots of Segregation: Native Policy in Colonial Natal, 1845–1910,* chapter 5.

66. Braatvedt, "Zulu Marriage Customs and Ceremonies."

67. The nature and specific workings of these political and institutional arrangements can only be touched on here. Scholars, for instance, debate the extent to which segregation was shaped by Shepstone's initiatives, the expansion of capitalism, the eugenics movement, or anthropologists' writings on culture. Nevertheless, few doubt the significance for the present day of the devolution of power to chiefs. On the relevance of Natal's history to the roots of segregation see Welsh, *The Roots of Segregation.* On segregation in the interwar years see Dubow, *Racial Segregation and the Origins of Apartheid in South Africa, 1919–36.* On the history of anthropology in South Africa see Hammond-Tooke, *Imperfect Interpreters: South Africa's Anthropologists, 1920–1990.*

68. Between 1960 and 1983 around 3.5 million people were forcibly removed from freehold areas, white farms, and urban (often informal) areas and unceremoniously dumped into what by then were becoming self-governing homelands. This history is outlined in detail in Platzky and Walker, *The Surplus People: Forced Removals in South Africa.* On the particular history of land and labor tenants, see McClendon, *Genders and Generations Apart: Labor Tenants and Customary Law in Segregation-Era South Africa, 1920s to 1940s.*

69. Jean Comaroff and John Comaroff, *Christianity, Colonialism, and Consciousness in South Africa;* John Comaroff and Jean Comaroff, *The Dialectics of Modernity on a South African Frontier.*

70. See Cope, *To Bind the Nation: Solomon kaDinuzulu and Zulu Nationalism, 1913–1933;* La Hausse de Lalouviere, *Restless Identities: Signatures of Nationalism, Zulu Ethnicity and*

History in the Lives of Petros Lamula (c. 1881–1948) and Lymon Maling (1889–c. 1936); Marks, *The Ambiguities of Dependence in South Africa: Class, Nationalism, and the State in Twentieth-Century Natal.*

71. For instance, Schapera, "Premarital Pregnancy and Native Opinion: A Note on Social Change."

72. Mager, *Gender and the Making of a South African Bantustan: A Social History of the Ciskei, 1945–1959*, 183.

73. On changes to inhlawulo and the decline of virginity testing see C. Dlamini, "Seduction in Zulu Law." On men's abandonment in Kenya see Thomas, *Politics of the Womb*, chapter 4.

4. Urban Respectability

1. Longmore, *The Dispossessed: A Study of the Sex-Life of Bantu Women in and around Johannesburg*, 52. I use the word "township" throughout this chapter. This is the English term most often used today to describe formal urban spaces previously designated for Africans. "Location" was a favored earlier word, and Sundumbili and other townships are still commonly referred to in isiZulu as *ilokishi.*

2. Krige, "Changing Conditions in Marital Relations and Parental Duties among Urbanized Natives"; Phillips, *The Bantu in the City: A Study of Cultural Adjustment on the Witwatersrand*; Hellman, *Rooiyard: A Sociological Survey of an Urban Native Slum Yard.* It should be noted that early urban ethnographies combined sweeping generalizations with often rich and varied accounts of specific places. They also broke new ground by moving away from anthropologists' conventional focus on Africans in rural societies.

3. Links between these writers and the South African Institute for Race Relations are discussed by Glaser in "Managing the Sexuality of Urban Youth: Johannesburg, 1920s–1960s."

4. Not all anthropologists, however, emphasized urban "promiscuity." Absolom Vilakazi, for instance, derided Longmore's study for generalizing from the "lower classes of African urban society." It was, he claimed, based on the common illusion that "city life is unsuitable and unwholesome for the Africans whose natural habitat is the [rural] reserves." Vilakazi, review of *The Dispossessed*, 949, 950. Vilakazi's comments had some similarities to the arguments made by urban anthropologists based at the Rhodes Livingstone Institute in Zambia. For these (white) anthropologists, Africans' urban adaption demonstrated their readiness for political rights. See Ferguson, *Expectations of Modernity: Myths and Meanings of Urban Life on the Zambian Copperbelt.*

5. See particularly Deborah Posel, *The Making of Apartheid, 1948–1961: Conflict and Compromise.*

6. However, many historical accounts have, in effect, questioned linear accounts of "family decline." Important recent writings on gender in urban areas include Glaser, *Bo-tsotsi: The Youth Gangs of Soweto, 1935–1976*; Eagle, "A Study of African Women's Access to Housing in the Durban Area"; Deborah Posel, *The Making of Apartheid*; Robinson, *The Power of Apartheid: State, Power, and Space in South African Cities*; Mager, *Gender and the Making of a South African Bantustan.* The latter includes a particularly relevant exploration of state paternalism in Zwelitsha, a model township in the Eastern Cape. On how colonial policy promoted "industrial man" elsewhere in the continent, see F. Cooper, "Industrial Man Goes to Africa." Delius and Glaser adopt a different approach to challenge the "family decline" model; they show that in precolonial society "a great

deal of sex took place outside of marriage." Delius and Glaser, "The Myths of Polygamy: A History of Extra-Marital and Multi-partnership Sex in South Africa," 85.

7. The first formal urban areas built for Africans were constructed in the wake of the 1923 Native Urban Areas Act, well before the period of the greatest housing expansion, the 1950s–1960s. A large literature on urban policy in South Africa now exists. In addition to the above references, for a recent critical review, see Mbembe and Nutall, *Johannesburg: The Elusive Metropolis*. On contestations within the state over urban policy see Deborah Posel, *The Making of Apartheid*. On illegal shack settlements in Johannesburg, see Stadler, "Birds in the Cornfield: Squatter Movements in Johannesburg." On modernist plans see Parnell and Mabin, "Rethinking Urban South Africa." On respectability in urban South Africa see Goodhew, *Respectability and Resistance: A History of Sophiatown*. Other references are given within this chapter.

8. Key texts include Maré and Hamilton, *An Appetite for Power: Buthelezi's Inkatha and South Africa;* Waetjen, *Workers and Warriors: Masculinity and the Struggle for Nation in South Africa*. Both are vital sources on Inkatha in KwaZulu-Natal.

9. In using the phrase "welfare paternalism" I draw from Belinda Bozzoli's work. She argues that welfare paternalism characterized earlier townships but was replaced by a more aggressive "racial modernism" in the 1970s. Key to this shift was a change in the governance of townships from local authorities to the central state. Sundumbili township differs from the townships that Bozzoli discusses because it was located in the homeland of KwaZulu and not a "white" area; I am also more concerned with the links between the township and the area's dominant employer, the SAPPI paper mill, and therefore connections between employment, housing, and a gendered form of paternalism that endured into the late 1970s. Despite these differences, I think that the concept of welfare paternalism captures important features of the early period of the township. See Bozzoli, "Why Were the 1980s 'Millenarian'? Style, Repertoire, Space and Authority in South Africa's Black Cities"; Bozzoli, *Theatres of Struggle and the End of Apartheid*.

10. I conducted eighty interviews with sixty elderly informants living in Sundumbili. The Ulundi archives, where the KwaZulu papers are held, did not have an organized cataloguing system when I visited (in 2002 and 2003). I was fortunate to be allowed access in 2003 to Sundumbili's records, which can be found in the township administration buildings. However, these were not organized or catalogued in any discernable fashion. I have done my best to indicate where each source can be found.

11. It should be noted that apartheid urban segregation was implemented in different ways across the country. For instance, in Durban, Indians were the largest group removed as a consequence of the 1950 Group Areas Act. Kuper, Watts, and Davies, *Durban: A Study in Race Ecology.*

12. Three houses were also built for coloureds who had been living at Mangete. Stubbings and Pepper, *Mandini*, 32, 55.

13. Freund argues that by the 1960s both market gardening and sugar cane production had become economically residual for Indians. The Indian peasantry, descended from indentured laborers who worked on Natal's sugar cane plantations from the nineteenth century, dwindled in the twentieth century as a consequence of massive state support for white agriculture; many Indians moved into industrial work, largely in Durban, after World War II. For more background on the Indian working class in Natal see Freund, *Insiders and Outsiders: The Indian Working Class of Durban, 1910–1990.*

14. See Robinson, *The Power of Apartheid*, on the spatiality of social control in African urban areas.

15. Parnell and Mabin, "Rethinking Urban South Africa."

16. *Zululand Times,* "'Gezinsila' and 'Sundumbili' New Bantu Townships for Zululand." The swimming pool and tennis courts were never built but discussed repeatedly, as noted in the minutes of the Sundumbili meeting on May 4, 1972, held at SAPPI (KwaZulu Archives, Ulundi, 9/4/14/1).

17. Parnell and Mabin, "Rethinking Urban South Africa," 57.

18. Although Sundumbili was built on "reserve" land, in other cases authorities could manipulate boundaries so that townships in areas previously designated as white were now in newly created homelands. KwaMashu, for instance, found itself in KwaZulu in 1977.

19. *Zululand Times,* "'Gezinsila' and 'Sundumbili' New Bantu Townships for Zululand."

20. Although such anti-Indian sentiments were not uncommon in the area, leaders of African and Indian political organizations did sometimes cooperate in the 1960s, according to ANC leader Albert Luthuli, who lived in nearby Groutville. Conversely, the wish for a purely African liberation movement was a central reason for the Pan African Congress's split from the ANC in 1959. See Luthuli, *Let My People Go: An Autobiography.* On the intersecting lives of Africans and Indians in Natal see Soske, "'Wash me black again': African Nationalism, the Indian Diaspora, and KwaZulu-Natal, 1945–1979."

21. Deborah Posel, *The Making of Apartheid,* outlines the difficulties of administering influx controls.

22. Mandela, *No Easy Walk to Freedom,* 98.

23. Marks, *The Ambiguities of Dependence in South Africa.* This book contains a chapter on John Dube.

24. Bhabha, "Of Mimicry and Man: The Ambivalence of Colonial Discourse."

25. Calderwood, "Native Housing in South Africa," 18. The NE 51/9 houses were slightly bigger than the NE 51/6 houses also built in townships, which had a living space of forty-one square meters and no inside toilet.

26. Deborah Posel, "Marriage at the Drop of a Hat: Housing and Partnership in South Africa's Urban African Townships, 1920s–1960s," 60.

27. See, for instance, Robinson, *The Power of Apartheid.*

28. Letters from superintendent [for] personnel and training, SAPPI, to Bantu affairs commissioner, Eshowe, May 27, 1971, and August 17, 1971 (Sundumbili Township Records, N13/1/14).

29. Edwards, "Cato Manor, June 1959: Men, Women, Crowds, Violence, Politics and History," 122; see also Deborah Posel, *The Making of Apartheid.*

30. On apartheid and "heteropatriarchy" see Elder, *Hostels, Sex and the Apartheid Legacy: Malevolent Geographies.*

31. Edwards, "Cato Manor, June 1959," 118, 119; see also Louw, "Mkhumbane and New Traditions of (Un)African Same-Sex Weddings."

32. *Ilanga laseNatal,* "Amadoda Azishadisile Enye Ingumfazi" (Men Married Each Other, One Was a Wife).

33. Gilbert and Crankshaw, "Comparing South African and Latin American Experience: Migration and Housing Mobility in Soweto." It should be noted too that the state's strong interest in the viability of homeland townships (also called R293s) led it to subsidize basic services such as water in these settlements.

34. See, for instance, Gaitskell, "Wailing for Purity: Prayer Unions, African Mothers and Adolescent Daughters, 1912–1940."

35. Stubbings and Pepper, *Mandini,* 41.

36. Ibid., 38.

37. Brown, "Facing the 'Black Peril': The Politics of Population Control in South Africa."

38. Kuzwayo, "The Emergence of the African Woman as a Potent Economic Force" (Cullen Archives, Hellman Collection, A1419). Wilson and Mafeje captured these forms of distinction in Cape Town's Langa township in the 1960s. Wilson and Mafeje, *Langa: A Study of Social Groups in an African Township*. See also Brandel-Syrier, *"Coming Through": The Search for a New Cultural Identity*. Clive Glaser's *Bo-Tsotsi* provides rich details on urban youth style from the 1930s to the 1970s.

39. *Zululand Times*, "Domestic Science Course for Girls."

40. Some of these details are described in the court case pertaining to the rape of a four-year-old girl that took place in Manda Farm. *Rex v. Mkwanyana* (National Archives of South Africa, Durban, 1/MTU 1/1/1/1/2, 268/62).

41. Natal was the only province where customary marriages were registered; in the other three provinces that also constituted South Africa at this time it was impossible to determine marital status. Even in Natal, however, men could show the authorities a marriage certificate and then cohabit with a different woman. On the state's longstanding deliberations about whether to register customary marriages, see Deborah Posel, "State, Power and Gender: Conflict over the Registration of African Customary Marriage in South Africa, c. 1910–1970." For an overview of housing legislation, see Eagle, "A Study of African Women's Access to Housing in the Durban Area."

42. Letter from administrative manager, SAPPI, to township superintendent, February 8, 1968 (Sundumbili Township Records, N13/2/4/10).

43. This is discussed in a letter from the Sundumbili Township superintendent to the Eshowe Bantu affairs commissioner, January 23, 1970 (Sundumbili Township Records, N13/2/8/2).

44. Mayer, *Townsmen or Tribesmen: Conservatism and the Process of Urbanization in a South African City*. Mayer's account of East London recognized the sexual conservatism among "Red" migrants who were "encapsulated" in networks that ensured that they maintained a commitment to their rural home.

45. On similar anti-Indian feelings among Africans in Natal see Soske, "'Wash me black again.'" The use of words like "visitors" for Indians and not whites reveals how Africans' consciousness of Indians was formed in relation to white rule that ingrained itself through not only violent oppression but institutions such as schools and churches that could signal "modernity."

46. Ardington, "Decentralized Industry, Poverty and Development in Rural KwaZulu," 16.

47. See for instance Maré and Hamilton, *An Appetite for Power*. One way that the state sought to legitimate the homeland project was to embed ethnicity in everyday life, including by establishing distinct ethnic radio stations. See Nixon, *Homelands, Harlem, and Hollywood: South African Culture and the World Beyond*.

48. See Buthelezi, "Funeral of Prince Nhlanhla Ka Nonjombo Ka Dinuzulu: Address by Prince Mangosuthu Buthelezi, MP."

49. Thanks to Daniel Magaziner for this information (personal communication, November 4, 2008).

50. Interview with Rev. Mzoneli, Durban, March 13, 2003.

51. Hassim, "Black Women in Political Organisations: A Case Study of the Inkatha Women's Brigade, 1976 to Present," 7.

52. Buthelezi Commission, *The Requirements for Stability and Development in Kwazulu and Natal*, 2:294.

53. Simons, *African Women.*

54. Select committee report on the legal disabilities of Zulu women. With covering note for executive councillor for justice—KwaZulu, stamped March 24, 1975 (KwaZulu Cabinet Agenda and Minutes: 1981, KwaZulu Archives, Ulundi), 32.

55. See Hassim, "Black Women in Political Organisations," 93–95; Eagle, "A Study of African Women's Access to Housing in the Durban Area."

56. See Todes and Walker, "Women and Housing Policy in South Africa."

57. Hassim, "Black Women in Political Organisations," 125.

58. An assessment of the Interim Report on Community Development in Sundumbili (Sundumbili Township Records, SAPPI: Meetings, KwaZulu Archives, Ulundi).

59. See especially Bonnin, "Space, Place and Identity: Political Violence in Mpumalanga Township, KwaZulu-Natal, 1987–1993."

60. Baskin and Bissell, "Sundumbili General Strike of March 1982," 30.

61. Ardington, "Decentralized Industry, Poverty and Development," 9.

62. Special meeting held on 17/10/80. Office of the Manager, Sundumbili: Shortage of accommodation to unmarried girls employed in this area (Sundumbili Township Records, Interior 7/7/3).

63. Undated letter to KwaZulu Government (but reply written in 1983) with lead author Mr. Khumalo (Sundumbili Township Records, 7/5/3/14/1).

64. Ardington, "Decentralized Industry, Poverty and Development," 28.

65. When debating reforms to customary law, the KwaZulu Legislative Assembly questioned whether ilobolo should remain at ten cattle (plus one for the bride's mother), which had been the maximum payment (and de facto standard payment) under colonial law. In the end, it did not suggest any radical changes, although it recommended that ilobolo be interpreted more flexibly and be a matter of custom and not legislation. See Hassim, "Black Women in Political Organizations," 89. In practice, the customary payment is still widely thought of as eleven cattle.

66. The first installment of the series was *Drum,* "Everything You Ever Wanted to Know about Sex," 38–39.

67. Krige's study of a Pretoria township noted illegitimacy rates of 40–60%; in 1934 she wrote that illegitimacy is one "of the most striking symptoms of social disintegration and economic disorder." Krige, "Changing Conditions," 4. Yet Moeno pointed to subsequent marriages between parents to argue that high rates of urban illegitimacy could not be regarded as evidence of breakdown of the institution of marriage. Moeno, "Illegitimacy in an African Urban Township in South Africa: An Ethnographic Note."

68. These references were given in chapter 3.

69. For instance, Schuster, *New Women of Lusaka;* Wa Karanja, "'Outside Wives' and 'Inside Wives' in Nigeria."

70. Pauw notes that gift giving in couples in an East London township was generally reciprocal. Pauw, *The Second Generation: A Study of the Family among Urbanized Bantu in East London,* 116, 134. Similarly, Levin reports mainly reciprocal gifts in Langa township: "During courtship men try to win the favor of girls by giving them presents such as slabs of chocolate, jewelry, and scarves. Women, in turn, are said to give their boyfriends presents, such as ties and socks." Levin, "Marriage in Langa Native Location," 22. It appears that, compared to today at least, gifts were relatively unimportant in premarital relations.

71. On the shortage of township housing in the 1980s, see Bekker and Humphries, *From Control to Confusion: The Changing Role of Administration Boards in South Africa, 1971–1983.* On the transfer of townships' administration from municipalities to semi-auton-

omous administration boards in the 1970s, see Bozzoli, *Theatres of Struggle.* White-run municipalities tended to redistribute local finances in poorer African areas, but administration boards were expected to ensure that black areas were financially self-sufficient. Most of KwaZulu's townships were run on an agency basis by administration boards from the 1970s and faced a large cash shortfall. Authorities were forced to increase rent in homeland townships in order to balance their books, just as they had done in the South African townships.

72. When Redhill and Island were built in 1980, there was an outcry over their high rents and poor housing. According to complainants, ten roofs had been blown off houses that were only four years old. Moreover, the houses built in Redhill and Island were rented at R34, compared to R14.40 for those in the first sections of the township. Letter from Sundumbili Town Council to Department of the Interior, KwaZulu, March 28, 1984 (Sundumbili Township Records, Interior 7/7/3).

73. The 1969 figures are from South African Pulp & Paper Industries Limited, Tugela Mill. Sundumbili Township: Points for Discussion. 13.5.69 (KwaZulu Archives, Ulundi, N/13/1/2 (9) box 20); the 1983 figures are from Ardington, "Decentralized Industry, Poverty and Development," 9. The 1991 figures are calculated from Survey Completed for the Bureau of Market Research, Information on Housing: February 1992 (Sundumbili Township Records, Interior, 12/1/1) (number of houses) and a letter from the township manager to Postmaster, Mandini, June 13, 1991 (Sundumbili Township Records, Interior, 12/1/1) (population).

74. Ardington, "Decentralized Industry, Poverty and Development," 76.

75. Khumalo, *Touch My Blood,* 95, 110.

76. In 1983, only 6% of Sundumbili was electrified, but the proportion grew rapidly in the 1980s. Ardington, "Decentralized Industry, Poverty and Development," 65.

77. Although see Crankshaw, *Race, Class and the Changing Division of Labour under Apartheid;* Seekings and Nattrass, *Class, Race, and Inequality in South Africa.*

78. J. Hofmeyr, "Black Wages: The Post-war Experience."

79. Taxis led to profits that averaged R3,640 a year, compared to another common informal activity—running a shop—which led to R1,336. Ardington, "Decentralized Industry, Poverty and Development," 57.

80. See Xaba, "Masculinity and Its Malcontents: The Confrontation between 'Struggle Masculinity' and 'Post-struggle Masculinity' (1990–1997)"; Waetjen, *Workers and Warriors.*

81. Dlamini, "The Construction, Meaning and Negotiation of Ethnic Identities in KwaZulu Natal," 479.

82. In describing the chief's role in the Isithebe area, I am drawing from numerous conversations with residents.

83. On their return, these men became integrated with the South African police force and the KwaZulu police force.

84. See Bonnin, "Space, Place and Identity."

85. Mhlongo, "Trouble across the Tugela River: Political Instability and Conflict Resolution in Mandini; A Comparative Study with Special Emphasis on the Political Culture of Pre- and Post-apartheid South Africa (1984–2001)," 99.

86. Bonnin, "Space, Place and Identity."

87. Although see Campbell, "Learning to Kill? Masculinity, the Family and Violence in Natal," for an early account of violence and family change.

88. Khumalo, *Touch My Blood,* 108.

89. Bozzoli, "Why Were the 1980s 'Millenarian'?" 102.

5. Shacks in the Cracks of Apartheid

1. Davis, *Planet of Slums.*

2. For example, Preston-Whyte, "Families without Marriage."

3. Spiegel, "Migration, Urbanisation and Domestic Fluidity: Reviewing Some South African Examples."

4. Crankshaw, "Squatting, Apartheid and Urbanisation on the Southern Witwatersrand"; Hindson and McCarthy, *Here to Stay: Informal Settlements in KwaZulu-Natal.*

5. The park was initially run by the Bantu Investment Corporation, and then by the Corporation for Economic Development (from 1978), the KwaZulu Finance Corporation (from 1984), and Ithala (from 1999).

6. Burton, "Industrial Restructuring and Changing Gender Relations: The Case of Isithebe in KwaZulu-Natal," 102.

7. Pickles and Woods, "Taiwanese Investment in South Africa."

8. Platzky, "The Development Impact of South Africa's Industrial Decentralization Policies: An Unforeseen Legacy," 225.

9. Bell, "Some Aspects of Industrial Decentralization in South Africa"; Hyslop and Tomlinson, "Industrial Decentralization and the New Dispensation."

10. Yawitch, "Women in Wage Labour," 87.

11. Cock, "Introduction," 3, 4. Although she does not define the term, "black" presumably refers to persons categorized as African, Indian, and coloured.

12. Ardington, "Decentralized Industry, Poverty and Development," 35.

13. Pudifin and Ward, "Working for Nothing: Gender and Industrial Decentralisation in Isithebe," 57.

14. Ibid., 67.

15. "Skwatta Kamp: The Mkhukhu Guys," an interview with two members of the group, available at http://www.yeahbo.net/skwatta.html (accessed March 14, 2007).

16. On the chief's claims that he did not take money see Ardington, "Decentralized Industry, Poverty and Development," 15. However, the verb *ukudayisa* (to sell) is typically used by residents in discussing these transactions, which can perhaps best be described as purchase of the permanent entitlement to land use. Importantly, prevailing customary practices helped to blur the meanings of these payments: to be granted the use of land in any tribal area, new residents typically engaged in ukukhonza (put oneself under authority) by offering the chief a symbolic gift.

17. The literature on the contested nature of land and its embroilment in struggles over meanings is now large. See for instance Berry, *No Condition Is Permanent: The Social Dynamics of Agrarian Change in Sub-Saharan Africa;* James, *Gaining Ground: "Rights" and "Property" in South African Land Reform;* Ntsebeza and Hall, *The Land Question in South Africa: The Challenge of Transformation and Redistribution.*

18. Interview with Tom Faernerdt, Ithala, Umlazi, November 2000.

19. On land in KwaZulu see in particular Surplus People Project, *The Surplus People: Forced Removals in South Africa,* vol. 4.

20. Hindson and McCarthy, *Here to Stay.*

21. In the wake of the 1976 Soweto uprising and the dramatic growth of unions in the 1970s, the government set up the Riekert Commission to consider urban reforms. The commission's main proposal was to widen existing differences between urban and rural inhabitants by giving urban "insiders" preferential access to work and resi-

dency, while the "outsiders" were to relocate to the homelands. The repeal of the pass laws signaled the complete failure of this reform strategy. See for instance Tomlinson and Addleson, *Regional Restructuring under Apartheid: Urban and Regional Policies in Contemporary South Africa*.

22. Mabin, "Struggle for the City: Urbanisation and Political Strategies of the South African State," 14.

23. Hindson and McCarthy, *Here to Stay*, 2.

24. On women's growing industrial employment in KwaZulu and Natal in the 1980s see Posel and Todes, "The Shift to Female Labour in KwaZulu/Natal." The enthusiasm of the leader of KwaZulu, Chief Buthelezi, for industrial decentralization was an important reason for its success in this homeland. In line with his argument that homelands were a step on the route to full independence for Africans, Chief Buthelezi quoted Karl Marx to argue that industrial growth could provide a material basis for eventual political freedom—a position eventually at sharp odds with the ANC's push for sanctions. Address by Mangosuthu Buthelezi at opening of Akulu factory, Isithebe, 26 May 1977 (Sundumbili Township Records, no file number).

25. For 1951, see Union of South Africa, *Population Census, 8th May, 1951*, vol. 7, table 8, 34–35; for 1960, see Republic of South Africa, Bureau of Statistics, *Population Census, 1960, Sample Tabulation, No. 8*, table 4.4, 90–91; for 1970, see Republic of South Africa, Department of Statistics, *South African Statistics 1974* (population under 15 calculated from table on pages 1.19 and 1.20; marital figures taken from table on page 1.21. I have assumed, on the basis of census data from other years, that the number of married people under 15 was also negligible in 1970); for 1980, see Republic of South Africa, Central Statistical Services, *Population Census 80, Report No. 02-80-12*, table 2, 18–23; for 1991, see Republic of South Africa, Central Statistical Services, *Population Census 1991, Report No. 03-01-22*, table 3.5, 66–67; and for 2001, see Republic of South Africa, Statistics South Africa, *Census 2001: Primary Tables Compared*, table 6.4, 31. The other categories used by census takers are never married, living together, widowed, separated, and divorced. With the exception of the 2001 data, all census reports were consulted in the library of Statistics South Africa, Pretoria.

A few caveats on marriage data are necessary. The simplest way to track changes to marriage would be to scrutinize marriage rates. However, in the apartheid era such figures were collected only for whites, Indians, and coloureds, leaving marital status, available in census data, as the most reliable proxy for marriage rates among Africans. Caution is also necessary because the 1980 and 1991 census data excluded the populations of "independent" homelands. For these reasons I have not sought to disaggregate the figures by sex or discuss them in detail; they are undoubtedly crude, but nevertheless the best statistical evidence I could find on decreasing marriage rates over time. On marriage statistics in South Africa see Budlender, Chobokoane, and Simelane, "Marriage Patterns in South Africa: Methodological and Substantive Issues." For a discussion of the reliability of South African census data regarding fertility see Moultrie and Timaeus, *Trends in South African Fertility between 1970 and 1998: An Analysis of the 1996 Census and the 1998 Demographic and Health Survey*.

26. Denis and Ntsimane, in a sample of thirty-three households caring for young children in the Natal Midlands, found a marital union in only one case; this was an Indian couple. See Denis and Ntsimane, "Absent Fathers: Why Do Men Not Feature in Stories of Families Affected by HIV/AIDS in KwaZulu-Natal?" Although statistical evidence shows that the decline began in the 1960s, qualitative accounts suggest that it was especially marked from the 1980s. Ardington and De Haas, for instance, note quite

high marriage rates in the early 1980s in a rural KwaZulu-Natal site and a KwaZulu-Natal township, respectively. Ardington, "Nkandla Revisited: A Longitudinal Study of the Strategies Adopted to Alleviate Poverty in a Rural Community"; De Haas, "Changing Patterns of Black Marriage and Divorce in Durban."

27. One study of discordant couples (in which only one partner is infected) in rural KwaZulu-Natal showed that in four out of ten cases it was the woman who was HIV positive. Lurie et al., "Who Infects Whom? HIV-1 Concordance and Discordance among Migrants and Non-migrant Couples in South Africa."

28. Muhwava and Nyirenda, "Demographic and Socio-economic Trends in the ACDIS," 9.

29. Kok et al., *Post-apartheid Patterns of Internal Migration in South Africa.*

30. This study uses 1993 data. Dorrit Posel, "Moving On: Patterns of Labour Migration in Post-apartheid South Africa."

31. Muhwava and Nyirenda, "Demographic and Socio-economic Trends in the ACDIS," 17. A demographic surveillance site in northeast South Africa (Agincourt) also recorded the increasing mobility of women, although apparently on a lesser scale than that recorded in Hlabisa (differences in the way the two surveys are constructed make comparisons difficult). See Kok and Collinson, *Migration and Urbanization in South Africa.* The Agincourt Demographic Surveillance System also found extremely strong links between migrants and their rural homes—60% of temporary migrants communicated with their rural home in the two weeks prior to one study. Collinson et al., "Highly Prevalent Circular Migration: Households, Mobility and Economic Status in Rural South Africa."

32. Using data from the Africa Centre, we randomly selected households to visit from among those recorded as having close links with Mandeni and those whose recent migration events had been linked to marriage.

33. Niehaus, "Disharmonious Spouses and Harmonious Siblings: Conceptualizing Household Formation among Urban Residents in QwaQwa."

34. On social differentiation see Sharp, "A World Turned Upside Down: Households and Differentiation in a South African Bantustan in the 1980s." See also Spiegel, "Changing Patterns of Migrant Labour and Rural Differentiation in Lesotho." The resultant social differentiation in rural Mandeni, rooted in the 1980s, was especially accentuated by the expansion of the smallholder sugar economy. In 1980, there were 1,500–2,000 small-scale growers in this area, but this number had risen to 9,000 by 2002, making up 22% of the local mill's total input. In 2002, 50% of these growers produced less than twenty tons of sugar per year (interview with Mr. Peckham, Matikulu Sugar Mill, September 10, 2002). While the best-off sugar growers were able to buy tractors, casual workers earned as little as R10 a day in 2002, according to informants.

35. See Spiegel, "Changing Patterns of Migrant Labour."

36. Figures are derived from 2001 census data relating to wards 10 and 16 of Mandeni, where Isithebe informal settlement is situated. Census 2001 Mandeni data, http://www.statssa.gov.za/census01/html/C2001Interactive.asp (accessed February 10, 2008).

37. This timeline coincides with the growth of informal settlements in present-day KwaZulu-Natal. It is supported by numerous conversations I have had and a relatively quick examination of the Zulu newspaper *Ilanga.* One early reference to imijondolo in *Ilanga,* in 1980, discussed the settlement of Malukazi, near Umlazi township, one of the first informal settlements to emerge in the 1970s in present-day KwaZulu-Natal.

Ilanga laseNatal, "Abasemjondolo Bafuna Umjondolo Wesikolo" (Shack Dwellers Want a School).

38. Another possible source of the word "umjondolo" is the salvaged packing crates for John Deere tractors that were sometimes used to build shacks. Pithouse, "'Our struggle is thought, on the ground, running': The University of Abahlali baseMjondolo."

39. See Hindson, "Orderly Urbanisation and Influx Control: From Territorial Apartheid to Regional Spatial Ordering in South Africa."

6. Postcolonial Geographies

1. On MERG see Marais, *South Africa: Limits to Change; The Political Economy of Transformation;* Padayachee, "Progressive Academic Economists and the Challenge of Development in South Africa's Decade of Liberation."

2. See Bond, *Elite Transition: From Apartheid to Neoliberalism in South Africa;* Freund, "South Africa: The End of Apartheid and the Emergence of the 'BEE Elite'"; Marais, *South Africa;* Padayachee, "Progressive Academic Economists."

3. Indeed, the powerful unions took some solace in the weak form of corporatism on offer. Industrial strategy took its lead from the Industrial Strategy Project, a research group whose final report was entitled *Improving Manufacturing Performance in South Africa.* Influenced by the "flexible specialization" approach that promoted a highly skilled, flexible workforce to cater to fragmenting markets, the ISP sought to raise productivity through a series of supply-side measures and greater competition as a consequence of trade liberalization. See Hunter, "'The Post-Fordist High Road? A South African Case Study."

4. These debates were partly framed through Mbeki's revisiting of the longstanding notion of a first and second economy. For discussions see Hart, "Post-apartheid Developments in Historical and Comparative Perspective."

5. For an overview of the South African economy from 1994 to 2004, see Padayachee, "The South African Economy, 1994–2004."

6. United Nations Development Programme, *South Africa Human Development Report 2003,* 282.

7. On labor market casualization see Kenny and Webster, "Eroding the Core: Flexibility and the Resegmentation of the South African Labour Market"; Von Holt and Webster, "Work Restructuring and the Crisis of Reproduction." Describing these trends among female cleaning staff, Bezuidenhout and Fakier say, "In a nutshell, cheap labor is being reproduced under new conditions as the burden of reproduction shifts onto households and communities in both urban and rural areas." Bezuidenhout and Fakier, "Maria's Burden," 479.

8. The number of South Africans receiving social grants increased from 2.6 million in 1999 to more than twelve million in 2007. See Mbeki's speech at the 2007 ANC conference for this and other "development" figures that are given a positive spin. Mbeki, "Opening Address and Political Report of the President of the African National Congress, Thabo Mbeki, to the 52nd National Conference of the ANC."

9. Under apartheid a similar child support grant had been given by the state mainly to parents of coloured and Indian children. Child maintenance laws designed to require payments from fathers to mothers were notoriously weak under apartheid (and, although strengthened after apartheid, still poorly enforced). See Lund, *Changing Social Policy: The Child Support Grant in South Africa.*

10. The importance of pensions to rural livelihoods, even at a much lower rate, was noted by Ardington and Lund, "Pensions and Development: Social Security as Complementary to Programmes of Reconstruction and Development."

11. For a critical assessment of the ANC's record of "delivery" in government see Hempson and O'Donovan, "Putting Numbers to the Scorecard: Presidential Targets and the State of Delivery."

12. A key text on the depoliticizing tendencies of discourses of "development" is Ferguson, *The Anti-politics Machine: "Development," Depoliticization, and Bureaucratic Power in Lesotho.* For an instructive recent study of development and the social technologies that engender a "will to improve," see Li, *The Will to Improve: Governmentality, Development, and the Practice of Politics.*

13. Republic of South Africa, Department of Labour, *Women in the South African Labour Market, 1995–2005,* 3, 20–24.

14. On the decline of informal opportunities for women see Rogerson, "Globalization or Informalization? African Urban Economies in the 1990s."

15. These figures use the broad definition of unemployment, which includes people deterred from actively seeking employment. Republic of South Africa, Department of Labour, *Women in the South African Labour Market,* 5.

16. Ibid., 18.

17. On new social inequalities caused by AIDS see particularly Marais, *Buckling.*

18. Habib and Padayachee, "Economic Policy and Power Relations in South Africa's Transition to Democracy," 259.

19. Seekings and Nattrass, "Class, Distribution and Redistribution in Post-apartheid South Africa"; Seekings and Nattrass, *Class, Race, and Inequality in South Africa.*

20. In 2005 South Africa's number of dollar millionaires increased by 15.9%, a figure surpassed only in South Korea, India, and Russia. South Africa.info, "South Africa's Dollar Millionaires on the Rise."

21. See Adam and Moodley, *Comrades in Business: Post-liberation Politics in South Africa;* Freund, "South Africa: The End of Apartheid."

22. "Black" here means Africans, coloureds, and Indians. Republic of South Africa, Department of Labour, *Commission for Employment Equity, 7th CEE Annual Report.* The *Mail & Guardian* was skeptical of the report's accuracy. Newmarch, "Equity: Is the Data Wrong?"

23. On "class compression" in the apartheid era see Crankshaw, "Class, Race and Residence in Black Johannesburg, 1923–1970."

24. On middle-class Africans remaining in townships see *Natal Mercury,* "Middle Classes Choose Township Lifestyle."

25. Housing programs were implemented through a one-off capital subsidy scheme. See Huchzermeyer, *Unlawful Occupation: Informal Settlements and Urban Policy in South Africa and Brazil.*

26. Desmond, "Apartheid: Dead or Alive."

27. Republic of South Africa, Department of Housing, *Mainstreaming Gender in the Housing and Human Settlement Sector.* The document was designed primarily as a guideline to assist institutions developing and implementing housing policy. It was prepared for the government by the Council for Scientific and Industrial Research.

28. Hempson and O'Donovan, "Putting Numbers to the Scorecard," 19; Pressly, "The Rise and Rise of South Africa's Shacks."

29. Official housing statistics are available at the Department of Housing's website, http://www.housing.gov.za/ (accessed August 2, 2008). Data on informal dwellings for 2007 is calculated from Republic of South Africa, Statistics South Africa, *Community Survey 2007 (Revised Version)*, 44, 46.

30. Pirouz, "Have Labour Market Outcomes Affected Household Structure in South Africa? A Preliminary Descriptive Analysis of Households."

31. For a discussion of the state's shift toward upgrading some inner-city informal settlements, as outlined in its Breaking New Ground strategy, see Huchzermeyer, "The New Instrument for Upgrading Informal Settlements in South Africa: Contributions and Constraints."

32. According to Naidoo, in 1990 ten large (mostly South African) clothing firms were present in the area. Naidoo, "Industrial Decentralization and Everyday Forms of Class Struggles: A Case Study of Isithebe (1988–1992)," 109. By 2009 most clothing firms were Taiwanese-owned.

33. The background to Taiwanese investment in KwaZulu-Natal is described in Hart, *Disabling Globalization: Places of Power in Post-apartheid South Africa*. The American Growth and Opportunity Act of 2000, which promotes exports from Africa to the U.S., is one reason why reasonable levels of employment were maintained in the clothing sector.

34. Some loopholes allowing for "individual contractors" in the clothing sector have now been closed. See Skinner and Valodia, "Labour Market Policy, Flexibility, and the Future of Labour Relations: The Case of KwaZulu-Natal Clothing Industry."

35. Employment figures for industrial decentralization areas are notoriously inaccurate, especially following the abolition of state subsidies in 1990 that had required companies to provide figures. The 2001 figures are my estimate based on a small survey conducted by a research assistant who went factory to factory asking workers themselves about employment numbers. A senior manager at Ithala, the institution that now runs the industrial park, concurred with these figures. Explaining firms' continued presence in the industrial park, some factory managers told me that the rent for factory spaces was still cheap, an indirect consequence of past subsidies, and labor costs were still lower in Isithebe than in large urban areas. This supports Platzky's argument that, although artificially created, industrial parks developed significant comparative advantages, especially in the form of cheap wages. See Platzky, "The Development Impact of South Africa's Industrial Decentralization Policies."

36. Interview with Patrick Vundla, South African Clothing and Textile Workers' Union (SACTWU), Isithebe, July 31, 2009.

37. See Hunter, "The Post-Fordist High Road?"

38. The 1996 census was the first after the end of apartheid, and data derived from it must be treated with special caution. Both 1996 and 2001 data are available through the interactive 2001 census tools available on the Web. Census 2001 Mandeni data, http://www.statssa.gov.za/census01/html/C2001Interactive.asp.

39. Pudifin and Ward report that in the mid-1980s women's wages were typically R18–R38 a week, while accommodation in the area could be R5 per month. Today, therefore, most people spend a higher proportion of their wages on rent. See Pudifin and Ward, "Working for Nothing," 46, 43.

40. These township imijondolo host a relatively educated population. Only 5% of the people over twenty in Sundumbili had had no schooling, and 42% had completed Standard 10 or higher. Figures are calculated from the 2001 census data for wards 13,

14, and 15 of Mandeni, in which most of Sundumbili is situated, but which also include some outlying informal areas. Census 2001 Mandeni data, http://www.statssa.gov.za/census01/html/C2001Interactive.asp.

41. Ardington, "Decentralized Industry, Poverty and Development," 21. This survey, we should note, had a small sample size.

42. Census 2001 Mandeni data, http://www.statssa.gov.za/census01/html/C2001Interactive.asp.

43. Interview with Norman Mhlungu, former Sundumbili township administrator, Mandini, July 1, 2003.

44. On the rise of social movements see Gibson, *Challenging Hegemony: Social Movements and the Quest for a New Humanism in Post-apartheid South Africa;* Ballard, Habib, and Valodia, *Voices of Protest: Social Movements in Post-apartheid South Africa.* The Centre for Civil Society offers much excellent material on these struggles: http://www.ukzn.ac.za/ccs.

45. Shongwe, "Kufanele Abazali Bajezise Izingane" (It Is Necessary for Parents to Punish Children).

46. See Lemon, "Redressing School Inequalities in the Eastern Cape, South Africa." Technically, students cannot be refused entry to their nearest public school because of an inability to pay. The vice-principal of the formerly white Mandini Academy told me in 2006 that around half of the students' parents had applied for fee exemptions. Interview with Mr. La Grange, Mandini Academy, April 20, 2006.

47. See Lemon, "Redressing School Inequalities."

48. Bertelsen, "Ads and Amnesia: Black Advertising in the New South Africa."

49. For a vivid account of ukuhlala in another KwaZulu-Natal township (and also a rich analysis of gender dynamics), see Motsemme, "'Loving in a Time of Hopelessness': On Township Women's Subjectivities in a Time of HIV/AIDS," 71.

50. YFm is a very popular radio station among youth. It was part of a partnership that led to the establishment of *Y Magazine.* See Nutall, "Stylizing the Self: The Y Generation in Rosebank, Johannesburg." On Kwaito and township culture see Steingo, "South African Music after Apartheid: Kwaito, the 'Party Politic,' and the Appropriation of Gold as a Sign of Success."

51. On drinking, consumption, cell phones, and sex in Soweto see Mbembe, Dlamini, and Khunou, "Soweto Now."

52. Wilson and Mafeje, *Langa,* 26.

53. This appraisal of Zola's fame is given by Lance Stehr of Ghetto Ruff records. See Inside Out Documentaries, "South Africa's Kwaito Generation," http://www.insideout.org/documentaries/kwaito/artists.asp (accessed January 20, 2010).

54. See for instance Matlwa, *Coconut: A Novel.*

55. Officers at Nyoni police station provided me with these figures in May 2006. Sexual violence is discussed in chapter 8.

7. Independent Women

1. For a rich exploration of women's strategies in renegotiating the "patriarchal bargain" in a shack settlement in Brazil, see Gregg, *Virtually Virgins: Sexual Strategies and Cervical Cancer in Recife, Brazil.*

2. Shota, "She's Got IT," 50.

3. Sboros, "Style Gurus Have Their Say in Fashion," 9.

4. N. Roberts, "Let's Three-Time Those Randy Dogs."

5. N. Roberts, "White's Not Always Right."

6. Henry, "Orgasms and Empowerment: *Sex and the City* and the Third Wave Feminism," 71.

7. Hlongwane, "R1m Lobolo for King's Daughter."

8. Goredema, "No Strings Sex" (my italics).

9. http://www.sondeza.com (accessed 1 September, 2008). By 2010 the word "black" had been dropped, so that the motto was simply "supplying what South Africa is deprived of" (accessed 19 January 2010).

10. These words were used in a reproductive health workshop that I attended at love-Life youth center in Sundumbili township. As an icebreaker, the moderator encouraged attendees to state different terms for genitalia: he collected fifteen names for men's and twenty-three for women's.

11. For instance, Krige, "Girls' Puberty Songs."

12. The letter was borrowed by my female research assistant, who was friends with the author. It was written by hand in capital letters.

13. Deborah Posel, "Sex, Death and the Fate of the Nation: Reflections on the Politicization of Sexuality in Post-apartheid South Africa," 131. In a climate when the government endorsed neo-liberal spending restraints, advertising also became an important source of revenue for the government broadcaster. See Barnett, "Broadcasting the Rainbow Nation: Media, Democracy, and Nation-Building in South Africa."

14. Ballantine, "Gender, Migrancy, and South African Popular Music in the Late 1940s and 1950s," 380.

15. A related term is *zenda zangishiya*. Meintjes describes a song by this title. Meintjes, *The Sound of Africa! Making Music Zulu in a South African Studio*, 44.

16. On contemporary disapproval of cohabitation, see Nkosi, "Kuyihlazo Ukukipita Kwendoda" (It's a Disgrace to Kipita with a Man); Shangase, "Yini Eyenza Intsha Yakithi Ikipite?" (What is This Thing Young People Do, Kipite?)." A more polite term is *ukuhlal-isana* (to stay together), and a slightly less common one is *umshado esikameleni* (bedroom marriage). Notably, the verb "ukukipita" was historically associated with informal accommodation, but now can be used to describe middle-class men and women living together in an urban area or suburb.

17. Carolyn Steedman provides a revealing and analogous account of how gendered and classed sentiments became attached to consumption in postwar Britain. "Changes in the market place, the growth of real income and the proliferation of consumer goods that marked the mid-1950s, were used by my [working-class] mother to measure out her discontent: there existed a newly expanding and richly endowed material world in which she was denied a place." Steedman, *Landscape for a Good Woman: A Story of Two Lives*, 36.

18. Nutall, "Stylizing the Self."

19. See, for instance, Barnes, *"We women worked so hard"*; L. White, *The Comforts of Home*; Gregg, *Virtually Virgins*.

20. Biyase, "A Simple Analysis of the Impact of Child Support Grant on the Fertility Rate in South Africa."

21. Brown, "Facing the 'Black Peril.'"

22. See Potts and Marks, "Fertility in Southern Africa: The Quiet Revolution," 191; Republic of South Africa, Department of Health, *South African Demographic and Health Survey 2003, Preliminary Report*, 7. The report acknowledges doubts about the accuracy of the 2003 figures, which found a fertility rate of 2 for African women.

23. Republic of South Africa, Department of Health, *South African Demographic and Health Survey 2003*, 11.

24. HSRC, *South African National Survey 2008*, 45.

25. Camlin, Garenne, and Moultrie, "Fertility Trend and Pattern in a Rural Area of South Africa in the Context of HIV/AIDS," 42.

26. Jane Guyer's article on "polyandrous motherhood" captures the economic benefits for women of having children with multiple fathers. See Guyer, "Alinear Identities and Lateral Networks: The Logic of Polyandrous Motherhood." We did not explore in detail the politics around the signing of a birth certificate and therefore the child's legal name. The main point I am trying to make is that women can position their child as part of its father's family in ways that would have been less accepted in the past.

27. "Ugwayi" literally means "tobacco"; the meaning "penis" comes through association with the long pipes smoked by isiXhosa-speaking women.

28. On women's approval of sugar daddies see also Setel, *A Plague of Paradoxes: AIDS, Culture, and Demography in Northern Tanzania*, chapter 4; Parikh, "Sugar Daddies and Sexual Citizenship in Uganda: Rethinking Third Wave Feminism." See also Luke on the sugar daddy stereotype in Kenya. Through a large survey, Luke showed that sugar daddy relationships were uncommon, although age asymmetry in relationships (women having relationships with men typically five or six years their senior) was common. Luke, "Confronting the 'Sugar Daddy' Stereotype: Age and Economic Asymmetries and Risky Sexual Behaviour in Urban Kenya."

29. For a contrasting account that looks at sex exchanges in Papua New Guinea see Wardlow, *Wayward Women: Sexuality and Agency in a New Guinea Society*, chapter 3. Wardlow's ethnography argues that women resist men's exchange of women for bride-wealth by exchanging sex for money and thus taking direct control of their bodies.

30. On "bodily labor" see Wacquant, "Pugs at Work: Bodily Capital and Bodily Labour among Professional Boxers."

31. See Scorgie, "Virginity Testing and the Politics of Sexual Responsibility: Implications for AIDS interventions," and Vincent, "Virginity Testing in South Africa: Re-traditioning the Postcolony." In 2005, virginity testing was banned for girls under the age of sixteen.

32. Scorgie, "Virginity Testing and the Politics of Sexual Responsibility," 60.

33. See *Mail & Guardian*, "No 'Sex Perverts' Allowed at Zulu Reed Dance."

34. Some people I knew in the area felt that this was a very high figure and suggested that Nomusa, from whom I received the information, might have exaggerated it.

8. Failing Men

1. Many scholars have noted that liquor offers a powerful gendered guide to South Africa's history. See, for instance, Crush and Ambler, *Liquor and Labor in Southern Africa*.

2. Moffett, "'These women, they force us to rape them': Rape as Narrative of Social Control in Post-apartheid."

3. For a fascinating study of "ritual haunts" in rural homesteads in KwaZulu-Natal, see H. White, "Ritual Haunts: The Timing of Estrangement in a Post-apartheid Countryside."

4. Interview quoted in Viljoen, "Masculine Ideals in Post-apartheid South Africa: The Rise of Men's Glossies, " 331.

5. Masemola, "Rebirth of the True Self," 25.

6. Shangase, "Amanyala Esimobeni" (Dirt in the Sugar Cane Fields); Shangase, "Ixhegu Lamanyala (71) Linukubeze Ingane eno 5" (A Dirty Old Man (71) Abuses a 5-Year-Old).

7. Against the barrage of stereotypes that position African men (and, more generally, men of African descent) as inherently violent, some studies of masculinities have sought to understand violence against the background of men's disempowerment. Some of the most relevant include Breckenridge, "The Allure of Violence: Men, Race and Masculinity on the South African Goldmines, 1900–1950"; Morrell, *Changing Men in Southern Africa*; Morrell, "Of Boys and Men: Masculinity and Gender in Southern African Studies"; Niehaus, "Masculine Domination in Sexual Violence: Interpreting Accounts of Three Cases of Rape in the South African Lowveld"; Silberschmidt, *Women Forget That Men Are the Masters* (on Kenya).

8. See Deborah Posel, "The Scandal of Manhood: 'Baby Rape' and the Politicization of Sexual Violence in Post-apartheid South Africa."

9. Wicks, "Order Sought over Ban." For South Africans' discussion of whether women should wear trousers, see Ngobese, "Women and the Wearing of Trousers."

10. The biggest collection I looked at was in the Supreme Court Records of the Durban Archives. I concentrated mainly on the start of this series, 1958 (RSC 1/480–1/516). The difficulty in tracking quantitative changes over time is due to the fact that the legal definition of rape, as well as women's ability to take cases to court, was not consistent. In addition, many cases were "scrutinized" by officials of the archives—in other words, selectively destroyed. See Glaser for examples of gang rape in Soweto township in the 1940s and 1950s. Glaser, *Bo-Tsotsi*.

11. Vetten, "Mbeki and Smith Both Got It Wrong." The word "jackrolling" comes from the name of a Soweto gang. Mokwena, "The Era of the Jackrollers: Contextualising the Rise of Youth Gangs in Soweto." On gang rape see Wood and Jewkes, "'Dangerous Love': Reflections on Violence among Xhosa Township Youth"; Vogelman and Lewis, "Gang Rape and the Culture of Violence in South Africa."

12. Wood, Lambert, and Jewkes, "'Injuries are beyond love': Physical Violence in Young South Africans' Sexual Relationships," 61.

13. Reid and Dirsuweit, "Understanding Systemic Violence: Homophobic Attacks in Johannesburg and Its Surrounds."

14. Halperin, *Saint Foucault: Towards a Gay Hagiography*. For an alternative critical reflection on the concept of "homophobia" see Herek, "Beyond 'Homophobia': Thinking about Sexual Prejudice and Stigma in the Twenty-first Century."

15. See particularly Hoad, Martin, and Reid, *Sex and Politics in South Africa*.

16. On post-apartheid same-sex identity see especially Donham, "Freeing South Africa: The 'Modernization' of Male-Male Sexuality in Soweto"; Reid, "'It's just a fashion!' Linking Homosexuality and 'Modernity' in South Africa." As anthropologist Don Donham has argued, Foucault's famous analysis of sexuality never imagined the transnational flows of persons, signs, commodities, and narratives that created sexual subjects in a country like South Africa. Donham, "Freeing South Africa."

17. See Epprecht, *Heterosexual Africa*; Hoad, *African Intimacies*.

18. Tshabalala, "Growing Anti-lesbian Violence," 7; see also Reid and Dirsuweit, "Understanding Systemic Violence."

19. Swarr and Nagar, "Dismantling Assumptions: Interrogating 'Lesbian' Struggles for Identity and Survival in India and South Africa." See also Oswin, "Producing

Homonormativity in Neoliberal South Africa: Recognition, Redistribution, and the Equality Project."

20. Hunter, "Beneath the 'Zunami': Jacob Zuma and the Gendered Politics of Social Reproduction in South Africa."

21. Zuma was forced to qualify his comments in the face of criticism. See de Lange, "Zuma's Demons Remain for Him to Bury."

22. We must be aware of the pitfalls of looking for a singular "indigenous" same-sex intimacy. Pointing to differences in the use of the word "isitabane," Ronald Louw notes that it was a derogatory term used in Cato Manor to mean an effeminate man who may or may not prefer sexual relations with other men; it could also be used to mean a hermaphrodite. Louw, "Mkhumbane and New Traditions," 292. In contemporary Soweto township, Donham notes that "isitabane" can mean "hermaphrodite"; see Donham, "Freeing South Africa."

23. See especially Boellstorff, *The Gay Archipelago: Sexuality and Nation in Indonesia*. This ethnography of Indonesia's "gay archipelago" shows that *gay* and *lesbi* people frequently married and, while influenced by the Western gay rights movement, were reluctant to seek identity-based recognition for same-sex relations.

24. In addition to the groundbreaking work of D. Donham, M. Epprecht, N. Hoad, G. Reid, N. Oswin, and A. Swarr cited earlier, see Reddy, Sandfort, and Rispel, *From Social Silence to Social Science: Same-Sex Sexuality, HIV and AIDS, and Gender in South Africa*.

9. All You Need Is Love?

1. Stone, *The Family, Sex and Marriage*.

2. Katz, "Vagabond Capitalism," 709–710.

3. Though I find the concept of the "gift" useful, it can, without care, focus too much attention on the moment of "exchange"; see the introduction for how I lay out a historical dialectical approach to intimacy. The reciprocal nature of gifts (as opposed to the single act of commodity exchange) is an analysis rooted in the work of Marcel Mauss, especially *The Gift: The Form and Reason for Exchange in Archaic Societies*. For useful discussions see Gregory, *Gifts and Commodities: Studies in Political Economy*; Parry and Bloch, *Money and the Morality of Exchange*; Piot, *Remotely Global*. The importance of love to creating and maintaining bonds is especially well described by Linda Rebhun in her work in Brazil. She describes how women evoke idioms of *amor* (love) to oblige men to help them; in exchange, women offer affection and sometimes sex. Rebhun, *The Heart Is Unknown Country*.

4. L. White, *The Comforts of Home*.

5. The term "romantic utopia" is taken from Illouz, *Consuming the Romantic Utopia*.

6. Groenewald, "Cell Firms Brace for SMS Frenzy."

7. Hochschild, *The Managed Heart: Commercialization of Human Feeling*. Hochschild's term describes employees selling their "emotional labor" in the growing service sector. Although most women in Mandeni are unemployed or working in factories, I believe that the term is still useful because gendered forms of emotional management are closely connected to men's advantaged position in the labor market. See also Brennan's use of the concept to understand sex tourism in the Dominican Republic. Brennan, *What's Love Got to Do with It? Transnational Desires and Sex Tourism in the Dominican Republic*.

8. Schapera, *Married Life in an African Tribe*, 46.

9. Beauvoir, *The Second Sex*, 642.

10. The South African version of the show's website (now defunct) was at http://
www.allyouneedislove.co.za (accessed June 10, 2003). Different versions of the show have
been broadcast in more than fifteen countries.

11. See Thomas, "Love, Sex, and the Modern Girl."

12. Mafikizolo, "Emlanjeni," *Kwela*, Columbia Europe CD (B0002W108M), 2003.

13. See Ashforth, *Witchcraft, Violence, and Democracy in South Africa*; Niehaus, "Death
before Dying: Understanding AIDS Stigma in the South African Lowveld."

14. As Deborah Durham notes, among kinship groups the obligation to provide care
is taken for granted, whereas caring for neighbors and friends can be constituted more
explicitly as being motivated by love. Durham, "Love and Jealousy in the Space of Death."

15. Rutenberg et al., "Falling Pregnant or Falling Positive: Adolescent Pregnancy and
HIV Infection in South Africa."

16. A study of sexual exchanges in three areas of Durban—Point Road (where
Thandi worked as a prostitute), near a truck stop (where men frequently return to
the same partner), and in a township (where male partners are usually positioned as
"boyfriends")—showed that condom use was inversely related to the commodification
(and "lovelessness") of the relationship. Preston-Whyte et al., "Survival Sex and HIV/
AIDS in an African City."

17. Giddens, *The Transformation of Intimacy*.

18. Evans, *Love: An Unromantic Discussion*, 143.

19. See Marais, *Buckling*, 64–70.

20. World Council of Churches, "Desmond Tutu: 'Caring and compassion will prevail over evil and injustice.'"

21. After the change in government in 1994 and with the need for reconciliation,
ubuntu was especially lauded as a kind of innate "African generosity." In contrast to
this static description of African personhood, Comaroff and Comaroff show how both
Tswana and Western conceptions of personhood are fluid. John Comaroff and Jean
Comaroff, "On Personhood: An Anthropological Perspective from Africa." For an analysis of personhood in the context of AIDS in Tanzania see Setel, *A Plague of Paradoxes*. On
personhood and morality in Botswana see Livingston, *Debility and the Moral Imagination
in Botswana*.

10. The Politics of Gender, Intimacy, and AIDS

1. Republic of South Africa, Office of the Presidency, "Address by Deputy President
Zuma at the Launch of the Public-Private Partnership in Support of loveLife."

2. LoveLife, *LoveLife 2002: Report on Activities and Progress*, inside cover.

3. Pettifor, Rees, Kleinschmidt, et al., "Young People's Sexual Health in South Africa:
HIV Prevalence and Sexual Behaviors from a Nationally Representative Household
Survey," 1527. The study also found that among men, HIV prevalence was 2–3% between
ages 15 and 19 and then steadily increased to 11–12% by ages 23–24 (1527).

4. LoveLife, *LoveLife 2002*, 53.

5. For these criticisms of loveLife see Parker, "Re-appraising Youth Prevention
in South Africa: The Case of loveLife." In 2005 the Global Fund to Fight AIDS,
Tuberculosis, and Malaria withdrew its support for loveLife because of concerns about
the organization's effectiveness in reducing HIV infection. In response, loveLife argued
that its emphasis on positive sexuality, including its endorsement of condoms, upset
"US-led right-wing ideology." See *Business Day*, "Fund Hits Back at loveLife's Charges."

6. One of the reasons why I felt that I fit in quite easily to the center was that I offered an immediate source of English and, center staff believed, a cosmopolitan outlook, possibly because I could report tidbits about Europe and "white" South Africa and knowledge of safe sex (dominant AIDS narratives positioned me, as a white person, as someone already practicing safe sex and knowledgeable about it). More generally, loveLife's approach to "race" was ambiguous. It included all racial groups in its advertisements, a mixing that reflected the organization's concern not to overtly associate AIDS with black South Africans. In practice, however, the youth centers' locations in former African areas and their preference for volunteers who spoke both English and a local language meant that nearly all volunteers were African.

7. LoveLife, description of "groundbreaker" volunteers, http://www.lovelife.org .za/youth/what/index.html (accessed January 22, 2010).

8. Bourdieu, *Distinction: A Social Critique of the Judgment of Taste.*

9. The estimated rates of infection in South Africans aged 15 to 19, according to government antenatal data, were 13.7% in 2006, 13.1% in 2007, and 14.1% in 2008. Republic of South Africa, Department of Health, *2008 National Antenatal Sentinel HIV and Syphilis Prevalence Survey, South Africa*, 8. However, see also HSRC, *South African National HIV Prevalence, Incidence, Behaviour and Communication Survey 2008: A Turning Tide among Teenagers?* As its title suggests, a major theme of this report is an apparent reduction in HIV prevalence among the young in recent years: among fifteen- to twenty-four-year-olds, it went from 9.3% in 2002, to 10.3% in 2005, to 8.7% in 2008.

10. For data suggesting that young people engaged in loveLife programs might have lower-than-average HIV prevalence, and a useful discussion of the difficulty of evaluating AIDS interventions, see Pettifor, MacPhail, et al., "Challenge of Evaluating a National HIV Prevention Programme: The Case of loveLife, South Africa." More generally, "life skills"–based HIV and AIDS education is now given in virtually all schools, and some research shows that this has affected sexual behavior. Magnani et al., "The Impact of Life Skills Education on Adolescent Sexual Risk Behaviors in KwaZulu-Natal, South Africa."

11. HIV prevalence in urban informal areas in 2005 was 17.6%; in 2008 it was 20.6%. HSRC, *South African National HIV Survey 2005;* the 2008 figures were provided to me by Professor Thomas Rehle. It is striking that the HSRC's widely anticipated 2008 household study (*South African National HIV Survey 2008*) did not, in its main report, provide data about high HIV prevalence in informal settlements; this was, in my view, one of the most important findings of the HSRC's 2002 and 2005 studies. The omission indicates the silence around questions of class and geography in discussions of HIV in South Africa.

12. For an incisive review of the politics surrounding ARVs in South Africa see Lawson, *Side Effects.* Nattrass provides a very good book-length history of treatment activism. Nattrass, *Mortal Combat: AIDS Denialism and the Struggle for Antiretrovirals in South Africa.*

13. The TAC's overall membership was still quite small, around 9,500 in 2004, a year in which South Africa had more than five million HIV positive people. Its effectiveness came from the way it deftly combined legal challenges, a media strategy based on highlighting universal health rights, grassroots mobilization, and international solidarity. Membership figures are taken from Friedman and Mottiar, "A Rewarding Engagement? The Treatment Action Campaign and the Politics of HIV/AIDS," 516.

14. Fassin, *When Bodies Remember: Experiences and Politics of AIDS in South Africa,* xv. Other works that seek to contextualize Mbeki's stance, although in a less supportive way than Fassin, include Hoad, *African Intimacies;* Mbali, "AIDS Discourses and the South African State: Government Denialism and Post-apartheid AIDS Policy-Making."

15. See Robins, "Re-Interpreting the 'Political Rationality' of President Mbeki's Position on AIDS."

16. Friedman and Mottiar quote Zackie Achmat as saying that, nationwide, around 80% of the TAC's members are unemployed, 70% are women, 70% are between fourteen and twenty-four, and 90% are African. Friedman and Mottiar, "A Rewarding Engagement?" 524.

17. Mbali, "TAC in the History of Patient-Driven AIDS Activism."

18. For instance, Emslie et al., "Men's Accounts of Depression: Reconstructing or Resisting Hegemonic Masculinity?"; Courtenay, "Constructions of Masculinity and Their Influence on Men's Well-Being: A Theory of Gender and Health."

19. Fanon, *The Wretched of the Earth*. Thanks to Lesley Lawson for informing me that a similar class pattern unfolded in Uganda, where the poorest people were more likely to be open about being HIV positive (personal communication, September 16, 2008).

20. Robins, "From 'Rights' to 'Ritual': AIDS Activism in South Africa."

21. For a nuanced and incisive account of why one man did not get tested for HIV in Mpondoland, see Steinberg, *Sizwe's Test: A Young Man's Journey through Africa's AIDS Epidemic*. Biehl's portrayal of how the poorest benefited least from AIDS treatment in Brazil is a vivid reminder of how class affects seemingly universal access. Biehl, *Will to Live: AIDS Therapies and the Politics of Survival*.

22. South African Press Association, "Government Ahead of ARV targets."

23. Biehl, *Will to Live*, 12.

24. Gibson, "Calling Everything into Question: Broken Promises, Social Movements and Emergent Intellectual Currents in Post-apartheid South Africa," 7. Critics argue that the TAC never fully opposed the state's neo-liberal macro-economic plan and that it depended on its respectability to attract international funds.

25. L. Walker, "Negotiating the Boundaries of Masculinity in Post-apartheid South Africa."

26. Robins, "'Brothers are doing it for themselves': AIDS, Sexual Politics and 'New Masculinities' after Apartheid." The South African Men's Forum and Men as Partners Network are other organizations promoting more respectable forms of manliness.

27. This isiZulu name for AIDS, *ingculaza*, was derived from the word for syphilis, *ugcunsula*. Showing the fluidity of the concept, there are in fact two words in circulation used for AIDS, *ingculaza* and *ingculazi*. The general term is widely thought to have been coined by Thokozani Nene, an announcer on the isiZulu radio station Ukhozi FM.

28. For instance, see "Ngafa" (I Died) on Shwi Nomtekhala's album *Wangisiza Baba*, and "Dadewethu" (Our Sister) on Shiyani Ngcobo's album *Introducing Shiyani Ngcobo*. I took Maskanda guitar lessons in 2004 with Shiyani Ngcobo as part of a community education group based at the University of KwaZulu-Natal; in that class, he sang a verse of "Dadewethu" that decried men for having too many lovers, although the album version describes a sister who had too many lovers and died of AIDS.

29. Interview with Qap's Mngadi, Durban, August 20, 2007.

30. Shozi, "Hhayi, Asibesabi, Siyabathanda" (No, We're Not Scared of Them, We Like Them).

31. Connell, *The Men and the Boys, 26–27*.

32. R. Roberts, *Fit to Govern: The Native Intelligence of Thabo Mbeki*.

33. Kark, "The Social Pathology of Syphilis in Africans."

34. Andersson and Marks, "Apartheid and Health in the 1980s"; Wisner, "Health and Health Care in South Africa"; Packard, *White Plague, Black Labor: Tuberculosis and the Political Economy of Health and Disease in South Africa*.

35. Wisner, "Health and Health Care in South Africa: The Challenge for a Majority Ruled State," 130.

36. Pithouse, "'Our struggle is thought, on the ground, running.'" See also the Abahlali website, at http://www.abahlali.org.

37. Interview with Sbu Zikode, August 2007. I am very grateful to Raj Patel for arranging and recording this interview.

38. On this case, see Abahlali baseMjondolo, "Victory in the Constitutional Court!" http://www.abahlali.org/node/5908 (accessed January 20, 2009).

39. Mthembu, "Development: Marchers Threaten Blockades."

40. Packard, "Post-colonial Medicine."

BIBLIOGRAPHY

ARCHIVAL MATERIAL
National Archives of South Africa, Durban

Catalogued Cases

Mxokozeli kaBobe v. Msincomkwenyana (1/ESH 2/1/1/2/1, 15/1905)
Rex v. Gumakwake (RSC II/1/42, 85/87)
Rex v. Mkwanyana (1/MTU 1/1/1/1/2, 268/62)
Vanganye v. Makanyezi (1/ESH 2/1/1/2/1, 1907)
Yibhepu v. Makwapa Xulu & Ratana Lutuli (1/ESH 2/1/1/2/1, 80/1937)
Supreme Court Criminal Records, 1958 (RSC 1/480–1/516)

Uncatalogued Civil Cases, Eshowe District

(Note: These were accessed from the strongroom in 2002–2003.)
Buthelezi v. Ntuli (66/66)
Majozi v. Khuzwayo (65/63)
Mtiyeni Vilakazi v. Matini Vilakazi (50/54)
Joena Zulu v. Tom Zulu (38/55)

Eshowe Magistrates' Court

Eshowe District Record Book, 30-4-72 (Note: This was made available for me to read in
2003.)

KwaZulu Archives, Ulundi

(Note: There is no catalogue for these files; an archivist helped me to find the documents
in 2002 and 2003.)
Minutes of the Sundumbili meeting on May 4, 1972, held at SAPPI (9/4/14/1).
Select committee report on the legal disabilities of Zulu women. With covering note
for executive councillor for justice—KwaZulu, stamped March 24, 1975 (KwaZulu
Cabinet Agenda and Minutes: 1981).
South African Pulp & Paper Industries Limited, Tugela Mill. Sundumbili Township:
Points for Discussion. May 13, 1969. (N/13/1/2 (9) box 20).

Sundumbili Township Records

(Note: There is no discernable cataloguing system for these records; some are simply
loose documents. They are held in the township administration building,
Sundumbili, and I accessed them in 2003.)
Address by Mangosuthu Buthelezi at opening of Akulu factory, Isithebe, May 26, 1977
(no file number).
An assessment of the Interim Report on Community Development in Sundumbili
(SAPPI: Meetings).

Letter from administrative manager, SAPPI, to township superintendent, February 8, 1968 (N13/2/4/10).

Letter from Sundumbili Township Council to Department of the Interior, KwaZulu, March 28, 1984 (Interior 7/7/3).

Letter from Sundumbili Township Council to the secretary, Department of the Interior, KwaZulu, September 11, 1980 (7/7/3).

Letter from Sundumbili township superintendent to Eshowe Bantu affairs commissioner, January 23, 1970 (N13/2/8/2).

Letter from township manager to postmaster, Mandini, June 13, 1991 (Interior, 12/1/1).

Letters from superintendent [of] personnel and training, SAPPI, to Bantu affairs commissioner, Eshowe, May 27, 1971, and August 17, 1971 (N13/1/14).

Special meeting held on October 17, 1980. Office of the Manager, Sundumbili: Shortage of accommodation to unmarried girls employed in this area (Interior 7/7/3).

Survey Completed for the Bureau of Market Research. Information on Housing: February 1992 (Interior, 12/1/1).

Undated letter to KwaZulu government (but reply written in 1983) with lead author Mr. Khumalo (7/5/3/14/1).

Cullen Library, University of the Witwatersrand

Kuzwayo, E. K. "The Emergence of the African Woman as a Potent Economic Force." Symposium on Opening Up Direct Lines of Commercial Communication between the Manufacturer and the Urban African Consumer, Johannesburg, April 17–19, 1968 (Hellman Collection, A1419).

SONGS

Arthur. "Sika Lekhekhe." *Sika.* EMI CD (6009509316074), 2005.

Mafikizolo. "Emlanjeni." *Kwela.* Columbia Europe CD (B0002W108M), 2003.

Ngcobo, Shiyani. "Dadewethu." *Introducing Shiyani Ngcobo.* World Music Network CD (B000285IL6), 2004.

Nomtekhala, Shwi. "Ngafa." *Wangisiza Baba.* Bula Music CD (CDBULA153), 2006.

INTERVIEWS WITH INFORMANTS ASSOCIATED WITH OR REPRESENTING INSTITUTIONS

Tom Faernerdt. Manager, Ithala. Umlazi, November 2000.

Mr. La Grange. Vice-principal, Mandini Academy. Mandini, April 20, 2006.

Norman Mhlungu. Former administrator, Sundumbili township. Mandini, July 1, 2003.

Qap's Mngadi. Freelance cartoonist with a daily cartoon in *Isolezwe.* Durban, August 20, 2007.

Reverend Mzoneli. Founder of Siwasivuka and a Lutheran priest. Durban, March 13, 2003.

Mr. Peckham. Manager, Matikulu Sugar Mill. Matigulu, September 10, 2002.

Patrick Vundla. Negotiator, South African Clothing and Textile Workers' Union, Isithebe, July 31, 2009.

Sbu Zikode. Chairperson, Abahlali baseMjondolo. Durban, August 2007.

OTHER SOURCES

Achmat, Zackie. "'Apostles of Civilised Vice': 'Immoral Practices' and 'Unnatural Vice' in South African Prisons and Compounds, 1890–1920." *Social Dynamics* 19, no. 2 (1993): 92–110.

Actuarial Society of Southern Africa. *Summary Statistics, ASSA2003*, 2005. http://assaaids.eu1.rentasite.co.za/ASSA2003-Model-3165.htm (accessed January 20, 2010).

Adam, Heribert, and Cogila Moodley. *Comrades in Business: Post-liberation Politics in South Africa*. Cape Town: Tafelberg, 1997.

Adams, Vincanne, and Stacy Leigh Pigg, eds. *Sex in Development: Science, Sexuality, and Morality in Global Perspective*. Durham, N.C.: Duke University Press, 2005.

Ahlberg, Beth. "Is There a Distinct African Sexuality? A Critical Response to Caldwell." *Africa* 64, no. 2 (1994): 220–242.

Amadiume, Ifi. *Male Daughters, Female Husbands: Gender and Sex in an African Society*. London: Zed, 1987.

Andersson, Neil, and Shula Marks. "Apartheid and Health in the 1980s." *Social Science & Medicine* 27, no. 7 (1988): 667–681.

Ardington, Elisabeth. "Decentralized Industry, Poverty and Development in Rural KwaZulu." Working Paper 10, Development Studies Unit, University of Natal, Durban, 1984.

———. "Nkandla Revisited: A Longitudinal Study of the Strategies Adopted to Alleviate Poverty in a Rural Community." Working Paper 16, Centre for Social and Development Studies, University of Natal, Durban, 1988.

Ardington, Elisabeth, and Frances Lund. "Pensions and Development: Social Security as Complementary to Programmes of Reconstruction and Development." *Development Southern Africa* 12, no. 4 (1995): 557–577.

Ashforth, Adam. *Witchcraft, Violence, and Democracy in South Africa*. Chicago: Chicago University Press, 2005.

Auvert, Bertran, Dirk Taljaard, Emmanuel Lagarde, Joëlle Sobngwi-Tambekou, and Rémi Sitta. "Randomized, Controlled Intervention Trial of Male Circumcision for Reduction of HIV Infection Risk: The ANRS 1265 Trial." *PLoS Med* 2, no. 11 (2005): e298: doi:10.1371/journal.pmed.0020298.

Bailey, Beth. *From Front Porch to Back Seat: Courtship in Twentieth-Century America*. Baltimore: Johns Hopkins University Press, 1988.

Bakker, Isabella, and Rachel Silvey, eds. *Beyond States and Markets: The Challenges of Social Reproduction*. London: Routledge, 2008.

Ballantine, Christopher. "Gender, Migrancy, and South African Popular Music in the Late 1940s and 1950s." *Ethnomusicology* 44, no. 3 (2000): 376–407.

Ballard, Richard, Adam Habib, and Imraan Valodia, eds. *Voices of Protest: Social Movements in Post-apartheid South Africa*. Pietermaritzburg: University of KwaZulu-Natal Press, 2006.

Barnes, Teresa. *"We women worked so hard": Gender, Urbanization and Social Reproduction in Colonial Harare, Zimbabwe, 1930–1956*. Cape Town: David Philip, 1999.

Barnett, Clive. "Broadcasting the Rainbow Nation: Media, Democracy, and Nation-Building in South Africa." *Antipode* 31, no. 3 (1999): 274–303.

Baskin, Jeremy, and Ian Bissell. "Sundumbili General Strike of March 1982." *South African Labour Bulletin*, no. 82 (1982): 26–33.

Beauvoir, Simone de. *The Second Sex*. Harmondsworth: Penguin Books, 1972.

Bekker, Simon, and Richard Humphries. *From Control to Confusion: The Changing Role of Administration Boards in South Africa, 1971–1983.* Pietermaritzburg: Shuter & Shooter, 1985.

Bell, R. T. "Some Aspects of Industrial Decentralization in South Africa." *South African Journal of Economics* 41, no. 4 (1973): 252–273.

Berry, Sara. *No Condition Is Permanent: The Social Dynamics of Agrarian Change in Sub-Saharan Africa.* Madison: University of Wisconsin Press, 1993.

Bertelsen, Eve. "Ads and Amnesia: Black Advertising in the New South Africa." In *Negotiating the Past: The Making of Memory in South Africa,* ed. Sarah Nuttall and Carli Coetzee, 221–241. Cape Town: Oxford University Press, 1998.

Bezanson, Kate. *Gender, the State, and Social Reproduction: Household Insecurity in Neo-liberal Times.* Toronto: University of Toronto Press, 2006.

Bezuidenhout, Andries, and Khayaat Fakier. "Maria's Burden: Contract Cleaning and the Crisis of Social Reproduction in Post-apartheid South Africa." *Antipode* 38, no. 3 (2006): 462–485.

Bhabha, Homi. "Of Mimicry and Man: The Ambivalence of Colonial Discourse." *October* 28, no. 1 (1984): 125–133.

Biehl, João. *Will to Live: AIDS Therapies and the Politics of Survival.* Princeton, N.J.: Princeton University Press, 2007.

Biyase, Me. "A Simple Analysis of the Impact of Child Support Grant on the Fertility Rate in South Africa." Paper delivered at the Biennial Conference of the Economic Society of South Africa: Development Perspectives: Is Africa Different? Durban, September 7–9, 2005.

Bledsoe, Caroline. *Women and Marriage in Kpelle Society.* Stanford, Calif.: Stanford University Press, 1980.

Boellstorff, Tom. *The Gay Archipelago: Sexuality and Nation in Indonesia.* Princeton, N.J.: Princeton University Press, 2005.

Bond, Patrick. *Elite Transition: From Apartheid to Neoliberalism in South Africa.* London: Pluto Press, 2000.

Bongaarts, John. "Late Marriage and the HIV Epidemic in Sub-Saharan Africa." *Population Studies* 61, no. 1 (2007): 73–83.

Bonner, Phillip. "'Desirable or Undesirable Basotho Women?' Liquor, Prostitution and the Migration of Basotho Women to the Rand, 1920–1945." In *Women and Gender in Southern Africa to 1945,* ed. Cherryl Walker, 221–250. Cape Town: David Philip, 1990.

Bonnin, Deborah. "Space, Place and Identity: Political Violence in Mpumalanga Township, KwaZulu-Natal, 1987–1993." Ph.D. thesis, Faculty of Humanities, University of the Witwatersrand, Johannesburg, 2007.

Bourdieu, Pierre. *Distinction: A Social Critique of the Judgment of Taste.* Cambridge, Mass.: Harvard University Press, 1984.

Bozzoli, Belinda. *Theatres of Struggle and the End of Apartheid.* Johannesburg: Wits University Press, 2004.

———. "Why Were the 1980s 'Millenarian'? Style, Repertoire, Space and Authority in South Africa's Black Cities." *Journal of Historical Sociology* 13, no. 1 (2000): 78–110.

———. *Women of Phokeng: Consciousness, Life Strategy, and Migrancy in South Africa, 1900–1983.* With Mmantho Nkotsoe. Portsmouth, N.H.: Heinemann, 1991.

Braatvedt, H. P. "Zulu Marriage Customs and Ceremonies." *South African Journal of Science* 24 (1927): 553–565.

Brandel-Syrier, Mia. *"Coming Through": The Search for a New Cultural Identity.* Johannesburg: McGraw-Hill, 1978.

Breckenridge, Keith. "The Allure of Violence: Men, Race and Masculinity on the South African Goldmines, 1900–1950." *Journal of Southern African Studies* 24, no. 4 (1998): 669–693.

———. "Love Letters and Amanuenses: Beginning the Cultural History of the Working Class Private Sphere in Southern Africa, 1900–1933." *Journal of Southern African Studies* 26, no. 2 (2000): 337–348.

Brennan, Denise. *What's Love Got to Do with It? Transnational Desires and Sex Tourism in the Dominican Republic.* Durham, N.C.: Duke University Press, 2004.

Brown, Barbara. "Facing the 'Black Peril': The Politics of Population Control in South Africa." *Journal of Southern African Studies* 13, no. 3 (1987): 256–273.

Brown, Wendy. "Suffering Rights as Paradoxes." *Constellations* 7, no. 2 (2000): 230–241.

Bryant, A. T. *A Zulu-English Dictionary with Notes on Pronunciation.* Marianhill: Marianhill Mission Press, 1905.

———. *The Zulu People as They Were before the White Man Came.* Pietermaritzburg: Shuter & Shooter, 1949.

Budlender, Debbie, Ntebaleng Chobokoane, and Sandile Simelane. "Marriage Patterns in South Africa: Methodological and Substantive Issues." *Southern African Journal of Demography* 9, no. 1 (2004): 1–26.

Bujra, Janet. "Women 'Entrepreneurs' of Early Nairobi." *Canadian Journal of African Studies* 9, no. 2 (1975): 213–234.

Burawoy, Michael, and Katherine Verdery. Introduction to *Uncertain Transition: Ethnographies of Change in the Postsocialist World,* ed. Michael Burawoy and Katherine Verdery, 1–17. Lanham, Md.: Rowman and Littlefield, 1998.

Burton, Patrick. "Industrial Restructuring and Changing Gender Relations: The Case of Isithebe in KwaZulu-Natal." Master's thesis, Urban and Regional Planning, University of Natal, Durban, 1999.

Business Day. "Fund Hits Back at loveLife's Charges." January 5, 2006. http://www.businessday.co.za/ (accessed January 20, 2008).

Buthelezi Commission. *The Requirements for Stability and Development in Kwazulu and Natal.* Vol. 2. Durban: H + H Publications, 1982.

Buthelezi, Mangosuthu. "Funeral of Prince Nhlanhla Ka Nonjombo Ka Dinuzulu: Address by Prince Mangosuthu Buthelezi, MP." June 23, 2007. http://www.ifp.org.za/Archive/Speeches/230607sp.htm (accessed August 2, 2008).

Calderwood, D. M. "Native Housing in South Africa." Ph.D. thesis, Architecture, University of the Witwatersrand, Johannesburg, 1955.

Caldwell, John, Pat Caldwell, and Pat Quiggin. "The Social Context of AIDS in Sub-Saharan Africa." *Population and Development Review* 15, no. 2 (1989): 185–234.

Camlin, Carol, Michel Garenne, and Tom Moultrie. "Fertility Trend and Pattern in a Rural Area of South Africa in the Context of HIV/AIDS." *African Journal of Reproductive Health* 8, no. 2 (2004): 38–54.

Campbell, Catherine. "Learning to Kill? Masculinity, the Family and Violence in Natal." *Journal of Southern African Studies* 18, no. 3 (1992): 614–628.

Carton, Benedict. *Blood from Your Children: The Colonial Origins of Generational Conflict in South Africa.* Charlottesville: University Press of Virginia, 2000.

Carton, Benedict, John Laband, and Jabulani Sithole, eds. *Zulu Identities: Being Zulu, Past and Present.* Pietermaritzburg: University of KwaZulu-Natal Press, 2008.

Castle, S., and M. Konate. "The Context and Consequences of Economic Transactions Associated with Sexual Relations among Malian Adolescents." Paper presented at the Third African Population Conference, Durban, South Africa, December 6–10, 1999.

Centers for Disease Control and Prevention, U.S. Department of Health and Human Services. "The Role of STD Prevention and Treatment in HIV Prevention." http://www.cdc.gov/std/hiv/stds-and-hiv-fact-sheet.pdf (accessed February 12, 2010).

Chanock, Martin. *Law, Custom and Social Order: The Colonial Experience in Malawi and Zambia.* Cambridge: Cambridge University Press, 1985.

Clement, Elizabeth. *Love for Sale: Courting, Treating, and Prostitution in New York City, 1900–1945.* Chapel Hill: University of North Carolina Press, 2006.

Cock, Jacklyn. "Introduction." *South African Labour Bulletin* 9, no. 3 (1983): 1–6.

Cohen, Jon. "HIV/AIDS: India Slashes Estimate of HIV-Infected People." *Science* 317, no. 5835 (2007): 179–181.

Cole, Jennifer. "Fresh Contact in Tamatave, Madagascar: Sex, Money, and Intergenerational Transformation." *American Ethnologist* 31, no. 4 (2004): 573–588.

Cole, Jennifer, and Lynn Thomas, eds. *Love in Africa.* Chicago: University of Chicago Press, 2009.

Colenso, John. *Zulu-English Dictionary.* Pietermaritzburg: Davis, 1878.

———. *Zulu-English Dictionary.* Pietermaritzburg: Davis, 1861.

Collinson, Mark, Stephen Tollman, Kathleen Kahn, and Samuel Clark. "Highly Prevalent Circular Migration: Households, Mobility and Economic Status in Rural South Africa." Paper presented at the Conference on African Migration, Johannesburg, June 4–7, 2003.

Comaroff, Jean, and John Comaroff. *Christianity, Colonialism, and Consciousness in South Africa.* Vol. 1 of *Of Revelation and Revolution.* Chicago: University of Chicago Press, 1991.

———. "Criminal Justice, Cultural Justice: The Limits of Liberalism and the Pragmatics of Difference in the New South Africa." *American Ethnologist* 31, no. 2 (2004): 188–204.

Comaroff, John. "The Discourse of Rights in Colonial South Africa: Subjectivity, Sovereignty, Modernity." In *Identities, Politics, and Rights,* ed. Austin Sarat and Thomas Kearns, 193–238. Ann Arbor: University of Michigan Press, 1995.

———, ed. *The Meaning of Marriage Payments.* London: Academic Press, 1980.

Comaroff, John, and Jean Comaroff. *The Dialectics of Modernity on a South African Frontier.* Vol. 2 of *Of Revelation and Revolution.* Chicago: University of Chicago Press, 1997.

———. "On Personhood: An Anthropological Perspective from Africa." *Social Identities* 7, no. 2 (2001): 267–283.

Connell, R. W. *Gender and Power: Society, the Person and Sexual Politics.* Cambridge: Polity Press in association with Blackwell, 1987.

———. *Masculinities.* Berkeley: University of California Press, 1995.

———. *The Men and the Boys.* Berkeley: University of California Press, 2000.

Connell, R. W., and James Messerschmidt. "Hegemonic Masculinity: Rethinking the Concept." *Gender and Society* 19, no. 6 (2005): 829–859.

Cooper, Barbara. "Women's Worth and Wedding Gift Exchange in Maradi, Niger, 1907–89." *Journal of African History* 36, no. 1 (1995): 121–140.

Cooper, Frederick. "Industrial Man Goes to Africa." In *Men and Masculinities in Modern Africa,* ed. Lisa Lindsay and Stephan Miescher, 128–137. Portsmouth, N.H.: Heinemann, 2003.

Cooper, Frederick, and Ann Stoler, eds. *Tensions of Empire: Colonial Cultures in a Bourgeois World*. Berkeley: University of California Press, 1997.

Cope, Nicholas. *To Bind the Nation: Solomon kaDinuzulu and Zulu Nationalism, 1913–1933*. Pietermaritzburg: University of KwaZulu-Natal Press, 1993.

Cornwall, Andrea. "Spending Power: Love, Money, and the Reconfiguration of Gender Relations in Ado-Odo, Southwestern Nigeria." *American Ethnologist* 29, no. 4 (2002): 963–980.

Cornwall, Andrea, and Maxine Molyneux. *The Politics of Rights: Dilemmas for Feminist Praxis*. London: Routledge, 2008.

Courtenay, Will. "Constructions of Masculinity and Their Influence on Men's Well-Being: A Theory of Gender and Health." *Social Science & Medicine* 50, no. 10 (2000): 1385–1401.

Crankshaw, Owen. "Class, Race and Residence in Black Johannesburg, 1923–1970." *Journal of Historical Sociology* 18, no. 4 (2005): 353–393.

———. *Race, Class and the Changing Division of Labour under Apartheid*. London: Routledge, 1997.

———. "Squatting, Apartheid, and Urbanisation on the Southern Witwatersrand." *African Affairs* 92, no. 366 (1993): 31–51.

Crush, Jonathan, and Charles Ambler, eds. *Liquor and Labor in Southern Africa*. Athens: Ohio University Press, 1992.

Davenport, T. R. H., and K. S. Hunt, eds. *The Right to the Land*. Cape Town: David Philip, 1974.

Davidson, Joyce, Liz Bondi, and Mick Smith, eds. *Emotional Geographies*. Aldershot: Ashgate, 2005.

Davis, Mike. *Planet of Slums*. New York: Verso, 2006.

De Haas, Mary. "Changing Patterns of Black Marriage and Divorce in Durban." Master's thesis, Department of Anthropology, University of Natal, Durban, 1984.

De Lange, Deon. "Zuma's Demons Remain for Him to Bury." *Natal Mercury*, March 28, 2008.

Delius, Peter, and Clive Glaser. "The Myths of Polygamy: A History of Extramarital and Multi-partnership Sex in South Africa." *South African Historical Journal* 50 (2004): 84–114.

Denis, Philippe, and Radikobo Ntsimane. "Absent Fathers: Why Do Men Not Feature in Stories of Families Affected by HIV/AIDS in KwaZulu-Natal?" Paper presented to the Masculinities Symposium, University of the Witwatersrand, Johannesburg, September 5–7, 2004.

Desmond, Cosmas. "Apartheid: Dead or Alive." *Mail & Guardian*, April 11, 2008.

Dlamini, C. R. M. "Seduction in Zulu Law." *Tydskrif vir Hedendaagse Romeins-Hollandse Reg* 47 (1984): 18–35.

Dlamini, Nombuso. "The Construction, Meaning and Negotiation of Ethnic Identities in KwaZulu Natal." *Social Identities* 4, no. 3 (1998): 473–497.

Doke, Clement, D. Malcolm, J. Sikakana, and Benedict Vilakazi. *English-Zulu, Zulu-English Dictionary*. Johannesburg: Witwatersrand University Press, 1990.

Doke, Clement, and Benedict Vilakazi. *Zulu-English Dictionary*. Johannesburg: Witwatersrand University Press, 1948.

Donham, Don. "Freeing South Africa: The 'Modernization' of Male-Male Sexuality in Soweto." *Cultural Anthropology* 13, no. 1 (1998): 3–21.

Drum. "Everything You Ever Wanted to Know about Sex." March 8, 1972.

Dubow, Saul. *Racial Segregation and the Origins of Apartheid in South Africa, 1919–36.* Basingstoke: Macmillan, 1989.

Dunkle, Kristin, Rachel Jewkes, Heather Brown, James McIntryre, and Sioban Harlow. "Transactional Sex among Women in Soweto, South Africa: Prevalence, Risk Factors and Association with HIV Infection." *Social Science & Medicine* 59, no. 8 (2004): 1581–1592.

Durham, Deborah. "Love and Jealousy in the Space of Death." *Ethnos* 67, no. 2 (2002): 155–179.

Eagle, Jane. "A Study of African Women's Access to Housing in the Durban Area." Master's thesis, Department of Town and Regional Planning, University of Natal, Durban, 1987.

Edwards, Iain. "Cato Manor, June 1959: Men, Women, Crowds, Violence, Politics and History." In *The People's City: African Life in Twentieth-Century Durban,* ed. Paul Maylam and Iain Edwards, 102–142. Pietermaritzburg: University of Natal Press, 1996.

Elder, Glen. *Hostels, Sex and the Apartheid Legacy: Malevolent Geographies.* Athens: Ohio University Press, 2003.

Emslie, Carol, Damien Ridge, Sue Ziebland, and Kate Hunt. "Men's Accounts of Depression: Reconstructing or Resisting Hegemonic Masculinity?" *Social Science & Medicine* 62, no. 9 (2006): 2246–2257.

Englund, Harri. *Prisoners of Freedom: Human Rights and the African Poor.* Berkeley: University of California Press, 2006.

Epprecht, Marc. *Heterosexual Africa? The History of an Idea from the Age of Exploration to the Age of AIDS.* Athens: Ohio University Press, 2008.

———. *Hungochani: The History of a Dissident Sexuality in Southern Africa.* Montreal: McGill-Queen's University Press, 2004.

Epstein, Helen. *The Invisible Cure: Africa, the West, and the Fight against AIDS.* New York: Picador, 2007.

Evans, Mary. *Love: An Unromantic Discussion.* Cambridge: Polity Press, 2003.

Fanon, Frantz. *Black Skin, White Masks.* London: Macgibbon & Kee, 1968.

———. *The Wretched of the Earth.* Harmondsworth: Penguin Books, 1963.

Farmer, Paul. *Infections and Inequalities: The Modern Plagues.* Berkeley: University of California Press, 1999.

Farmer, Paul, Philippe Bourgois, Nancy Scheper-Hughes, Didier Fassin, Linda Green, H. K. Heggenhougen, Laurence Kirmayer, and Loic Wacquant. "An Anthropology of Structural Violence." *Current Anthropology* 45, no. 3 (2004): 305–325.

Fassin, Didier. *When Bodies Remember: Experiences and Politics of AIDS in South Africa.* Berkeley: University of California Press, 2007.

Ferguson, James. *The Anti-politics Machine: "Development," Depoliticization, and Bureaucratic Power in Lesotho.* Cambridge: Cambridge University Press, 1990.

———. *Expectations of Modernity: Myths and Meanings of Urban Life on the Zambian Copperbelt.* Berkeley: University of California Press, 1999.

———. *Global Shadows: Africa in the Neoliberal World Order.* Durham, N.C.: Duke University Press, 2006.

Foucault, Michel. *The History of Sexuality.* Vol. 1, *An Introduction.* New York: Pantheon Books, 1978.

———. *The History of Sexuality.* Vol. 2. *The Use of Pleasure.* Vintage: New York, 1990.

———. *The History of Sexuality.* Vol. 3. *The Care of The Self.* Vintage: New York, 1988.

Freed, Louis. *The Problem of European Prostitution in Johannesburg: A Sociological Survey.* Cape Town: Juta, 1949.

Freund, Bill. *Insiders and Outsiders: The Indian Working Class of Durban, 1910–1990.* Portsmouth, N.H.: Heinemann, 1995.

———. "South Africa: The End of Apartheid and the Emergence of the 'BEE Elite.'" *Review of African Political Economy* 34, no. 114 (2007): 661–678.

Friedman, Steven, and Shauna Mottiar. "A Rewarding Engagement? The Treatment Action Campaign and the Politics of HIV/AIDS." *Politics and Society* 33, no. 4 (2005): 511–565.

Fynn, Henry Francis. *The Diary of Henry Francis Fynn.* Compiled and edited by James Stuart and D. Malcolm. Pietermaritzburg: Shuter & Shooter, 1986.

Gaitskell, Deborah. "Wailing for Purity: Prayer Unions, African Mothers and Adolescent Daughters, 1912–1940." In *Industrialisation and Social Change in South Africa: African Class Formation, Culture and Consciousness, 1870–1930,* ed. Shula Marks and Richard Rathbone, 338–357. Harlow, Essex: Longman, 1982.

Geschiere, Peter. *The Modernity of Witchcraft: Politics and the Occult in Postcolonial Africa.* Charlottesville: University Press of Virginia, 1997.

Gibson, Nigel. "Calling Everything into Question: Broken Promises, Social Movements and Emergent Intellectual Currents in Post-apartheid South Africa." Introduction to *Challenging Hegemony: Social Movements and the Quest for a New Humanism in Post-apartheid South Africa,* ed. Nigel Gibson, 1–53. Trenton: Africa World Press, 2006.

———, ed. *Challenging Hegemony: Social Movements and the Quest for a New Humanism in Post-apartheid South Africa.* Trenton: Africa World Press, 2006.

Gibson-Graham, J. K. *The End of Capitalism (As We Knew It): A Feminist Critique of Political Economy.* Cambridge: Blackwell, 1996.

Giddens, Anthony. *The Transformation of Intimacy: Sexuality, Love, and Eroticism in Modern Societies.* Stanford, Calif.: Stanford University Press, 1992.

Gilbert, Alan, and Owen Crankshaw. "Comparing South African and Latin American Experience: Migration and Housing Mobility in Soweto." *Urban Studies* 36, no. 13 (1999): 2375–2400.

Gillis, John. "From Ritual to Romance: Toward an Alternative History of Love." In *Emotions and Social Change: Towards a New Psychohistory,* ed. Carol Stearns and Peter Stearns, 87–121. New York: Holmes and Mier, 1988.

Glaser, Clive. *Bo-Tsotsi: The Youth Gangs of Soweto, 1935–1976.* Portsmouth, N.H.: Heinemann, 2000.

———. "Managing the Sexuality of Urban Youth: Johannesburg, 1920s–1960s." *International Journal of African Historical Studies* 38, no. 2 (2005): 307–327.

Goodhew, David. *Respectability and Resistance: A History of Sophiatown.* Westport, Conn.: Praeger, 2004.

Goredema, Prudence. "No-Strings Sex." *True Love,* http://www.women24.com/Content/LoveAndSex/SexAndSizzle/2418/a08c75455ade41218d2698b87cc805ad/26-06-2009-10-06/No-strings_sex (accessed January 20, 2010).

Gregg, Jessica. *Virtually Virgins: Sexual Strategies and Cervical Cancer in Recife, Brazil.* Stanford, Calif.: Stanford University Press, 2003.

Gregory, C. A. *Gifts and Commodities: Studies in Political Economy.* London: Academic Press, 1982.

Groenewald, Anneli. "Cell Firms Brace for SMS Frenzy." December 21, 2007. http://www.hellkom.co.za/news/local/view.php?id=3317 (accessed April 23, 2008).

Gunner, Liz, and Mafika Gwala. *Musho: Zulu Popular Praises.* Johannesburg: Witwatersrand University Press, 1994.

Gupta, Akhil, and James Ferguson. *Culture, Power, Place: Explorations in Critical Anthropology.* Durham, N.C.: Duke University Press, 1997.

Guy, Jeff. "An Accommodation of the Patriarchs: Theophilus Shepstone and the Foundations of the System of Native Administration in Natal." Paper presented at the Conference on Masculinities in Southern Africa, University of Natal, Durban, July 2–4, 1997.

———. "Analyzing Pre-capitalist Societies in Southern Africa." *Journal of Southern African Studies* 14, no. 1 (1987): 18–37.

———. *The Destruction of the Zulu Kingdom: The Civil War in Zululand, 1879–1884.* London: Longman, 1979.

———. *The Heretic: A Study of the Life of John William Colenso, 1814–1883.* Pietermaritzburg: University of KwaZulu-Natal Press, 1983.

———. "Love and Violence, Sex and Fertility, in the Zulu Kingdom." Paper presented for the workshop of the Project on the History of Sex in Southern Africa (POSH), University of Natal, Durban, October 4, 2003.

Guyer, Jane. "Alinear Identities and Lateral Networks: The Logic of Polyandrous Motherhood." In *Nuptiality in Sub-Saharan Africa,* ed. Caroline Bledsoe and Gilles Pison, 231–252. Oxford: Clarendon Press, 1994.

———. "Household and Community in African Studies." *African Studies Review* 24, nos. 2–3 (1981): 87–137.

Guyer, Jane, and Pauline Peters. "Conceptualizing the Household: Issues of Theory and Policy in Africa." *Development and Change* 18, no. 2 (1987): 197–214.

Habib, Adam, and Vishnu Padayachee. "Economic Policy and Power Relations in South Africa's Transition to Democracy." *World Development* 28, no. 2 (2000): 245–263.

Halberstam, Judith. *Female Masculinity.* Durham, N.C.: Duke University Press, 1998.

Halperin, David. *How to do the History of Homosexuality.* Chicago: University of Chicago Press, 2002.

———. *Saint Foucault: Towards a Gay Hagiography.* New York: Oxford University Press, 1995.

Halperin, Daniel, and Helen Epstein. "Concurrent Sexual Partnerships Help to Explain Africa's High HIV Prevalence: Implications for Prevention." *Lancet* 364, no. 9428 (2004): 4–6.

Hamilton, Carolyn. *Terrific Majesty: The Power of Shaka Zulu and the Limits of Historical Invention.* Cambridge, Mass.: Harvard University Press, 1998.

Hammond-Tooke, David. *Imperfect Interpreters: South Africa's Anthropologists, 1920–1990.* Johannesburg: Witwatersrand University Press, 1997.

Hanretta, Sean. "Women, Marginality and the Zulu State: Women's Institutions and Power in the Early Nineteenth Century." *Journal of African History* 39, no. 3 (1998): 389–415.

Hansen, Karen. "Getting Stuck in the Compound: Some Odds against Social Adulthood in Lusaka." *Africa Today* 51, no. 4 (2005): 3–16.

Hart, Gillian. *Disabling Globalization: Places of Power in Post-apartheid South Africa.* Berkeley: University of California Press, 2002.

———. "Post-apartheid Developments in Historical and Comparative Perspective." In *The Development Decade? Economic and Social Change in South Africa 1994–2004,* ed. Vishnu Padayachee, 13–32. Cape Town: HSRC Press, 2006.

Harvey, David. *Spaces of Hope.* Edinburgh: Edinburgh University Press, 2000.

Hassim, Shireen. "Black Women in Political Organisations: A Case Study of the Inkatha Women's Brigade, 1976 to Present." Master's thesis, African Studies, University of Natal, Durban, 1990.

———. *Women's Organizations and Democracy in South Africa: Contesting Authority.* Madison: University of Wisconsin Press, 2006.

Heald, Suzette. "The Power of Sex: Some Reflections on the Caldwells' 'African Sexuality' Thesis." *Africa* 65, no. 4 (1995): 489–505.

Health Systems Trust. *South African Health Review, 2003/4.* Durban: Health Systems Trust, 2004.

Hellman, Ellen. *Rooiyard: A Sociological Survey of an Urban Native Slum Yard.* Cape Town: Oxford University Press, 1948.

Hempson, David, and Michael O'Donovan. "Putting Numbers to the Scorecard: Presidential Targets and the State of Delivery." In *State of the Nation, 2005–2006,* ed. Sakhela Buhlungu, John Daniel, Roger Southall, and Jessica Lutchman, 11–45. Cape Town: HSRC Press, 2005.

Henry, Astrid. "Orgasms and Empowerment: *Sex and the City* and the Third Wave Feminism." In *Reading Sex and the City,* ed. Kim Akass and Janet McCabe, 65–83. New York: I. B. Tauris, 2004.

Herek, Gregory M. "Beyond Homophobia: Thinking about Sexual Stigma and Prejudice in the Twenty-first Century." *Sexuality Research and Social Policy* 1, no. 2 (2004): 6–24. Available at Social Science Research Network: http://ssrn.com/abstract=1142860.

Hindson, Doug. "Orderly Urbanisation and Influx Control: From Territorial Apartheid to Regional Spatial Ordering in South Africa." In *Regional Restructuring under Apartheid: Urban and Regional Policies in Contemporary South Africa,* ed. Richard Tomlinson and Mark Addleson, 74–105. Johannesburg: Ravan, 1987.

Hindson, Doug, and Jeff McCarthy. *Here to Stay: Informal Settlements in KwaZulu-Natal.* Dalbridge: Indicator, 1994.

Hirsch, Jennifer. *A Courtship after Marriage: Sexuality and Love in Mexican Transnational Families.* Berkeley: University of California Press, 2003.

Hirsch, Jennifer, and Holly Wardlow, eds. *Modern Loves: The Anthropology of Romantic Courtship and Companionate Marriage.* Ann Arbor: University of Michigan Press, 2006.

Hlongwane, Agiza. "R1m Lobolo for King's Daughter." *Sunday Tribune,* April 19, 2009.

Hoad, Neville. *African Intimacies: Race, Homosexuality, and Globalization.* Minnesota: University of Minnesota Press, 2007.

Hoad, Neville, Karen Martin, and Graeme Reid. *Sex and Politics in South Africa.* Cape Town: Double Storey Books, 2005.

Hobsbawm, Eric, and Terence Ranger, eds. *The Invention of Tradition.* Cambridge: Cambridge University Press, 1983.

Hochschild, Arlie. *The Managed Heart: Commercialization of Human Feeling.* Berkeley: University of California Press, 1983.

Hofmeyr, Isabel. *"We spend our years as a tale that is told": Oral Historical Narratives in a South African Chiefdom.* Portsmouth, N.H.: Heinemann, 1994.

Hofmeyr, Julian. "Black Wages: The Post-war Experience." In *The Political Economy of South Africa,* ed. Nicoli Nattrass and Elisabeth Ardington, 129–147. Cape Town: Oxford University Press, 1990.

Horwitz, Simonne. "Migration and HIV/AIDS: A Historical Perspective." *South African Historical Journal* 45, no. 1 (2001): 103–123.

Houlbrook, Matt. *Queer London: Perils and Pleasures in the Sexual Metropolis, 1918–1957.* Chicago: University of Chicago Press, 2005.

HSRC. See Human Science Research Council.

Huchzermeyer, Marie. "The New Instrument for Upgrading Informal Settlements in South Africa: Contributions and Constraints." In *Informal Settlements: A Perpetual Challenge,* ed. Marie Huchzermeyer and Aly Karam, 41–61. Cape Town: University of Cape Town Press, 2006.

———. *Unlawful Occupation: Informal Settlements and Urban Policy in South Africa and Brazil.* Trenton: Africa World Press, 2004.

Human Science Research Council (HSRC). *Nelson Mandela/HSRC Study of HIV/AIDS: South African National HIV Prevalence, Behavioural Risks and Mass Media; Household Survey, 2002.* Cape Town: HSRC Press, 2002.

———. *South African National HIV Prevalence, HIV Incidence, Behaviour and Communication Survey, 2005.* Cape Town: HSRC Press, 2005.

———. *South African National HIV Prevalence, Incidence, Behaviour and Communication Survey, 2008: A Turning Tide among Teenagers?* Cape Town: HSRC Press, 2009.

Hunter, Mark. "Beneath the 'Zunami': Jacob Zuma and the Gendered Politics of Social Reproduction in South Africa." *Antipode,* forthcoming.

———. "The Changing Political Economy of Sex in South Africa: The Significance of Unemployment and Inequalities to the Scale of the AIDS Pandemic." *Social Science & Medicine* 64, no. 3 (2007): 689–700.

———. "Cultural Politics and Masculinities: Multiple-Partners in Historical Perspective in KwaZulu-Natal." *Culture, Health & Sexuality* 7, no. 4 (2005): 389–403.

———. "The Materiality of Everyday Sex: Thinking beyond Prostitution." *African Studies* 61, no. 1 (2002): 99–120.

———. "The Post-Fordist High Road? A South African Case Study." *Journal of Contemporary African Studies* 18, no. 1 (2000): 67–90.

Hyslop, Jon. "White Working-Class Women and the Invention of Apartheid: 'Purified' Afrikaner Nationalist Agitation for Legislation against 'Mixed' Marriages, 1934–9." *Journal of African History* 36, no. 1 (1995): 57–81.

Hyslop, Jon, and Richard Tomlinson. "Industrial Decentralization and the New Dispensation." *South African Labour Bulletin* 10, no. 3 (1984): 114–122.

Ilanga laseNatal. "Abasemjondolo Bafuna Umjondolo Wesikolo." January 21–23, 1980.

———. "Amadoda Azishadisile Enye Ingumfazi." September 19, 1970.

Iliffe, John. *The African AIDS Epidemic: A History.* Athens: Ohio University Press, 2006.

Illouz, Eva. *Consuming the Romantic Utopia.* Berkeley: University of California Press, 1997.

Industrial Strategy Project. *Improving Manufacturing Performance in South Africa: The Report of the Industrial Strategy Project.* Cape Town: University of Cape Town Press, 1995.

Isolewze. "Ngangingenankinga ngelobolo: JZ." April 6, 2006. http://www.isolezwe.co .za/index.php?fArticleId=3191647 (accessed August 5, 2008).

It's My Life. Directed by Brian Tilley. VHS tape. Icarus Films, Brooklyn: NY, 2002.

James, Deborah, *Gaining Ground: "Rights" and "Property" in South African Land Reform.* Milton Park: Routledge-Cavendish, 2007.

Jankowiak, William. *Romantic Passion: A Universal Experience?* New York: Columbia University Press, 1995.

Jeeves, Alan. "Migrant Workers and Epidemic Malaria on the South African Sugar Estates, 1906–1948." In *White Farms, Black Labour: The State and Agrarian Change in Southern Africa, 1910–1950,* ed. Alan Jeeves and Jonathan Crush, 114–136. Oxford: James Currey, 1997.

Jeffreys, M. "Lobolo Is Child-Price." *African Studies* 10, no. 4 (1951): 145–183.

Jochelson, Karen. *The Colour of Disease: Syphilis and Racism in South Africa, 1880–1950.* Houndmills: Palgrave, 2001.

Jochelson, Karen, Monyaola Mthibeli, and Jean-Patrick Leger. "Human Immunodeficiency Virus and Migrant Labour in South Africa." *International Journal of Health Services* 21, no. 1 (1991): 157–173.

Kandiyoti, Deniz. "Bargaining with Patriarchy." *Gender and Society* 2, no. 3 (1988): 274–290.

Kark, Sidney. "The Influence of Urban-Rural Migration on Bantu Health and Disease." *Leech* 21, no. 1 (1950): 23–37.

———. "The Social Pathology of Syphilis in Africans." *South African Medical Journal* 23 (1949): 77–84.

Katz, Cindi. "Vagabond Capitalism and the Necessity of Social Reproduction." *Antipode* 33, no. 4 (2001): 709–728.

Kaufman, Carol, and Stavros Stavrou. "'Bus Fare Please': The Economics of Sex and Gifts among Young People in Urban South Africa." *Culture, Health & Sexuality* 6, no. 5 (2004): 377–391.

Kempadoo, Kamala, and Jo Doezema. *Global Sex Workers: Rights, Resistance, and Redefinition.* New York: Routledge, 1998.

Kenny, Bridget, and Edward Webster. "Eroding the Core: Flexibility and the Resegmentation of the South African Labour Market." *Critical Sociology* 24, no. 3 (1998): 216–243.

Khumalo, Fred. *Touch My Blood: The Early Years.* Roggebaai, South Africa: Umuzi, 2006.

Köhler, Max. *Marriage Customs in Southern Natal.* Union of South Africa, Department of Native Affairs. Ethnological Publications, vol. 4. Edited by N. J. V. Warmelo. Pretoria: Government Printers, 1933.

Kok, Pieter, and Mark Collinson. *Migration and Urbanization in South Africa.* Pretoria: Statistics South Africa, 2006.

Kok, Pieter, Michael O'Donovan, Oumar Bouare, and Johan Van Zyl. *Post-apartheid Patterns of Internal Migration in South Africa.* Cape Town: HSRC Press, 2003.

Koopman, Adrian. "The Praises of Young Zulu Men." *Theoria* 70 (1987): 41–54.

Krige, Eileen. "Changing Conditions in Marital Relations and Parental Duties among Urbanized Natives." *Africa* 9, no. 1 (1936): 1–23.

———. "Girls' Puberty Songs and Their Relation to Fertility, Health, Morality and Religion among the Zulu." *Africa* 38, no. 2 (1968): 173–197.

———. *The Social System of the Zulus.* Pietermaritzburg: Shuter & Shooter, 1936.

Kuper, Leo, Hilston Watts, and Ron Davies. *Durban: A Study in Race Ecology.* London: Jonathan Cape, 1958.

La Hausse de Lalouviere, Paul. *Restless Identities: Signatures of Nationalism, Zulu Ethnicity and History in the Lives of Petros Lamula (c. 1881–1948) and Lymon Maling (1889–c. 1936).* Pietermaritzburg: University of KwaZulu-Natal Press, 2000.

Laslett, Barbara, and Johanna Brenner. "Gender and Social Reproduction: Historical Perspectives." *Annual Reviews in Sociology* 15, no. 1 (1989): 381–404.

Lawson, Lesley. *Side Effects: The Story of AIDS in South Africa.* Cape Town: Double Storey Books, 2008.

LeClerc-Madlala, Suzanne. "Transactional Sex and the Pursuit of Modernity." *Social Dynamics* 29, no. 2 (2003): 213–233.

Lefebvre, Henri. *The Production of Space.* Oxford: Basil Blackwell, 1991.

Lemon, Anthony. "Redressing School Inequalities in the Eastern Cape, South Africa." *Journal of Southern African Studies* 30, no. 2 (2004): 269–290.

Levin, Ruth. "Marriage in Langa Native Location." Master's thesis, Anthropology, University of Cape Town, 1947.

Li, Tania. *The Will to Improve: Governmentality, Development, and the Practice of Politics.* Durham, N.C.: Duke University Press, 2007.

Lipset, David. "Modernity without Romance?" *American Ethnologist* 31, no. 2 (2004): 205–224.

Little, Kenneth, and Anne Price. "Some Trends in Modern Marriage among West Africans." *Journal of the International African Institute* 37, no. 4 (1967): 407–423.

Livingston, Julie. *Debility and the Moral Imagination in Botswana.* Bloomington: Indiana University Press, 2005.

Longmore, Laura. *The Dispossessed: A Study of the Sex-Life of Bantu Women in Urban Areas in and around Johannesburg.* London: Jonathan Cape, 1959.

Louw, Ronald. "Mkhumbane and New Traditions of (Un)African Same-Sex Weddings." In *Changing Men in Southern Africa,* ed. Robert Morrell, 287–296. Pietermaritzburg: University of KwaZulu-Natal Press, 2001.

LoveLife. *LoveLife 2002: Report on Activities and Progress.* http://www.lovelife.org.za/corporate/research/lovelife_2002_report.pdf (accessed July 24, 2008).

Luke, Nancy. "Confronting the 'Sugar Daddy' Stereotype: Age and Economic Asymmetries and Risky Sexual Behaviour in Urban Kenya." *International Family Planning Perspectives* 31, no. 1 (2005): 6–14.

Lund, Frances. *Changing Social Policy: The Child Support Grant in South Africa.* Cape Town: HSRC Press, 2007.

Lurie, Mark, Brian Williams, Khangelani Zuma, David Mkaya-Mwamburi, Geoff Garnett, Michael Sweat, Joel Gittelsohn, and Salim Abdool Karim. "Who Infects Whom? HIV-1 Concordance and Discordance among Migrants and Non-migrant Couples in South Africa." *AIDS* 17, no. 15 (2000): 2245–2252.

Luthuli, Albert. *Let My People Go: An Autobiography.* New York: McGraw Hill, 1962.

Mabin, Alan. "Struggle for the City: Urbanisation and Political Strategies of the South African State." *Social Dynamics* 15, no. 1 (1989): 1–28.

Macfarlane, Alan. *Marriage and Love in England: Modes of Reproduction, 1300–1840.* Oxford: Blackwell, 1986.

MacGaffey, Janet. "Evading Male Control: Women in the Second Economy in Zaire." In *Patriarchy and Class: African Women in the Home and Workforce,* ed. Sharon Stichter and Jane Parpart, 161–176. Boulder, Colo.: Westview, 1988.

Mager, Anne. *Gender and the Making of a South African Bantustan: A Social History of the Ciskei, 1945–1959.* Portsmouth, N.H.: Heinemann, 1999.

Magnani, Robert, Kate MacIntyre, Ali Mehyrar Karim, Lisanne Brown, Paul Hutchinson, Carol Kaufman, Naomi Rutenburg, Kelly Hallman, Julian May, Anthea Dallimore, and Transition Study Team. "The Impact of Life Skills Education on Adolescent Sexual Risk Behaviors in KwaZulu-Natal, South Africa." *Journal of Adolescent Health* 36, no. 4 (2005): 289–304.

Mahala, Siphiwo. *When a Man Cries.* Pietermaritzburg: University of KwaZulu-Natal Press, 2007.

Mail & Guardian. "No 'Sex Perverts' Allowed at Zulu Reed Dance." September 5, 2007. http://www.mg.co.za/article/2007-09-05-no-sex-perverts-allowed-at-zulu-reed-dance (accessed January 20, 2010).

Mama, Amina. "Demythologising Gender in Development: Feminist Studies in African Contexts." *IDS Bulletin* 35, no. 4 (2004): 121–124.

Mamdani, Mahmood, ed. *Beyond Rights Talk and Culture Talk: Comparative Essays on the Politics of Rights and Culture.* Cape Town: David Phillips, 2000.

———. *Citizen and Subject: Contemporary Africa and the Legacy of Late Colonialism.* Princeton, N.J.: Princeton University Press, 1996.

Mandela, Nelson. *No Easy Walk to Freedom.* London: Little, Brown, 1994.

Manicom, Linzi. "Constituting 'Women' as Citizens: Ambiguities in the Making of Gendered Political Subjects in Post-apartheid South Africa." In *(Un)Thinking Citizenship: Feminist Debates in Contemporary South Africa*, ed. Amanda Gouws, 21–52. Cape Town: University of Cape Town Press, 2005.

Mann, Kristin, and Richard Roberts. *Law in Colonial Africa.* Portsmouth, N.H.: Heinemann, 1991.

Marais, Hein. *Buckling: The Impact of Aids in South Africa.* Pretoria: University of Pretoria, 2005.

———. *South Africa: Limits to Change; The Political Economy of Transformation.* London: Zed, 2001.

Maré, Gerhard, and Georgina Hamilton. *An Appetite for Power: Buthelezi's Inkatha and South Africa.* Johannesburg: Ravan Press, 1987.

Marks, Shula. *The Ambiguities of Dependence in South Africa: Class, Nationalism, and the State in Twentieth-Century Natal.* Baltimore: Johns Hopkins University Press, 1986.

———. "Patriotism, Patriarchy and Purity: Natal and the Politics of Zulu Ethnic Consciousness." In *The Creation of Tribalism in Southern Africa*, ed. Leroy Vail, 215–240. Berkeley: University of California Press, 1991.

Marx, Karl. *Economical and Philosophical Manuscripts of 1844.* Buffalo: Prometheus Books, 1987.

Masemola, Thami. "Rebirth of the True Self." *BLINK*, November 2004, 24–27.

Massey, Doreen. *Space, Place and Gender.* Cambridge: Polity Press, 1994.

Matlwa, Kopano. *Coconut: A Novel.* Auckland Park, South Africa: Jacana Media, 2007.

Mauss, Marcel. *The Gift: The Form and Reason for Exchange in Archaic Societies.* London: Routledge, 1989.

Mayer, Philip. "The Origin and Decline of Two Rural Resistance Ideologies." In *Black Villagers in an Industrial Society*, ed. Philip Mayer, 1–80. Cape Town: Oxford University Press, 1980.

———. *Townsmen or Tribesmen: Conservatism and the Process of Urbanization in a South African City.* With contributions by Iona Mayer. 2nd ed. Cape Town: Oxford University Press, 1971.

Mbali, Mandisa. "AIDS Discourses and the South African State: Government Denialism and Post-apartheid AIDS Policy-Making." *Transformations* 54 (2004): 104–122.

———. "TAC in the History of Patient-Driven AIDS Activism." In *Challenging Hegemony: Social Movements and the Quest for a New Humanism in Post-apartheid South Africa*, ed. Nigel Gibson, 129–156. Trenton: Africa World Press, 2006.

Mbali, Mandisa, and Mark Hunter. "Yesterday's Stereotypes Are a Thing of the Past." *Sunday Tribune*, October 17, 2004.

Mbeki, Thabo. "Opening Address and Political Report of the President of the African National Congress, Thabo Mbeki, to the 52nd National Conference of the ANC," December 16, 2007. http://www.anc.org.za/ancdocs/history/mbeki/2007/tm1216.html (accessed January 20, 2010).

Mbembe, Achille. *On the Postcolony.* Berkeley: University of California Press, 2001.

Mbembe, Achille, Nsizwa Dlamini, and Grace Khunou. "Soweto Now." *Public Culture* 16, no. 3 (2004): 499–506.

Mbembe, Achille, and Sarah Nutall, eds. *Johannesburg: The Elusive Metropolis.* Durham, N.C.: Duke University Press, 2008.

McClendon, Thomas. *Genders and Generations Apart: Labor Tenants and Customary Law in Segregation-Era South Africa, 1920s to 1940s.* Portsmouth, N.H.: Heinemann, 2002.

McClintock, Anne. *Imperial Leather: Race, Gender, and Sexuality in the Colonial Conquest.* London: Routledge, 1995.

McDowell, Linda. *Gender, Identity and Place: Understanding Feminist Geographies.* Minneapolis: University of Minnesota Press, 1999.

Meintjes, Louise. *The Sound of Africa! Making Music Zulu in a South African Studio.* Durham, N.C.: Duke University Press, 2003.

Mhlongo, Nhlaka. "Trouble across the Tugela River: Political Instability and Conflict Resolution in Mandini; A Comparative Study with Special Emphasis on the Political Culture of Pre- and Post-apartheid South Africa (1984–2001)." Master's thesis, University of Durban Westville (draft version given to author by Mhlongo in 2003).

Miller, Peter, and Nikolas Rose. *Governing the Present: Administering Economic, Social and Personal Life.* Cambridge: Polity Press, 2008.

Mitchell, Colin. "Death City." *Drum,* November 20, 1997.

Mitchell, Katharyne, Sallie Marston, and Cindi Katz. "Introduction: Life's Work; An Introduction, Review and Critique." *Antipode* 35, no. 3 (2003): 415–442.

Moeno, Ntlantla. "Illegitimacy in an African Urban Township in South Africa: An Ethnographic Note." *African Studies* 36, no. 1 (1977): 43–47.

Moffett, Helen. "'These women, they force us to rape them': Rape as Narrative of Social Control in Post-apartheid." *Journal of Southern African Studies* 32, no. 1 (2006): 129–144.

Mohanty, Chandra. "Under Western Eyes: Feminist Scholarship and Colonial Discourse." In *The Postcolonial Studies Reader,* ed. Bill Ashcroft, Gareth Griffiths, and Helen Tiffin, 333–358. New York: Routledge, 1995.

Mokwena, Steve. "The Era of the Jackrollers: Contextualising the Rise of Youth Gangs in Soweto." Paper presented to the Centre for the Study of Violence and Reconciliation, Johannesburg, 2001.

Moodie, Dunbar. *Going for Gold: Men, Mines and Migration.* Berkeley: University of California Press, 1994.

Moore, Henrietta, and Megan Vaughan. *Cutting Down Trees: Gender, Nutrition, and Agricultural Change in the Northern Province of Zambia, 1890–1990.* Portsmouth, N.H.: Heinemann, 1994.

Morrell, Robert. *Changing Men in Southern Africa.* Pietermaritzburg: University of KwaZulu-Natal Press, 2001.

———. "Of Boys and Men: Masculinity and Gender in Southern African Studies." *Journal of Southern African Studies* 24, no. 4 (1998): 605–630.

———, ed. *Political Economy and Identities in KwaZulu-Natal: Historical and Social Perspectives.* Durban: Indicator Press, 1996.

Morris, Martina, and Mirjam Kretzschmar. "Concurrent Partnerships and the Spread of AIDS." *AIDS* 11, no. 5 (1997): 681–683.

Motsemme, Nthabiseng. "'Loving in a Time of Hopelessness': On Township Women's Subjectivities in a Time of HIV/AIDS." *African Identities* 5, no. 1 (2007): 61–87.

Moultrie, Tom, and Ian Timaeus. *Trends in South African Fertility between 1970 and 1998: An Analysis of the 1996 Census and the 1998 Demographic and Health Survey.* Cape Town: Medical Research Council, 2002.

Mthembu, Bongani. "Development: Marchers Threaten Blockades." *Natal Witness,* November 26, 2008. http://www.witness.co.za/index.php?showcontent&global [_id]=16630 (accessed August 20, 2009).

Mudimbe, V. Y. *The Invention of Africa: Gnosis, Philosophy, and the Order of Knowledge.* Bloomington: Indiana University Press, 1988.

Muhwava, William, and Makandwe Nyirenda. "Demographic and Socio-economic Trends in the ACDIS." Monograph no 2. Mtubatuba: Africa Centre for Population Studies, 2008.

Murray, Colin. *Families Divided: The Impact of Migrant Labour in Lesotho.* Cambridge: Cambridge University Press, 1981.

Murray, Stephen, and Will Roscoe. *Boy-Wives and Female-Husbands: Studies in African Homosexualities.* New York: St. Martin's Press, 1998.

Nagar, Richa, Vicky Lawson, Linda McDowell, and Susan Hanson. "Locating Globalization: Feminist (Re)Readings of the Subjects and Spaces of Globalization." *Economic Geography* 78, no. 3 (2002): 257–284.

Naidoo, Laila. "Industrial Decentralization and Everyday Forms of Class Struggles: A Case Study of Isithebe (1988–1992)." Master's thesis, Department of Sociology, University of Natal, Durban, 1997.

Natal Mercury. "Middle Classes Choose Township Lifestyle." July 25, 2008.

Nattrass, Nicoli. *Mortal Combat: AIDS Denialism and the Fight for Antiretrovirals in South Africa.* Pietermaritzburg: University of KwaZulu-Natal Press, 2007.

———. "Poverty, Sex, and HIV." *AIDS and Behavior* 13, no. 5 (2009): 833–840. Published online on April 16, 2009, doi: 10.1007/s10461-009-9563-9.

Newmarch, Jocelyn. "Equity: Is the Data Wrong?" *Mail & Guardian,* May 18–24, 2007.

Ngobese, Nokulunga. "Women and the Wearing of Trousers." *Natal Witness,* August 16, 2007.

Niehaus, Isak. "Death before Dying: Understanding AIDS Stigma in the South African Lowveld." *Journal of Southern African Studies* 33, no. 4 (2007): 845–860.

———. "Disharmonious Spouses and Harmonious Siblings: Conceptualizing Household Formation among Urban Residents in QwaQwa." *African Studies* 53, no. 1 (1994): 115–135.

———. "Masculine Domination in Sexual Violence: Interpreting Accounts of Three Cases of Rape in the South African Lowveld." In *Men Behaving Differently: South African Men since 1994,* ed. Graeme Reid and Liz Walker, 65–88. Cape Town: Double Storey Books, 2005.

Nixon, Rob. *Homelands, Harlem, and Hollywood: South African Culture and the World Beyond.* New York: Routledge, 1994.

Nkosi, Deli. "Kuyihlazo Ukukipita Kwendoda." *Isolezwe,* September 1, 2004.

Ntsebeza, Lungisile, and Ruth Hall, eds. *The Land Question in South Africa: The Challenge of Transformation and Redistribution.* Cape Town: HSRC Press, 2007.

Nutall, Sarah. "Stylizing the Self: The Y Generation in Rosebank, Johannesburg." *Public Culture* 16, no. 3 (2004): 430–452.

Oswin, Natalie. "Producing Homonormativity in Neoliberal South Africa: Recognition, Redistribution, and the Equality Project." *Signs: Journal of Women in Culture and Society* 32, no. 3 (2007): 649–669.

Oyewumi, Oyeronke. *The Invention of Women: Making an African Sense of Western Gender Discourses.* Minneapolis: University of Minnesota Press, 1997.

Packard, Randall. "Post-colonial Medicine." In *Medicine in the Twentieth Century,* ed. Roger Cooter and John Pickstone, 97–112. Amsterdam: Harwood Academic Publishers, 2000.

———. *White Plague, Black Labor: Tuberculosis and the Political Economy of Health and Disease in South Africa.* Berkeley: University of California Press, 1989.

Packard, Randall, and Paul Epstein. "Epidemiologists, Social Scientists, and the Structure of Medical Research on AIDS in Africa." *Social Science & Medicine* 33, no. 7 (1991): 771–794.

Padayachee, Vishnu. "Progressive Academic Economists and the Challenge of Development in South Africa's Decade of Liberation." *Review of African Political Economy* 25, no. 77 (1998): 431–451.

———. "The South African Economy, 1994–2004." *Social Research: An International Quarterly of Social Sciences* 72, no. 3 (2005): 549–580.

Padilla, Mark, Jennifer Hirsch, Miguel Munoz-Laboy, Robert Sember, and Richard Parker, eds. *Love and Globalization: Transformations of Intimacy in the Contemporary World.* Nashville, Tenn.: Vanderbilt University Press, 2007.

Parikh, Shanti. "The Political Economy of Marriage and HIV: The ABC Approach, 'Safe' Infidelity, and Managing Moral Risk in Uganda." *American Journal of Public Health* 97, no. 7 (2007): 1198–1209.

———. "Sugar Daddies and Sexual Citizenship in Uganda: Rethinking Third Wave Feminism." *Black Renaissance/Renaissance noire* 5, no. 2 (2004): 75–99.

Parker, Richard. "Sexuality, Culture, and Power in HIV/AIDS Research." *Annual Review of Anthropology* 30 (2001): 163–179.

Parker, Richard, Regina Maria Barbosa, and Peter Aggleton. *Framing the Sexual Subject: The Politics of Gender, Sexuality, and Power.* Berkeley: University of California Press, 2000.

Parker, Warren. "Re-appraising Youth Prevention in South Africa: The Case of loveLife." Paper presented at the South African AIDS Conference in Durban, August 2003. http://www.cadre.org.za/files/reappraising_youth.pdf (accessed August 22, 2009).

Parle, Julie, and Fiona Scorgie. "Bewitching Zulu Women: Umhayizo, Gender, and Witchcraft in Natal." Paper presented to the History and African Studies Seminar, University of Natal, Durban, October 24, 2001.

Parnell, Susan, and Alan Mabin. "Rethinking Urban South Africa." *Journal of Southern African Studies* 21, no. 1 (1995): 39–61.

Parpart, Jane. "Sexuality and Power on the Zambian Copperbelt." In *Patriarchy and Class: African Women in the Home and Workforce,* ed. Sharon Stichter and Jane Parpart, 115–138. Boulder, Colo.: Westview, 1988.

Parry, Jonathan, and Maurice Bloch, eds. *Money and the Morality of Exchange.* Cambridge: Cambridge University Press, 1989.

Pauli, Julia, and Michael Schnegg. "'Blood tests with the eyes': Negotiating Conjugal Relations during the HIV/AIDS Crisis in Rural Namibia." Paper presented to the International ACACIA Conference, Königswinter, Germany, October 1–3, 2003.

Pauw, Berthold. *The Second Generation: A Study of the Family among Urbanized Bantu in East London.* Cape Town: Oxford University Press, 1964.

Petchesky, Rosalind. *Global Prescriptions: Gendering Health and Human Rights.* London: Zed, 2003.

Pettifor, Audrey, Michael Hudgens, Brooke Levandowski, Helen Rees, and Myron Cohen. "Highly Efficient HIV Transmission to Young Women in South Africa." *AIDS* 21, no. 7 (2007): 861–865.

Pettifor, Audrey, Catherine MacPhail, Stefano Bertozzi, and Helen Rees. "Challenge of Evaluating a National HIV Prevention Programme: The Case of loveLife, South Africa." *Sexually Transmitted Infections* 83, Suppl. 1 (2007): 70–74. doi: 10.1136/sti.2006.023689.

Pettifor, Audrey, Helen Rees, Immo Kleinschmidt, Annie Steffenson, Catherine MacPhail, Lindiwe Hlongwa-Madikizela, Kerry Vermaak, and Nancy Padian. "Young People's Sexual Health in South Africa: HIV Prevalence and Sexual Behaviors from a Nationally Representative Household Survey." *AIDS* 19, no. 14 (2005): 1525–1534.

Pettifor, Audrey, Helen Rees, Annie Steffenson, Lindiwe Hlongwa-Madikizela, Catherine MacPhail, Kerry Vermaak, and Immo Kleinschmidt, *HIV and Sexual Behaviour among Young South Africans: A National Survey of 15–24-Year-Olds.* Johannesburg: Reproductive Health Research Unit, University of Witwatersrand, 2004.

Phillips, Ray. *The Bantu in the City: A Study of Cultural Adjustment on the Witwatersrand.* Lovedale: Lovedale Press, 1938.

Pickles, John, and Jeff Woods. "Taiwanese Investment in South Africa." *African Affairs* 88, no. 353 (1989): 507–528.

Pigg, Stacy Leigh, and Vincanne Adams, "Introduction: The Moral Object of Sex." In *Sex in Development: Science, Sexuality, and Morality in Global Perspective*, ed. Vincanne Adams and Stacy Leigh Pigg, 1–38. Durham, N.C.: Duke University Press, 2005.

Piot, Charles. *Remotely Global: Village Modernity in West Africa.* Chicago: University of Chicago Press, 1999.

Pirouz, Farah. "Have Labour Market Outcomes Affected Household Structure in South Africa? A Preliminary Descriptive Analysis of Households." Paper presented at the Conference on African Development and Poverty Reduction, Cape Town, October 13–15, 2004.

Pithouse, Richard. "'Our struggle is thought, on the ground, running': The University of Abahlali baseMjondolo." Research Report 40, Centre for Civil Society, University of KwaZulu-Natal, 2006.

Platzky, Laurine. "The Development Impact of South Africa's Industrial Decentralization Policies: An Unforeseen Legacy." Ph.D. thesis, Institute of Social Studies, The Hague, 1995.

Platzky, Laurine, and Cheryl Walker. *The Surplus People: Forced Removals in South Africa.* Johannesburg: Ravan Press, 1985.

Posel, Deborah. *The Making of Apartheid, 1948–1961: Conflict and Compromise.* Oxford: Clarendon Press, 1991.

———. "Marriage at the Drop of a Hat: Housing and Partnership in South Africa's Urban African Townships, 1920s–1960s." *History Workshop Journal* 61, no. 1 (2006): 57–76.

———. "The Scandal of Manhood: 'Baby Rape' and the Politicization of Sexual Violence in Post-apartheid South Africa." *Culture, Health & Sexuality* 7, no. 3 (2005): 239–252.

———. "Sex, Death and the Fate of the Nation: Reflections on the Politicization of Sexuality in Post-apartheid South Africa." *Africa* 75, no. 2 (2004): 125–153.

———. "State, Power and Gender: Conflict over the Registration of African Customary Marriage in South Africa, c. 1910–1970." *Journal of Historical Sociology* 8, no. 3 (1995): 223–256.

Posel, Dorrit. "Moving On: Patterns of Labour Migration in Post-apartheid South Africa." In *Africa on the Move: African Migration and Urbanisation in Comparative Perspective,* ed. Marta Tienda, Sally Findley, and Stephen Tollman, 217–231. Johannesburg: Witwatersrand University Press, 2006.

Posel, Dorrit, and Alison Todes. "The Shift to Female Labour in KwaZulu/Natal." *South African Journal of Economics* 63, no. 2 (1995): 225–246.

Postero, Nancy. *Now We Are Citizens: Indigenous Politics in Postmulticultural Bolivia.* Stanford, Calif.: Stanford University Press, 2007.

Potts, Deborah, and Shula Marks. "Fertility in Southern Africa: The Quiet Revolution." *Journal of Southern African Studies* 27, no. 2 (2001): 189–205.

Powdermaker, Hortense. *Copper Town: Changing Africa; The Human Situation on the Rhodesian Copperbelt.* New York: Harper & Row, 1962.

Pred, Allan. *Even in Sweden: Racisms, Racialized Spaces, and the Popular Geographical Imagination.* Berkeley: University of California Press, 2000.

Pressly, Donwald. "The Rise and Rise of South Africa's Shacks." *Mail & Guardian,* January 6, 2006.

Preston-Whyte, Eleanor. "Families without Marriage." In *Social System and Tradition in Southern Africa: Essays in Honour of Eileen Krige,* ed. John Argyle and Eleanor Preston-Whyte, 53–85. Oxford: Oxford University Press, 1978.

Preston-Whyte, Eleanor, Christine Varga, Herman Oosthuizen, Rachel Roberts, and Frederick Blose. "Survival Sex and HIV/AIDS in an African City." In *Framing the Sexual Subject: The Politics of Gender, Sexuality, and Power,* ed. Richard Parker, Regina Maria Barbosa, and Peter Aggleton, 165–190. Berkeley: University of California Press, 2000.

Pudifin, Colette, and Sarah Ward. "Working for Nothing: Gender and Industrial Decentralization in Isithebe." Master's thesis, Department of Town and Regional Planning, University of Natal, Durban, 1986.

Radcliffe-Brown, A. R. Introduction to *African Systems of Kinship and Marriage,* ed. A. R. Radcliffe-Brown and Daryll Forde, 1–85. London: Oxford University Press, 1962.

Ratele, Kopano. "Ruling Masculinity and Sexuality." *Feminist Africa* 6 (2006): 48–64.

Rebhun, Linda-Anne. *The Heart Is Unknown Country: Love in the Changing Economy of Northeast Brazil.* Stanford, Calif.: Stanford University Press, 1999.

Reddy, Vasu, Theo Sandfort, and Laetitia Rispel, eds. *From Social Silence to Social Science: Same-Sex Sexuality, HIV and AIDS, and Gender in South Africa.* Cape Town: HSRC Press.

Reid, Graeme. "'It's just a fashion!' Linking Homosexuality and 'Modernity' in South Africa." *Etnofoor* 16, no. 2 (2003): 7–23.

Reid, Graeme, and Teresa Dirsuweit. "Understanding Systemic Violence: Homophobic Attacks in Johannesburg and Its Surrounds." *Urban Forum* 13, no. 3 (2002): 99–126.

Republic of South Africa. Bureau of Statistics. *Population Census, 1960, Sample Tabulation, No. 8.* Pretoria: Bureau of Statistics, 1965.

———. Central Statistical Service. *Population Census 80, Report No. 02-80-12.* Pretoria: Central Statistical Service, 1985.

———. Central Statistical Service. *Population Census 1991, Report No. 03-01-22.* Pretoria: Central Statistical Service, 1992.

———. Department of Health. *2008 National Antenatal Sentinel HIV and Syphilis Prevalence Survey, South Africa.* Pretoria: Department of Health. http://www.doh.gov.za/docs/reports/ (accessed January 29, 2010).

————. Department of Health. *South African Demographic and Health Survey 2003, Preliminary Report*. Pretoria: Department of Health. http://www.doh.gov.za/facts/index.html (accessed 1 June 2008).

————. Department of Housing. *Mainstreaming Gender in the Housing and Human Settlement Sector*. Pretoria: Department of Housing, 2006. http://www.housing.gov.za/Content/Gender%20Guidelines/Gender_2006_p1-25.pdf (accessed September 4, 2007).

————. Department of Labour. *Commission for Employment Equity, 7th CEE Annual Report, 2007*. Pretoria: Department of Labour, 2007.

————. Department of Labour. *Women in the South African Labour Market, 1995–2005*. Pretoria: Republic of South Africa, 2006.

————. Department of Statistics. *South African Statistics 1974*. Pretoria: Department of Statistics, 1974.

————. Office of the Presidency. "Address by Deputy President Zuma at the Launch of the Public-Private Partnership in Support of loveLife." July 19, 2001. http://www.thepresidency.gov.za/main.asp?include=former%5Fdeputy/sp/2001/sp0719.htm (accessed August 26, 2009).

————. Statistics South Africa. *Census 2001: Primary Tables South Africa: Census '96 and 2001 Compared*. Pretoria: Statistics South Africa, 2001.

————. Statistics South Africa. *Community Survey 2007 (Revised Version)*. Pretoria: Statistics South Africa, October 24, 2007. http://www.statssa.gov.za/publications/P0301/P0301.pdf (accessed October 10, 2008).

————. Statistics South Africa. *Stages in the Lifestyle of South Africans*. Pretoria: Statistics South Africa, 2005.

Roberts, Nomakula. "Let's Three-Time Those Randy Dogs." *Sunday World*, March 21, 2004.

————. "White's Not Always Right." *Sunday World*, April 19, 2009.

Roberts, Ronald Suresh. *Fit to Govern: The Native Intelligence of Thabo Mbeki*. Johannesburg: STE Publishers, 2007.

Robins, Steven. "'Brothers are doing it for themselves': AIDS, Sexual Politics and 'New Masculinities' after Apartheid." In *The Politics of AIDS: Globalization, the State and Civil Society*, ed. Maj-Lis Follér and Håkan Thörn, 156–176. New York: Palgrave Macmillan, 2008.

————. "From 'Rights' to 'Ritual': AIDS Activism in South Africa." *American Anthropologist* 108, no. 2 (2006): 312–323.

————. "Re-interpreting the 'Political Rationality' of President Mbeki's Position on AIDS." Review of *When Bodies Remember: Experiences and Politics of AIDS in South Africa*, by Didier Fassin. *Journal of Southern African Studies* 34, no. 2 (2008): 468–470.

————. "Sexual Politics and the Zuma Rape Trial." *Journal of Southern African Studies* 34, no. 2 (2008): 411–427.

Robinson, Jennifer. *The Power of Apartheid: State, Power, and Space in South African Cities*. Oxford: Butterworth-Heinemann, 1996.

Robinson, Vicky, Rapule Tabane, and Ferial Haffajee. "23 Days That Shook Our World." *Mail & Guardian*, April 28–May 4, 2006.

Rogerson, Christian. "Globalization or Informalization? African Urban Economies in the 1990s." *The Urban Challenge in Africa: Growth and Management of Its Large Cities*, ed. Carole Rakodi, 337–370. New York: United Nations University Press, 1997.

Rosner, Victoria, and Geraldine Pratt, eds. *The Global and the Intimate*. New York: Feminist Press at CUNY, 2006.

Rutenberg, Naomi, Carol Kaufman, Kate Macintyre, Lisanne Brown, and Cathrien Alons-Kehus. "Falling Pregnant or Falling Positive: Adolescent Pregnancy and HIV Infection in South Africa." Paper presented at the annual meeting of the Population Association of America, March 23–25, Los Angeles, 2000.

Sangtin Writers and Richa Nagar. *Playing with Fire: Feminist Thought and Activism through Seven Lives in India*. Minneapolis: University of Minnesota Press, 2006.

Sboros, Marika. "Style Gurus Have Their Say in Fashion." *Cape Argus*, September 13, 2004.

Schapera, Isaac. *Married Life in an African Tribe*. London: Faber & Faber, 1940.

———. *Migrant Labour and Tribal Life: A Study of Conditions in the Bechuanaland Protectorate*. Oxford: Oxford University Press, 1947.

———. "Premarital Pregnancy and Native Opinion: A Note on Social Change." *Africa 6*, no. 1 (1933): 59–89.

Schoepf, Brooke, Claude Schoepf, and Joyce Millen. "Theoretical Therapies, Remote Remedies: SAPs and the Political Ecology of Poverty and Health in Africa." In *Dying for Growth: Global Inequality and the Health of the Poor*, ed. Jim Yong Kim, Joyce Millen, Alec Irwin, and John Gershman, 91–126. Monroe, Maine: Common Courage Press, 2000.

Schuster, Ilsa. *New Women of Lusaka*. Palo Alto, Calif.: Mayfield, 1979.

Scorgie, Fiona. "Virginity Testing and the Politics of Sexual Responsibility: Implications for AIDS Interventions." *African Studies 61*, no. 1 (2002): 55–75.

Scott, Joan. *Gender and the Politics of History*. New York: Columbia University Press, 1999.

Seekings, Jeremy, and Nicoli Nattrass. "Class, Distribution and Redistribution in Post-apartheid South Africa." *Transformation 50* (2002): 1–30.

———. *Class, Race, and Inequality in South Africa*. New Haven, Conn.: Yale University Press, 2005.

Selikow, Terry-Ann, Bheki Zulu, and Eugene Cedras. "The Ingagara, the Regte and the Cherry: HIV/AIDS and Youth Culture in Contemporary Urban Townships." *Agenda 53* (2002): 22–32.

Setel, Philip. *A Plague of Paradoxes: AIDS, Culture, and Demography in Northern Tanzania*. Chicago: University of Chicago Press, 1999.

Shangase, Nonhlanhla. "Amanyala Esimobeni." *Umafrika*, May 16–22, 2003.

———. "Ixhegu Lamanyala (71) Linukubeze Ingane eno 5." *Umafrika*, January 31–February 6, 2003.

———. "Yini Eyenza Intsha Yakithi Ikipite?" *Isolezwe*, September 1, 2004.

Sharp, John. "A World Turned Upside Down: Households and Differentiation in a South African Bantustan in the 1980s." *African Studies 53*, no. 1 (1994): 71–88.

Shongwe, Vincent. "Kufanele Abazali Bajezise Izingane." Letter to editor. *Isolezwe*, May 17, 2007.

Shorter, Edward. *The Making of the Modern Family*. New York: Basic Books, 1975.

Shota, Babalwa. "She's Got IT." *Elle*, October 2004, 50–54.

Shozi, C. B. "Hhayi, Asibesabi, Siyabathanda." Letter to editor. *Isolezwe*, August 2, 2003.

Silberschmidt, Margrethe. *Women Forget That Men Are the Masters: Gender Antagonism and Socio-economic Change in Kisii District, Kenya*. Uppsala: Nordic Institute of African Studies, 1999.

Simons, Jack. *African Women: Their Legal Status in South Africa*. London: C. Hurst, 1968.

Skinner, Caroline, and Imraan Valodia. "Labour Market Policy, Flexibility, and the Future of Labour Relations: The Case of KwaZulu-Natal Clothing Industry." *Transformation 50* (2002): 56–76.

Smith, Daniel. "Love and the Risk of HIV: Courtship, Marriage, and Infidelity in Southeastern Nigeria." In *Modern Loves: The Anthropology of Romantic Courtship and Companionate Marriage,* ed. Jennifer Hirsch and Holly Wardlow, 135–156. Ann Arbor: University of Michigan Press, 2006.

Smith, Robert. *Labour Resources of Natal.* Cape Town: Oxford University Press, 1950.

Soske, Jon. "'Wash me black again': African Nationalism, the Indian Diaspora, and KwaZulu-Natal, 1945–1979." Ph.D. thesis, Department of History, University of Toronto, 2009.

SouthAfrica.info. "South Africa's Dollar Millionaires on the Rise." July 10, 2006. http://www.southafrica.info/business/success/world-wealth-200606.htm (accessed July 24, 2007).

South African Press Association. "Government Ahead of ARV targets." January 29, 2009. http://70.84.171.10/~etools/newsbrief/2009/news0129.txt (accessed May 22, 2009).

Spiegel, Andrew "Changing Patterns of Migrant Labour and Rural Differentiation in Lesotho." *Social Dynamics* 6, no. 2 (1981): 1–13.

———. "Migration, Urbanisation and Domestic Fluidity: Reviewing Some South African Examples." *African Anthropology* 2, no. 2 (1995): 90–113.

———. "Polygamy as Myth: Towards Understanding Extramarital Relations in Lesotho." In *Tradition and Transition in Southern Africa: Festschrift for Philip and Iona Mayer,* ed. Andrew Spiegel and Pat McAllister, 145–166. London: Transaction Publishers, 1991.

Stadler, A. W. "Birds in the Cornfield: Squatter Movements in Johannesburg." *Journal of Southern African Studies* 6, no. 1 (1979): 93–123.

Standing, Hilary. "AIDS: Conceptual and Methodological Issues in Researching Sexual Behaviour in Sub-Saharan Africa." *Social Science & Medicine* 34, no. 5 (1992): 475–483.

Steedman, Carolyn. *Landscape for a Good Woman: A Story of Two Lives.* New Brunswick: Rutgers University Press, 1986.

Steinberg, Jonny. *Sizwe's Test: A Young Man's Journey through Africa's AIDS Epidemic.* New York: Simon & Schuster, 2008.

Steingo, Gavin. "South African Music after Apartheid: Kwaito, the 'Party Politic,' and the Appropriation of Gold as a Sign of Success." *Popular Music & Society* 28, no. 3 (2005): 333–357.

Stillwaggon, Eileen. *AIDS and the Ecology of Poverty.* Oxford: Oxford University Press, 2006.

Stoler, Ann Laura. *Race and the Education of Desire: Foucault's "History of Sexuality" and the Colonial Order of Things.* Durham, N.C.: Duke University Press, 1995.

Stone, Lawrence. *The Family, Sex and Marriage in England, 1500–1800.* Harmondsworth: Penguin Books, 1979.

Stones, C., and J. Philbrick. "Attitudes toward Love among Xhosa University Students in South Africa." *Journal of Social Psychology* 129, no. 4 (1989): 573–575.

Stubbings, Moira, and Ione Pepper. *Mandini.* Mandini: Women's Institute, 1977.

Sundkler, Bengt. *Bantu Prophets in South Africa.* London: Butterworth Press, 1948.

Surplus People Project. *The Surplus People: Forced Removals in South Africa.* Vol. 4, Natal. Cape Town: Surplus People Project, 1983.

Susser, Ida. *AIDS, Sex, and Culture: Global Politics and Survival in Southern Africa.* Malden, Mass.: Wiley-Blackwell, 2009.

Swarr, Amanda, and Richa Nagar. "Dismantling Assumptions: Interrogating 'Lesbian' Struggles for Identity and Survival in India and South Africa." *Signs: Journal of Women in Culture and Society* 29, no. 2 (2004): 491–516.

Swidler, Ann. *Talk of Love: How Culture Matters.* Chicago: University of Chicago Press, 2001.

Swidler, Ann, and Susan Watkins. "Ties of Dependence: AIDS and Transactional Sex in Rural Malawi." *Studies in Family Planning* 38, no. 3 (2007): 147–162.

Terreblanche, Christine. "Poor Love Zuma, Study Finds." *Natal Mercury,* June 24, 2007.

Thomas, Lynn. "Love, Sex, and the Modern Girl in 1930s Southern Africa." In *Love in Africa,* ed. Jennifer Cole and Lynn Thomas, 31–57. Chicago: University of Chicago Press, 2009.

———. *Politics of the Womb: Women, Reproduction, and the State in Kenya.* Berkeley: University of California Press, 2003.

Thornton, Robert. *Unimagined Community: Sex, Networks, and AIDS in Uganda and South Africa.* Berkeley: University of California Press, 2008.

Todes, Alison, and Norah Walker. "Women and Housing Policy in South Africa: A Discussion of Durban Case Studies." *Urban Forum* 3, no. 2 (1992): 115–138.

Tomlinson, Richard, and Mark Addleson, eds. *Regional Restructuring under Apartheid: Urban and Regional Policies in Contemporary South Africa.* Johannesburg: Ravan Press, 1987.

Treichler, Paula. "AIDS, Africa, and Cultural Theory." *Transition* 51 (1991): 86–103.

Tshabalala, Thembelihle. "Growing Anti-lesbian Violence." *Mail & Guardian,* May 16, 2008.

Turner, Noleen. "Representations of Masculinity in the Contemporary Oral Praise Poetry of Zulu Men." *South African Journal of African Language* 19, no. 3 (1999): 196–203.

UNAIDS. *2008 Report on the Global AIDS Epidemic.* Geneva: UNAIDS, 2008.

———. *AIDS Epidemic Update, December 2009.* Geneva: UNAIDS, 2009.

UNHABITAT. *State of the World's Cities 2008/2009: Harmonious Cities.* London: Earthscan, 2008.

Union of South Africa. *Population Census, 8th May, 1951.* Vol. 7. Pretoria: Government Printer, 1959.

United Nations Development Programme. *South Africa Human Development Report 2003.* Oxford: Oxford University Press, 2003.

Vail, Leroy. *The Creation of Tribalism in Southern Africa.* Berkeley: University of California Press, 1991.

Valentine, David. *Imagining Transgender: An Ethnography of a Category.* Durham, N.C.: Duke University Press, 2007.

Vance, Carol. "Anthropology Rediscovers Sexuality: A Theoretical Comment." *Social Science & Medicine* 33, no. 8 (1991): 875–84.

Vandewiele, M., and J. Philbrick. "Attitudes of Senegalese Students toward Love." *Psychological Reports* 52, no. 3 (1983): 915–918.

Van Onselen, Charles. *Studies in the Social and Economic History of the Witwatersrand, 1886–1914.* 2 vols. Johannesburg: Ravan Press, 1982.

Vaughan, Megan. *Curing Their Ills: Colonial Power and African Illness.* Cambridge: Polity Press, 1991.

Vetten, Lisa. "Mbeki and Smith Both Got It Wrong." *Mail & Guardian,* October 29–November 4, 2004.

———. "Violence against Women in South Africa." In *State of the Nation: South Africa 2007,* ed. Sakhela Buhlungu, John Daniel, Roger Southall, and Jessica Lutchman, 425–447. Cape Town: HSRC Press, 2007.

Vilakazi, Absolom. Review of *The Dispossessed: A Study of the Sex-Life of Bantu Women in Urban Areas in and around Johannesburg*, by Laura Longmore. *American Anthropologist* 65, no. 4 (1963): 948–950.

———. *Zulu Transformations: A Study of the Dynamics of Social Change*. Pietermaritzburg: University of KwaZulu-Natal Press, 1962.

Viljoen, Stella. "Masculine Ideals in Post-apartheid South Africa: The Rise of Men's Glossies." In *Power, Politics and Identity in South African Media*, ed. Adrian Hadland, Eric Louw, Simphiwe Sesanti, and Herman Wasserman, 312–42. Cape Town: HSRC Press, 2008.

Vincent, Louise. "Virginity Testing in South Africa: Re-traditioning the Postcolony." *Culture, Health, and Sexuality* 8, no. 1 (2006): 17–30.

Vogelman, Lloyd, and Sharon Lewis. "Gang Rape and the Culture of Violence in South Africa." Unpublished paper, Centre for the Study of Violence and Reconciliation, Johannesburg, 1993.

Von Holdt, Karl, and Edward Webster. "Work Restructuring and the Crisis of Reproduction: A Southern Perspective." In *Beyond the Apartheid Workplace: Studies in Transition*, ed. Karl von Holdt and Edward Webster, 3–40. Pietermaritzburg: University of KwaZulu-Natal Press, 2005.

Wacquant, Loic. "Pugs at Work: Bodily Capital and Bodily Labour among Professional Boxers." *Body and Society* 1, no. 1 (1995): 65–93.

Waetjen, Thembisa. *Workers and Warriors: Masculinity and the Struggle for Nation in South Africa*. Urbana: University of Illinois Press, 2004.

Wa Karanja, Wambui. "'Outside Wives' and 'Inside Wives' in Nigeria: A Study of Changing Perceptions in Marriage." In *Transformations of African Marriage*, ed. David Parkin and David Nyamwaya, 247–261. Manchester: Manchester University Press, 1987.

Walker, Cherryl. "Gender and the Development of the Migrant Labour System, c. 1850–1930: An Overview." In *Women and Gender in Southern Africa to 1945*, ed. Cherryl Walker, 168–196. Cape Town: David Philip, 1990.

Walker, Liz. "Negotiating the Boundaries of Masculinity in Post-apartheid South Africa." In *Men Behaving Differently: South African Men since 1994*, ed. Liz Walker and Graeme Reid, 161–182. Cape Town: Double Storey Books, 2005.

Wardlow, Holly. *Wayward Women: Sexuality and Agency in a New Guinea Society*. Berkeley: University of California Press, 2006.

Webb, Colin, and John Wright, eds. *The James Stuart Archive of Recorded Evidence Relating to the History of the Zulu and Neighbouring Peoples*. Vols. 1–5. Pietermaritzburg: University of KwaZulu-Natal Press, 1976–2001.

———, eds. *A Zulu King Speaks: Statements Made by Cetshwayo kaMpande on the History and Customs of His People*. Pietermaritzburg: University of KwaZulu-Natal Press, 1978.

Weeks, Jeffrey. *Sex, Politics, and Society: The Regulation of Sexuality since 1800*. London: Longman, 1989.

Welsh, David. *The Roots of Segregation: Native Policy in Colonial Natal, 1845–1910*. London: Oxford University Press, 1971.

White, Hylton. "Ritual Haunts: The Timing of Estrangement in a Post-apartheid Countryside." In *Producing African Futures: Ritual and Reproduction in a Neoliberal Age*, ed. Brad Weiss, 141–166. Boston: Brill, 2004.

White, Luise. *The Comforts of Home: Prostitution in Colonial Nairobi*. Chicago: University of Chicago Press, 1990.

White, Luise, Stephan Miescher, and David William Cohen. *African Words, African Voices: Critical Practices in Oral History*. Bloomington: Indiana University Press, 2001.

Wicks, Jeff. "Order Sought over Ban." *Natal Mercury*, March 11, 2008.

Wieringa, Saskia. "Women Marriages and Other Same-Sex Practices: Historical Reflections on African Women's Same-Sex Relations." In *Tommy Boys, Lesbian Men and Ancestral Wives*, ed. Ruth Morgan and Saskia Wieringa, 281–308. Johannesburg: Jacana Media, 2005.

Wilson, Monica Hunter. *Reaction to Conquest: Effects of Contact with Europeans on the Pondo of South Africa*. Oxford: Oxford University Press, 1936.

Wilson, Monica, and Archie Mafeje. *Langa: A Study of Social Groups in an African Township*. Cape Town: Oxford University Press, 1963.

Wisner, Ben. "Health and Health Care in South Africa: The Challenge for a Majority Ruled State." *Antipode* 23, no. 1 (1991): 121–136.

Wood, Katherine, and Rachel Jewkes. "'Dangerous Love': Reflections on Violence among Xhosa Township Youth." In *Changing Men in Southern Africa*, ed. Robert Morrell, 317–336. Pietermaritzburg: University of KwaZulu-Natal Press, 2001.

Wood, Kate, Helen Lambert, and Rachel Jewkes. "'Injuries are beyond love': Physical Violence in Young South Africans' Sexual Relationships." *Medical Anthropology* 27, no. 1 (2008): 43–69.

World Council of Churches. "Desmond Tutu: 'Caring and compassion will prevail over evil and injustice.'" May 20, 2008. http://www.oikoumene.org/en/news/news-management/eng/a/article/1722/desmond-tutu-caring-and.html?tx_ttnews%5Bcat%5D=138&cHash=239ebe5c27 (accessed October 24, 2008).

Wright, John. "Control of Women's Labour in the Zulu Kingdom." In *Before and after Shaka*, ed. J. Peires, 82–99. Grahamstown: Institute for Social and Economic Research, 1983.

Xaba, Thokozani. "Masculinity and Its Malcontents: The Confrontation between 'Struggle Masculinity' and 'Post-struggle Masculinity' (1990–1997)." In *Changing Men in Southern Africa*, ed. Robert Morrell, 105–124. Pietermaritzburg: University of KwaZulu-Natal Press, 2001.

Yawitch, Joanne. "Women in Wage Labour." *South African Labour Bulletin* 9, no. 9 (1983): 82–93.

Zelizer, Viviana. *The Purchase of Intimacy*. Princeton, N.J.: Princeton University Press, 2005.

Zembe, Yanga, Loraine Townsend, Cathy Mathews, Mickey Chopra, Anna Mia Elkstrom, Anna Thorson, Susanne Stromdahl, and Heidi O'Bra. "Transactional Sex amongst Young Women at High Risk of HIV in the Western Cape." Paper presented to the South African AIDS Conference, Durban, March 31–April 3, 2009.

Zikode, Sbu. "The Third Force." Research Report 40. In *Yonk' Indawo Umzabalazo Uyasivumela: New Work from Durban*. Research Reports 2006, Centre for Civil Society, University of KwaZulu-Natal, 2006.

Zululand Times. "'Gezinsila' and 'Sundumbili' New Bantu Townships for Zululand." June 21, 1962.

———. "Domestic Science Course for Girls." June 13, 1963.

INDEX

MARK HUNTER is Assistant Professor of Geography in the Department of Social Sciences, University of Toronto Scarborough, and Research Associate in the School of Development Studies, University of KwaZulu-Natal. A graduate of the University of Sussex, the University of KwaZulu-Natal, and the University of California, Berkeley, he has published extensively on AIDS and South Africa.